The Nation's Health

Jones and Bartlett Publishers Series in Health

AIDS: Science and Society, Fan

Basic Epidemiological Methods and Biostatistics: A Practical Guidebook, Page/Cole/Timmreck

Basic Law for the Allied Health Professions, Cowdrey/Drew

Bioethics: An Introduction to the History, Methods, and Practice, Jecker/Jonsen/Pearlman

Clinical Decision Making: From Theory to Practice, Eddy

Community Health Promotion Ideas That Work: A Field-Book for Practitioners, Kreuter et al.

EMPOWER: To Plan and Organize Programs for Mammography Screening, Gold et al.

Essential Medical Terminology, Second Edition, Stanfield

Essentials for Health and Wellness, Edlin/Golanty/McCormack Brown

Grant Application Writer's Handbook, Reif-Lehrer

Handbook of Planning and Program Development for Health Promotion, Aging, Social and Health Services, Timmreck

Health Education: A Cognitive-Behavioral Approach, Read

Health and Wellness, Fifth Edition, Edlin/Golanty/McCormack Brown

Health Policy and Nursing: Crisis and Reform in the US Health Care Delivery System, Second Edition, Harrington/Estes

Health Services Cyclopedic Dictionary, Third Edition, Timmreck

Healthy Children 2000, U.S. Department of Health and Human Services

Health People 2000, U.S. Department of Health and Human Services

Healthy People 2000: Midcourse Review and 1995 Revisions, U.S. Department of Health and Human Services

Healthy People 2000: Summary Report, U.S. Department of Health and Human Services

An Introduction to Epidemiology, Timmreck

Introduction to the Health Professions, Stanfield

Introduction to Human Disease, Fourth Edition, Crowley

Managing Stress: Principles and Practice for Health and Wellbeing, Second Edition, Seaward

Mastering the New Medical Terminology Through Self-Instructional Modules, Stanfield

Mathematics for Health Professionals, Third Edition, Whistler

Medical Ethics, Second Edition, Veatch

New Dimensions in Women's Health, Alexander/LaRosa

Statistics: An Interactive Text for the Health and Life Sciences, Krishnamurty et al.

Teaching Health Science: Elementary and Middle School, Fourth Edition

Web Sites for Health Professionals, Kittleson

Women's Health: A Relational Perspective Across the Life Cycle, Lewis/Bernstein

World Health Organization's Women's Health and Development: A Global Challenge, McElmurray/Norr

❖ The Nation's Health

Fifth Edition

Edited by

Philip R. Lee
Carroll L. Estes

Institute for Health Policy Studies
School of Medicine
and
Institute for Health and Aging
School of Nursing
University of California
San Francisco

Liz Close

Associate Editor
Department of Nursing
School of Natural Sciences
Sonoma State University

Jones and Bartlett Publishers
Sudbury, Massachusetts
Boston   London   Singapore

Editorial, Sales, and Customer Service Offices
Jones and Bartlett Publishers
40 Tall Pine Drive
Sudbury, MA 01776
508-443-5000

Jones and Bartlett Publishers International
Barb House, Barb Mews
London W6 7PA
UK

Library of Congress Cataloging-in-Publication Data
The nation's health / edited by Philip R. Lee. Carroll L. Estes : Liz
   Close. assoc. ed. — 5th ed.
      p.   cm. — (The Jones and Bartlett series in health sciences)
      Includes bibliographical references and index.
      ISBN 0-7637-0405-9 (pbk.)
      1. Public health—United States.   2. Medical policy—United
      States.   3. Health care reform—United States.   I. Lee, Philip R.
      (Philip Randolph), 1924-   .   II. Estes, Carroll L.   III. Close,
      Liz.   IV. Series.
      RA445.N38   1997   97-5162
      362.1'0973—dc21   CIP

Vice President, Editorial: Joseph E. Burns
Production Administrator: Anne S. Noonan
Manufacturing: Jenna Sturgis
Editorial Production Service: The Clarinda Company
Typesetting: The Clarinda Company
Cover Design: Hannus Design Associates
Cover photo: © Mark Wieland Photography
Printing and Binding: Malloy Lithographing
Cover Printing: Coral Graphics
Photo credits: Page 3 © John C Lei Studios/Stock Boston; page 37 © Peter Southwick/Stock Boston; page 55 © Bob Daemmrich/Stock Boston; page 67 © John Griffin/The Imageworks; page 153 © Billy Barnes/Stock Boston; page 195 © Bob Daemmrich/The Imageworks; page 237 © Beringer-Dratch/The Picture Cube; page 273 © Frank Siteman/Stock Boston; page 323 © S. Agricola/The Imageworks; page 377 © Michael Weisbrot/Stock Boston

Printed in the United States of America
00 99 98 97   10 9 8 7 6 5 4 3 2 1

❖ Contents

❖ Preface

The nation's health is a high priority for the people and for policy makers as it has been for over 200 years. This volume—edited by two top health policy analysts—includes a practical, in-depth guide to the factors affecting the health of Americans and the role of public health and medical care in assuring the nation's health.

Health care reform was the top domestic priority when the fourth edition was published. President Clinton's proposal to provide universal health insurance and contain the rapidly rising costs of care was never acted on by Congress after more than two years of debate and discussion. Despite the failure of Congress to act on health care reform, progress has been made in a host of areas affecting health: tobacco, immunization, HIV/AIDS, environmental health (e.g., water, pesticides), dietary guidelines, physical activity, and food safety. There are a continuing set of questions related to health care, including those related to managed competition, capitation, global budgets, the medical-industrial complex, rationing of care, specialist versus generalist practice of medicine, and the role and supply of nurses. An overriding question: is it possible to expand access to care and at the same time control relentlessly rising costs?

Other important questions addressed in this volume are: what is the relationship of socioeconomic class to health? How important is preventive care? Why do Americans spend over twice as much per capita for health care as most other industrial countries and yet rank far behind in infant mortality and life expectancy? And how do we eliminate medical care that is wasteful, inefficient, and unnecessary?

In this book, a number of the nation's leading health policy experts look at the complex web of issues, policies, controversies, hazards, and proposed solutions that surround the health care system.

The fifth edition of *The Nation's Health* represents part of a multidisciplinary program for advanced training and education in health policy and health services research that is conducted by the Institute for Health Policy Studies, School of Medicine, and the Institute for Health and Aging, School of Nursing, University of California, San Francisco.

Philip Lee, Emeritus Professor of Social Medicine on the UCSF faculty, served as Assistant Secretary for Health, U.S. Department of Health and Human Services, in the administration of President Bill Clinton from July 1, 1993 until January 31, 1997. In this role, he took part in the national effort to restate the nation's health care agenda in response to many of the problems and issues described in this book and in keeping with many of its themes.

Professor Carroll Estes is Professor of Sociology in the School of Nursing and Director of the Institute for Health & Aging, UCSF. She is also Social Science Research Analyst for the Social Security Administration, past President of the Gerontological Society of America, and served as a member of the "Notch" Commission dealing with Social Security retirement benefits.

Special appreciation goes to Professor Liz Close for her important role in the entire process, from all phases of manuscript development and review to final publication. She is Professor and Chair, Department of Nursing, Sonoma State University and an affiliated faculty Professor, Institute for Health & Aging, and was previously Professor, Division of Nursing, California State University, Dominguez Hills.

Although *The Nation's Health* is a project of the Institute for Health Policy Studies and the Institute for Health and Aging, UCSF, the views expressed are those of the authors only and do not necessarily reflect those of the University of California.

❖ Introduction

In this volume, we have attempted to provide a clear view of the factors affecting the health of people who live in the United States. The emphasis of the fifth edition of *The Nation's Health* is the precarious set of circumstances faced by the nation's public health and health care systems in the mid-1990s as we stand on the verge of the 21st century. We intend this textbook to represent a range of views about factors affecting health status, the current state of public health and health care, and the future of the health system with particular emphasis on the current issues and proposals for change.

During the past 20 years, there has been continued improvement in the health of the nation. At the same time, the number of uninsured has grown, technology has proliferated, costs have risen relentlessly, and the foundations of the public health system have been weakened. Today, in view of the failure of Congress to enact the major health care reforms proposed by President Clinton in 1993, more and more people are looking for incremental reforms in health care policy at the federal level, while managed care is being pushed aggressively by employers and a highly profitable insurance industry. The problems of the public health infrastructure are beginning to attract serious attention.

Expenditures for health will soon reach over one trillion dollars representing more than 14 percent of the gross national product (GNP). Only one percent of these expenditures is for core public health, while over 85 percent is spent for health care. It is estimated that, unfettered by government action, health care costs will surpass $1.7 trillion, or 18 percent of the GNP, by the year 2000. The rise in personal health care expenditures can be broken into four components: general inflation; medical care price inflation above general inflation; population growth; and a group of other factors, including increases in volume and intensity of services. Population growth accounted for the least (9%) and general inflation accounted for the most (30%) of the increase in the past 20 years, medical care price inflation (profits) accounted for 17 percent of the increase, and growth in the volume and intensity of services for approximately 28 percent. These components have been affected by an array of factors, including: increased patient complexity; a tendency in the delivery system toward specialization rather than primary care; concentration of physicians and hospitals in certain urban areas that leads to excess capacity and low productivity; unnecessary and inappropriate care, which some analysts estimate may be as high as 25 percent of health care services; the practice of defensive medicine to avoid the threat of malpractice suits; and, finally, excessive administrative costs.

Rising costs are exacerbated by the fact that the U.S. system insulates both providers and consumers through the cushion of third-party payers, thus avoiding incentives to seek or provide care in a cost-effective manner. A number of failures in the health care market have vastly influenced the way insurance companies try to cope with the rising cost of health care services. In order to contain their costs, employers often shift costs to employees and benefits are reduced or eliminated.

While some economists and policymakers characterize the past decade as a period of increased competition and deregulation, during the same period public programs were exposed to growing regulation. This was particularly important in the Medicare and Medicaid programs, which pay for approximately 33 percent of all acute health care benefits. In order to control costs, the federal government devised ingenious schemes to limit spending, most notably through the Medicare prospective payment system for hospitals, which was introduced in 1983, and the Medicare fee schedule for physicians that went into effect in 1992. These events have slowed the rate of increase in medicare costs in recent years. With the efforts in the private sector to stimulate competition and require more and more patients to fit into managed care plans, cost increases have slowed dramatically in 1994 and 1995, but the trends in health care costs for the future is unknown. Nevertheless, health care costs are the highest of any nation in the world and have consistently risen well above the rate of general inflation for 50 years.

Compounding the problem of rising costs and the move to more and more managed care has been a deterioration in access to care. Greater and greater numbers of people across all socioeconomic levels have found it difficult or impossible to obtain health insurance coverage, thus expanding the ranks of the uninsured to over 41 million (up from 37 million when the fourth edition of *The Nation's Health* was published). More than 60 million Americans have been found to lack health insurance at one point in time during the year. Those who hold the purse-strings—third-party payers—have come to dictate treatment plans and hospital stays, as coverage has become increasingly limited. In many cases, people with chronic health problems cannot obtain health benefits. This circumstance is called a *preexisting condition,* and in recent years it has become common for insurance companies to exclude coverage for illnesses people are under treatment for at the time they apply for coverage. It has also been difficult for people to carry their coverage from job to job. As a result of these problems, Congress, in late 1996, enacted the Health Insurance Portability and Accountability Act (Kennedy-Kassenbaum) to provide for portability of health insurance and limit exclusions because of preexisting conditions. As Medicaid eligibility shrank in relation to a growing need and other charity care began to decline, the political system effectively turned its back on the working poor. In the past, cost shifting by hospitals from the insured to the uninsured was common, but this has become increasingly difficult in the era of managed care. Welfare reform enacted and signed into law in 1996 denied medical care to millions of legal and illegal immigrants and increased state discretion over eligibility and benefits for welfare programs. The impact on the Medicaid population is unclear and likely to be worrisome.

Soaring costs and the depletion of financial support for the uninsured and underinsured are a deadly combination existing side by side with the world's most sophisticated and high-priced health care technology. Serious problems remain that require the combined efforts of public health and health care. Issues that have begun to be dealt with in a more systematic manner include tobacco use, immunization, HIV/AIDS, food safety, newly emerging infections, unintended pregnancy (including adolescent pregnancy), and environmental health. Problems that require particular attention in the near future include the disparity in health status related to socioeconomic status. These particularly affect minorities. Infant mortality, related to access to prenatal and maternity care, is considerably higher for blacks than for whites, largely because of the continuing prevalence of low-birth weight infants among blacks. Infant mortality is higher for the poor than for the rich, and it is higher in the United States than in 21 other countries. Sophisticated treatments such as coronary artery bypass graft surgery, coronary angioplasty, and total hip replacement are less available to many poor people, even when insured. Other services often unavailable to the poor are preventive services and management of chronic conditions. These services are critical to good health, as is prenatal care.

At the same time that the health care delivery crisis is playing out, a number of health and social problems are sweeping the nation, decimating the lives of many and cutting at the heart of the health care system. At issue are the epidemics of violence, substance abuse, AIDS, homelessness, and unintended pregnancy, all of them devastatingly expensive in terms of human life, and each with a very high price tag. Concurrently, the number of chronically ill elderly continues to increase, highlighting the lack of provision in our system for serving their special needs.

For many sick people, medicine is the key to life and well being, and thus doctors and hospitals become the arbiters of our most precious commodities. This fact, coupled with the high cost of services and the insulation provided by third-party payers, means that health care does not operate according to classical market principles.

Most observers and participants agree that there is need for fundamental change and restructuring of the health care system. In 1993, President Clinton proposed a restructuring of the nation's health care system through a proposal that would provide comprehensive health insurance coverage to all Americans. It was designed to be phased in gradually by the year 2000. The plan was debated in Congress, but eventually was not enacted. The failure of this approach to comprehensive reform has led to a good deal of soul searching about how to best address the serious health problems confronting the nation. The biggest change in the fifth edition of *The*

Nation's Health from those that have gone before is the emphasis on public health and the greater emphasis on the determinants of health as the basis for health policy.

Many contributors to this volume argue that the nation is confronted by an outmoded personal health care system that is the result of failed policies and continued technological expansion at the expense of the provision of sound basic care for all and effective nationwide programs of disease prevention, health protection, and health promotion. Those who are well insured are the beneficiaries of a comprehensive delivery system. Those who suffer most from a lack of adequate public health protection and access to personal health care are children, some of whom are unable to obtain even basic care, including immunizations; the disabled and those who suffer from debilitating chronic illness; and, across all age groups and geographic areas, the working poor.

Throughout the 1980s and 1990s, the nation also experienced an increase in the number and types of corporate for-profit providers and insurers, including managed care plans. In addition, there are major conversions of nonprofit health entities to for-profit corporations such as Blue Cross of California that have raised serious questions of the disposition and control of assets as well as access to care. This hotly debated phenomenon has resulted in the proprietary ownership of many hospitals, surgicenters, urgent care centers, clinical laboratories, and imaging facilities. Hospitals and other providers have become increasingly competitive and, as a result, they have begun to operate more like businesses, using techniques such as advertising, marketing, specialization, and productivity monitoring. The effects of this trend are just beginning to be understood.

The irony is that at a time when the working poor have been victimized by society's disparities, a large segment of society has come to expect access to almost unlimited medical care. Along with the benefits of high-priced care come the pitfalls of overtreatment, overprescribing, unnecessary surgery, and neglect of emphasis on sound preventive measures. Thus, issues related to quality of care are being examined anew. Measuring the effects of medical interventions is a complex and imprecise science. Increasingly, clinicians are asked to interpret medical findings that they are ill-equipped to evaluate. This causes vastly differing treatments from one clinician to another, and the end result is that new issues related to inappropriate care are being investigated today.

In this book, we critically examine the nation's health, the determinants of health, and the roles of public health (population based intervention) and personal health care in protecting and assuring the health of the population. Rather than merely emphasizing the care of the sick, the financing of care, and public health, we look at the complex web of issues, policies, controversies, hazards, problems, and proposed solutions to protect and promote the nation's health. While acknowledging the inevitability of death, we would like to explore a means to greater health and longevity

for everyone. Despite changes in health behaviors, environmental improvements, and the advances of science, medical care, and public health that
have contributed to increased life expectancy and reduced mortality, on the
verge of the 21st century, America faces critical issues if it is to maintain
its leadership role in science and to become a world leader in public health
and health care.

❖ Acknowledgments

❖ Chapter 1

Thomas McKeown. (1978). Determinants of health. Abridged from HUMAN NATURE MAGAZINE, April 1978. Copyright © 1978 by Harcourt Brace & Company. Reprinted by permission of the publisher.

Nancy E. Adler, Thomas Boyce, Margaret A. Chesney, Susan Folkman, and Leonard Syme. (1993) Socioeconomic inequalities in health: No easy solution. *Journal of the American Medical Association* 269(24): 3140-3145. Copyright 1993, American Medical Association.

Vicente Navarro. (1990). Race or class versus race and class: Mortality differentials in the United States. *The Lancet, 336*:1238-1240. © by the Lancet Ltd. 1990.

❖ Chapter 2

J. Michael McGinnis and Philip R. Lee. (1995). Healthy People 2000 at mid decade. *Journal of the American Medical Association, 273*(14): 1123-1129.

❖ Chapter 3

Institute of Medicine (IOM). (1988). The Future of Public Health: Summary and Recommendations. Washington DC: National Academy Press. Adapted with permission from *The Future of Public Health.* Copyright 1988 by the National Academy of Sciences. Courtesy of the National Academy Press, Washington, D.C.

❖ Chapter 4

David A. Kessler, Ann M. Witt, Philip S. Barnett et al. (September 26, 1996). "The Food and Drug Administration's Regulation of Tobacco Products," *The New England Journal of Medicine*, Volume 335(13), 1996, pp. 988-994. Copyright 1996, *Massachusetts Medical Society.* Reprinted by permission of *The New England Journal of Medicine.*

Marion Nestle. "Dietary Guidance for the 21st Century: New Approaches," *Journal of Nutrition Education*, Volume 27(5), 1995, pp. 272-275. Reprinted by permission of the publisher.

U.S. Department of Health and Human Services. (1996). Surgeon General's Report on Physical activity and health.

Bortz, IV, W. M., and Bortz II, W. M. 1996. How fast do we age? Exercise performance over time as a biomarker. *Journal of Gerontology: MEDICAL SCIENCES, 51A*(5): M223-M225. Copyright © The Gerontological Society of America.

Ann Marie Kimball, Seth Berkley, Elizabeth Ngugi, and Helen Gayle. (1995). International aspects of AIDS/HIV epidemic. *Annual Review of Public Health, 16*:253-282. Reprinted by permission of the publisher.

Stephen B. Thacker, Donna F. Stroup, R. Gibson Parrish, and Henry A. Anderson. (1996). Surveillance in environmental public health: Issues, systems, and sources. Abridged from *American Journal of Public Health*, Volume 86(5), 1996, pp. 633-637. Copyright 1996 by the American Public Health Association. Reprinted by permission of the publisher.

Ruth Hubbard and R. C. Lewontin. "Sounding Board: Pitfalls of genetic testing." *The New England Journal of Medicine*, Volume 334(18), 1996, pp. 1192-1194. Copyright 1996, *Massachusetts Medical Society*. Reprinted by permission of *The New England Journal of Medicine*.

❖ Chapter 5

United Nations. (1996). Fourth World Congress on Women—Strategic objectives and Actions: Women and health. The Beijing Declaration and The Platform for Action (New York: United Nations Department of Public Information), 56-73. DPI/1766/wom, February 1996.

Jacques E. Rossouw, Loretta P. Finnigan, William R. Harlan, Vivian W. Pinn, Carolyn Clifford, and Joan A. McGowan. 1995. The evolution of the Women's Health Initiative: Perspectives from the NIH. *Journal of the American Medical Women's Association, 50*(2): 50-55. Reprinted by permission of the publisher.

Carroll L. Estes and Liz Close. "Public policy and long term care." In R. P. Abcles, H. C. Gift & M. G. Ory (Eds.), *Aging and quality of life* (pp. 310-335). New York: Springer. Copyright 1993 by Springer Publishing Company. Reprinted by permission of the Springer Publishing Company.

❖ Chapter 6

Carroll L. Estes. (1992). Privatization, the Welfare State, and Aging: The Reagan-Bush Legacy. Abridged from a paper presented at the 21st Annual Conference of the British Society of Gerontology, University of Kent at Canterbury, September 19, 1992. Reprinted by permission of the author.

Nestle, M. 1993. Food lobbies, the food pyramid, and U.S. nutrition policy. *International Journal of Health Services*, 23(3): 483-496. Copyright Baywood Publishing Company, Incorporated. Reprinted by permission of the publisher.

Stanton A. Glantz. "Preventing tobacco use—the youth access trap." *American Journal of Public Health*, Volume 86, 1996, pp. 156-158. Copyright 1996 by the American Public Health Association. Reprinted by permission of the publisher.

Carroll L. Estes and Karen W. Linkins. Race to the bottom? The challenge facing long term care. Reprinted by permission of the authors.

❖ Chapter 7

Linda H. Aiken. (1995). The registered nurse workforce: Infrastructure for health care reform. *Statistical Bulletin, 76*(3): 2-9. Reprinted by permission of the publisher.

Claire M. Fagin. (1996). Improving nursing practice, education, and research. *Journal of Nursing Administration, 26*(3): 30-37.

Charlene Harrington. (1996). Nurse staffing: Developing a political action agenda for change. *Nursing Policy Forum* 2(3): 14-16, 24-27.

❖ Chapter 8

Karen Donelan, Robert J. Blendon, Craig A. Hill, Catherine Hoffman, Diane Rowland, Martin Frankel, and Drew Altman. (1996). Whatever happened to the health insurance crisis in the United States? *Journal of the American Medical Association,* 276(16): 1346-1350. Copyright 1996, American Medical Association.

Marilyn Moon and Karen Davis. "Preserving and strengthening Medicare." *Health Affairs,* Volume 14(4), 1995, pp. 31-46. Reprinted with permission of the publisher.

The Kaiser Commission on the Future of Medicaid. "Policy Brief: Medicaid and Long-Term Care." 1996. Washington, DC The Kaiser Commission on the Future of Medicaid. Abridged and reprinted with permission of the publisher.

Bruce C. Vladeck. "Medicaid 1115 demonstrations: Progress through partnership." *Health Affairs,* Volume 14(1), 1995, pp. 217-220. Reprinted with permission of the publisher.

Jerome P. Kassirer. (1994). Academic medical centers under siege. *New England Journal of Medicine,* Volume 331(20), 1994, pp. 1370-1371. Copyright 1994, Massachusetts Medical Society. Reprinted by permission of *The New England Journal of Medicine.*

❖ Chapter 9

Alain C. Enthoven and Richard Kronick. 91991). "Universal health insurance through incentive reform." Abridged from *Journal of the American Medical Association,* Volume 265(19), 1991, pp. 2532-2536. Copyright 1991, American Medical Association.

Harold S. Luft. "Modifying Managed Competition to Address Cost and Quality." *Health Affairs,* Volume 15(1), 1996, pp. 23-48. Reprinted with permission of the publisher.

John Rother. "Consumer Protection in Managed Care: A Third-Generation Approach." *Generations,* Volume 20(2), 1996, pp. 42-46. Reprinted with permission from *Generations,* 833 Market Street, Suite 511, San Francisco, CA 94103. Copyright 1996, American Society on Aging. Requests for permissions call (415) 974-9600; *e-mail:* nainaa@asa.asaging.org.

Allen W. Immershein and Carroll L. Estes. "From Health Services to Medical Markets: The Commodity Transformation of Medical Production and the Nonprofit Sector." *International Journal of Health Services,* Volume 26(2), 1996, pp. 221-238. Copyright Baywood Publishing Company, Incorporated. Reprinted by permission of publisher and authors.

❖ Chapter 10

Robert H. Brook, Caren J. Kamberg, and Elizabeth A. McGlynn. (1996). Health system reform and quality. *Journal of the American Medical Association,* 276(6) 476-480. Copyright 1996, American Medical Association.

David L. Sackett, William C. Rosenberg, J. A. Muir Gray, R. Brian Haynes, and W. Scott Richardson. (1996). "Evidence based medicine: What it is and what it isn't." *British Medical Journal*, Volume 312, 1996, pp. 71-72. Reprinted with permission of the BMJ Publishing Group.

John E. Wennberg. (1993) Future directions for small area variations. *Medical Care*, 31(5) YS75-80, Supplement. Reprinted by permission of the publisher.

Karen Davis. (1996). Incremental coverage of the uninsured. *Journal of the American Medical Association*, 276(10): 831-832. Copyright 1996, American Medical Association.

❖ PART I
Health

❖ Chapter 1
Determinants of Health

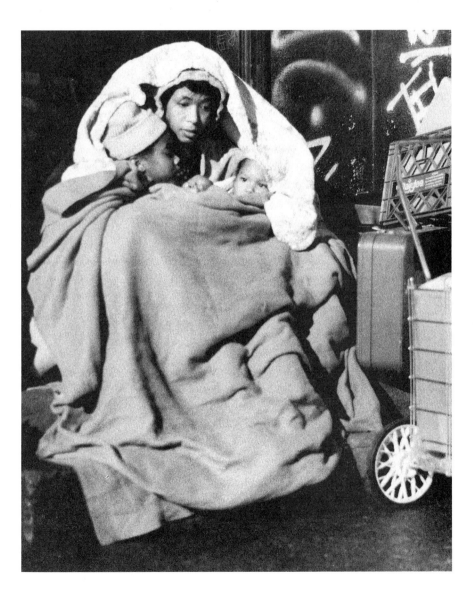

Since the 18th century, there has been a dramatic improvement in the health and life span of Americans. This largely reflects a general improvement in the socioeconomic status of the population, improvements in nutrition, changes in reproductive behavior, and advances in environmental sanitation (e.g., chlorination of water supplies, pasteurization of milk). Until the last 60 years, improvements in medical care had relatively little impact on the decline in mortality. The decline in mortality was largely due to the decline in mortality from tuberculosis, diarrheal diseases, (e.g., cholera), and other infections (e.g., small pox). Particularly important were declines in infant and maternal mortality (McKeown, 1978).

In the 20th century the pattern of morbidity and mortality changed dramatically with the decline in infectious disease and the rise of chronic cardiovascular diseases and cancer as the major causes of death. Pneumonia and influenza remained as major killers, particularly among the elderly. Infant and maternal morbidity declined steadily in the first half of the 20th century.

The introduction of the sulfonamides in the 1930s began the era of modern medical care with the development of a number of antimicrobial agents that were effective in treating a broad spectrum of infectious diseases including tuberculosis. From the mid-1950s to the mid-1960s, little progress was made in reducing infant mortality or increasing life expectancy. Beginning in the mid-1960s, however, and continuing into the 1990s, America's health improved. Following the implementation of Medicaid, which provided low income women and children health insurance, the expansion of the Women, Infants, and Children (WIC) program by the Department of Agriculture; and the rapid improvements in neonatal intensive care, infant deaths gradually dropped to about one half the 1965 level. The life expectancy of those born in 1979 rose more than three years over that of 1965. By 1995, life expectancy was at its highest level ever.

Today the leading causes of death are diseases of the heart, malignant neoplasms, cerebrovascular disease, unintentional injuries, chronic obstructive pulmonary disease, pneumonia and influenza, diabetes mellitus, chronic liver disease and cirrhosis, atherosclerosis, and suicides. Among those ages 25–44 years, acquired immunodeficiency syndrome (AIDS) has become the leading cause of death. These causes result in part from socioeconomic conditions, the ways we choose to live, and the environments we create. Management of these problems requires different strategies than those for the infectious diseases that were the leading killers during the early part of this century. We often cannot rely on the cures of modern medicine but must combine these with broad public health measures. Today, ensuring good health and controlling disease requires a focus on (1) socioeconomic factors (e.g., income, education, work), (2) individual behavior and the factors that influence health-related behaviors, (3) environment, (4) human biology, and (5) access to health care. The Centers for Disease Control and Prevention (CDC) of the U.S. Public Health Service has analyzed the relative importance of four of these factors to the ten leading causes of premature mortality in the United States (U.S. Department of Health and Human Services, 1980). Although socioeconomic factors influence all other determinants of health, except human biology, the CDC did not explicitly include socioeconomic status as a determinant of health. The first analysis was done in 1977 (U.S. Department of Health and Human Services) and it was repeated in 1990 (U.S. Department of Health and Human Services). By allocating the contributing factors of premature mortality to the four major determinants of health, the results were: personal behavior/life style contributed approximately 47 percent; environmental factors contributed 16 percent, human biology (inherited and genetic factors) contributed 27 percent; and inadequacies in health care contributed 10 percent.

While it is likely that the CDC analysis still holds in its broad dimensions, recent studies by Bunker and his associates (Bunker, 1995; Bunker, Frazier, & Mosteller, 1994) suggest that personal medical care, particularly clinical preventive services, play a larger role than in the past. They estimated that medical care contributed 6 of the 30 years of increased life expectancy (17 percent) since the turn of the century and three of the seven years (43 percent) since 1950.

In addition, Newacheck, Jameson, and Halfon (1994), analyzing data from the National Health Interview Study, found that low income, uninsured children are less likely than non-poor insured children to receive timely physical and visual examinations and preventive dental care. Poor children with insurance use preventive services at about the same rate as non-poor children. The authors conclude:

> These findings suggest expanding the provision of insurance to all low income children could help to close the remaining gaps in the use of preventive services and, eventually to eliminate existing disparity in the preventable health problems described earlier (p. 232).

Not only does medical care contribute to reducing premature mortality and increased life expectancy, but it also contributes to the quality of life. These studies clearly illustrate the importance of both population based (public health) and individually directed (personal medical/health care) approaches to the reduction in premature mortality and morbidity.

The authors in chapter 1 analyze trends in morbidity and mortality during the 19th and 20th centuries with a view toward understanding the impact of health care and public health on the human life span and on the quality of life. These trends are of interest to policy makers and analysts as a means to understand the determinants of health and point the direction for future policy decisions. All analysts, however, do not draw the same conclusions from available data and thus the conclusions drawn and the forecasts vary.

Using primary data on death rates (mortality), the late British physician Thomas McKeown, in his 1978 seminal article "Determinants of Health," reviewed the reasons for the dramatic decline in the death rate since the eighteenth century. He noted that much of the decline in mortality took place before the introduction of specific medical interventions, such as antibiotics. Therefore, McKeown argued, improved nutrition, a safer, cleaner environment, and a change in sexual behavior (smaller family size) were more significant determinants of health than were improvements in medical care. He also suggested that for improvements in health we should look more toward changing our ways of living and personal health habits than to continued reliance on personal health care. These ideas were more fully developed in his book (McKeown, 1979).

In their article, "Producing Health, Consuming Health Care," reprinted in the fourth edition of *The Nation's Health* (1994), Evans and Stoddart present an analytic framework for understanding the determinants of health that they contend is more comprehensive and flexible than the traditional framework, which essentially defines health as absence of disease or injury and presents the health care system as a response or feedback mechanism to disease or injury. The authors' broad, complex framework encompasses meaningful categories that are responsive and sensitive to the ways in which a variety of factors interact to determine the health status of individuals and populations. The proposed framework has particular relevance to the current policy debate because it includes a definition of health that reflects the individual's experience as well as the perspective of the health care system; it encourages consideration of both behavioral and biological factors; and it acknowledges the economic trade-off involved in allocating scarce resources. These and other important ideas are discussed in depth in their recent book (Evans, Stoddart, and Marmor, 1994).

In "Health Inequalities and Social Class" included in the 4th Edition of *The Nation's Health* (1994), M. G. Marmot and associates present evidence drawn from the 1985–1988 Whitehall II study, concerning the degree and causes of differences in morbidity rates in a cohort of over 10,000 British civil servants. This was a follow-up to the original Whitehall study in 1967, which demonstrated an inverse relationship between employment grade and mortality. The importance of social class (socioeconomic status) to health is evident at every level—from the lowest socioeconomic group to the highest, with the highest social classes showing lower mortality than the next highest and so on down to the lowest social classes that have the highest mortality rates. Self-perceived health status and symptoms were also worse in workers in the lower status jobs. The inferences that can be drawn from these studies are far-reaching, including such factors as the influence on health and longevity of early life environment, leisure-time activity, social networks, housing circumstances, education, and control over the work environment. One of the most important findings relates to the diminished level of healthy behaviors practiced by those in the lower socioeconomic groups, which was reflected in the fact that fewer of those in lower status jobs believed that they could reduce their risk for a heart attack. This group also demonstrated a higher incidence of smoking, less vigorous exercise, more obesity, less healthy diet patterns, and more stressful life events. The study has many important policy implications, including the fact that people in lower socioeconomic groups are not benefiting from our vast knowledge about the close relationship between health status and behavioral factors. It also showed that these socioeconomic factors continue to have a strong influence in this population despite the availability of universal health care through the National Health Service in the United Kingdom.

In their paper on socioeconomic status and health in chapter 1, Adler and her colleagues (1993) build on the classic study by Marmot noted above and review the wealth of research that demonstrates a linear mortality gradient at all socioeconomic levels with a variety of diseases. These studies raise as many questions as they answer, including the impact of socioeconomic status (SES) on morbidity.

While a growing number of studies support the view that the relationship between health and socioeconomic status is a linear, not a threshold, phenomenon, the mechanisms underlying this relationship between SES and health are not clear. Many studies have focused on the behavioral characteristics of individuals of different occupations, educational levels, income and social class. Where one lives also makes a difference. In a recent study of mortality rates in poverty and nonpoverty areas Waitzman & Smith (1996) found in a younger group residing in the poverty area an all cause mortality rate 1.5 times those in the nonpoverty area. Income inequality has also been recognized as a factor in life expectancy in industrialized countries. Wilkinson (1992) demonstrated that those industrialized countries with a greater equality income distribution had a proportionately greater increase in life expectancy. In the United States, Kaplan and colleagues (1996) demonstrated a correlation between the household income of the less well off and all cause mortality. Income inequality was associated with higher rates of lower birth weights, homicide, violent crimes, work disability, smoking and sedentary life style. A number of studies demonstrate that access to health care alone (e.g., the National Health Services in the UK) does not overcome the profound effects of socioeconomic status on health. Indeed, the gap between the higher and lower socioeconomic groups has grown, particularly in the United States in the past 15 years, with potentially serious implications for the health of the general population.

The issues of race, class, and health status have been examined by Pappas (1994) and by Navarro (1990), each included in chapter 1. Although much of premature mortality in African Americans can be attributed to socioeconomic status, race does affect such problems as low birth weight, homicide, diabetes mellitus and access to medical care. Pappas also notes that the most important factor in the increasing difference in life expectancy between whites and blacks is related to the slower decline in heart disease mortality in blacks in recent decades. Navarro's (1990) analysis suggests the mortality differentials by social class are greater than mortality differentials due to race. Another under-studied area is whether (and how) social differences in health are greater or less for particular age groups across the life course. Such data are essential to formulating and targeting effective public health policies (Jefferys, 1996).

Taking a different approach that did not focus on socioeconomic status (SES), McGinnis and Foege (1993) found that approximately half of all deaths in 1990 could be attributed to the following factors (1) tobacco (400,000 deaths); (2) diet and sedentary activity patterns (300,000 deaths); (3) alcohol abuse (100,000 deaths); (4) microbial agents (90,000 deaths); (5) toxic agents (60,000 deaths); (6) firearms (35,000 deaths); (7) sexual behavior (30,000 deaths); (8) motor vehicles (20,000 deaths); and (9) illicit drug use (20,000 deaths). Here, again, we see the importance of personal behavior and environment.

❖ Determinants of Health

Thomas McKeown

Modern medicine is not nearly as effective as most people believe. It has not been effective because medical science and service are misdirected and society's investment in health is misused. At the base of this misdirection is a false assumption about human health. Physicians, biochemists, and the general public assume that the body is a machine that can be protected from disease primarily by physical and chemical intervention. This approach, rooted in 17th-century science, has led to widespread indifference to the influence of the primary determinants of human health—environment and personal behavior—and emphasizes the role of medical treatment, which is actually less important than either of the others. It has also resulted in the neglect of sick people whose ailments are not within the scope of the sort of therapy that interests the medical professions.

An appraisal of influences on health in the past suggests that the contribution of modern medicine to the increase of life expectancy has been much smaller than most people believe. Health improved, not because of steps when we are ill, but because we become ill less often. We remain well, less because of specific measures such as vaccination and immunization than because we enjoy a higher standard of nutrition, we live in a healthier environment, and we have fewer children.

The utmost in healing can be achieved when there is unity, when the internal spirit and the external physical shape perfect each other.
—The Yellow Emperor
China, 1000 BC

For some 300 years, an engineering approach has been dominant in biology and medicine and has provided the basis for the treatment of the sick. A mechanistic concept of nature developed in the 17th century led to the idea that a living organism, like a machine, might be taken apart and reassembled if its structure and function were sufficiently understood. Applied to medicine, this concept meant that understanding the body's response to disease would allow physicians to intervene in the course of disease. The consequences of the engineering approach to medicine are more conspicuous today than they were in the 17th century, largely because the resources of the physical and chemical sciences are so much greater. Medical education begins with the study of the structure and function of the body, continues with examination of disease processes, and ends with clinical instruction on selected sick people. Medical service is dominated by the image of the hospital for the acutely ill, where technological resources are concentrated. Medical research also reflects the mechanistic approach, concerning itself with problems such as the chemical basis of inheritance and the immunological response to transplanted tissues.

No one disputes the predominance of the engineering approach in medicine, but we must now ask whether it is seriously deficient as a conceptualization of the problems of human health. To answer this question, we must examine the determinants of human health. We must first discover why health improved in the past and then go on to ascertain the important influences on health today in the light of the change in health problems that has resulted from the decline of infectious diseases.

It is no exaggeration to say that health, especially the health of infants and young children, has been transformed since the 18th century (Figure 1). For the first time in history, a mother knows it is likely that all her children will live to maturity. Before the 19th century, only about three out of every 10 newborn infants lived beyond the age of 25. Of the seven who died, two or three never reached their first birthday, and five or six died before they were six. Today, in developed countries fewer than one in 20 children die before they reach adulthood.

The increased life expectancy, most evident for young children, is due predominantly, to a reduction of deaths from infectious diseases (Figure 2). Records from England and Wales (the earliest national statistics available) show that this reduction was the reason for the improvement in health before 1900 and it remains the main influence to the present day.

But when we try to account for the decline of infections, significant differences of opinion appear. The conventional view attributes the change

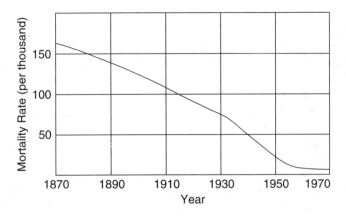

FIGURE 1 Infant mortality rate.

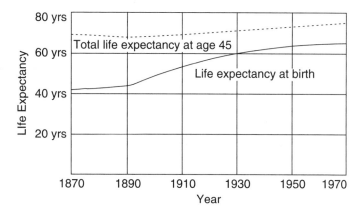

FIGURE 2 Life expectancy.

to an increased understanding of the nature of infectious disease and to the application of that knowledge through better hygiene, immunization, and treatment. This interpretation places particular emphasis on immunization against diseases like smallpox and polio, and on the use of drugs for the treatment of other diseases, such as tuberculosis, meningitis, and pneumonia. These measures, in fact, contributed relatively little to the total reduction of mortality; the main explanation for the dramatic fall in the number of deaths lies not in medical intervention but elsewhere.

Deaths from the common infections were declining long before effective medical intervention was possible. By 1900, the total death rate had dropped substantially, and over 90 percent of the reduction was due to a decrease of deaths from infectious diseases. The relative importance of the major influences can be illustrated by reference to tuberculosis. Although respiratory tuberculosis was the single largest cause of death in the mid-19th century, mortality from the disease declined continuously after 1938, when it was first registered in England and Wales as a cause of death.

Robert Koch identified the tubercle bacillus in 1882, but none of the treatments used in the 19th or early 20th centuries significantly influenced the course of the disease. The many drugs that were tried were worthless; so, too, was the practice of surgically collapsing an infected lung, a treatment introduced about 1920. Streptomycin, developed in 1947, was the first effective treatment, but by this time mortality from the disease had fallen to a small fraction of its level during 1848 to 1854. Streptomycin lowered the death rate from tuberculosis in England and Wales by about 50 percent, but its contribution to the decrease in the death rate since the early 19th century was only about 3 percent.

Deaths from bronchitis, pneumonia, and influenza also began to decline before medical science provided an effective treatment for these illnesses.

Although the death rate in England and Wales increased in the second half of the 19th century, it has fallen continuously since the beginning of the 20th. There is still no effective immunization against bronchitis or pneumonia, and influenza vaccines have had no effect on deaths. The first successful treatment for these respiratory diseases was a sulfa drug introduced in 1938, but mortality attributed to the lung infections was declining from the beginning of the 20th century. There is no reason to doubt that the decline would have continued without effective therapeutic measures, if at a far slower rate.

In the United States, the story was similar: Thomas Magill noted that "the rapid decline of pneumonia death rates began in New York State before the turn of the century and many years before the 'miracle drugs' were known." Obviously, drug therapy was not responsible for the total decrease in deaths that occurred since 1938, and it could have had no influence on the substantial reduction that occurred before then.

The histories of most other common infections, such as whooping cough, measles, and scarlet fever, are similar. In each of these diseases, mortality had fallen to a low level before effective immunization or therapy became available.

In some infections, medical intervention *was* valuable before sulfa drugs and antibiotics became available. Immunization protected people against smallpox and tetanus, antitoxin treatment limited deaths from diphtheria; appendicitis, peritonitis, and ear infections responded to surgery; Salvarsan was a long-sought "magic bullet" against syphilis; intravenous therapy saved people with severe diarrheas; and improved obstetric care prevented childbed fever.

But even if such medical measures had been responsible for the whole decline of mortality from these particular conditions after 1900 (and clearly they were not), they would account for only a small part of the decrease in deaths attributed to all infectious diseases before 1935. From that time, powerful drugs came into use and they were supplemented by improved vaccines. But mortality would have continued to fall even without the presence of these agents; and over the whole period since cause of death was first recorded, immunization and treatments have contributed much less than other influences.

The substantial fall in mortality was due in part to reduced contact with microorganisms. In developed countries, an individual no longer encounters the cholera bacillus, he is rarely exposed to the typhoid organism, and his contact with the tubercle bacillus is infrequent. The death rate from these infections fell continuously from the second half of the 19th century when basic hygienic measures were introduced: purification of water, efficient sewage disposal, and improved food hygiene—particularly the pasteurization of milk, the item in the diet most likely to spread disease.

Pasteurization was probably the main reason for the decrease in deaths from gastroenteritis and for the decline in infant mortality from about 1900.

In the 20th century, these essential hygienic measures were supported by improved conditions in the home, the work place, and the general environment. Over the entire period for which records exist, better hygiene accounts for approximately a fifth of the total reduction of mortality.

But the decline of mortality caused by infections began long before the introduction of sanitary measures. It had already begun in England and Wales by 1838, and statistics from Scandinavia suggest that the death rate had been decreasing there since the first half of the 18th century.

A review of English experience makes it unlikely that reduced exposure to microorganisms contributed significantly to the falling death rate in this earlier period. In England and Wales that was the time of industrialization, characterized by rapid population growth and shifts of people from farms into towns, where living and working conditions were uncontrolled. The crowding and poor hygiene that resulted provided ideal conditions for the multiplication and spread of microorganisms, and the situation improved little before sanitary measures were introduced in the last third of the century.

A further explanation for the falling death rate is that an improvement in nutrition led to an increase in resistance to infectious diseases. This is, I believe, the most credible reason for the decline of the infections, at least until the late 19th century, and also explains why deaths from airborne diseases like scarlet fever and measles have decreased even when exposure to the organisms that cause them remains almost unchanged. The evidence demonstrating the impact of improved nutrition is indirect, but it is still impressive.

Lack of food and the resulting malnutrition were largely responsible for the predominance of the infectious diseases, from the time when men first aggregated in large population groups about 10,000 years ago. In these conditions an improvement in nutrition was necessary for a substantial and prolonged decline in mortality.

Experience in developing countries today leaves no doubt that nutritional state is a critical factor in a person's response to infectious disease, particularly in young children. Malnourished people contract infections more often than those who are well fed and they suffer more when they become infected. According to a recent World Health Organization report on nutrition in developing countries, the best vaccine against common infectious diseases is an adequate diet.

In the 18th and 19th centuries, food production increased greatly throughout the Western world. The number of people in England and Wales tripled between 1700 and 1850 and they were fed on home-grown food.

In summary: The death rate from infectious diseases fell because an increase in food supplies led to better nutrition. From the second half of the 19th century this advance was strongly supported by improved hygiene and safer food and water, which reduced exposure to infection. With the exception of the smallpox vaccination, which played a small part in the total decline of mortality, medical procedures such as immunization and therapy had little impact on human health until the 20th century.

One other influence needs to be considered: a change in reproductive behavior, which caused the birth rate to decline. The significance of this change can hardly be exaggerated, for without it the other advances would soon have been overtaken by the increasing population. We can attribute the modern improvement in health to food, hygiene, and medical intervention in that order of time and importance—but we must recognize that it is to a modification of behavior that we owe the permanence of this improvement.

But it does not follow that these influences have the same relative importance today as in the past. In technologically advanced countries, the decline of infectious diseases was followed by a vast change in health problems, and even in developing countries advances in medical science and technology may have modified the effects of nutrition, sanitation, and contraception. In order to predict the factors likely to affect our health in the future, we need to examine the nature of the problems in health that exist today.

Because today's problems are mainly with noncommunicable diseases, physicians have shifted their approach. In the case of infections, interest centers on the organisms that cause them and on the conditions under which they spread. In noninfective conditions, the engineering approach established in the 17th century remains predominant and attention is focused on how a disease develops rather than on why it begins. Perhaps the most important question now confronting medicine is whether the commonest health problems—heart disease, cancer, rheumatoid arthritis, cerebrovascular disease—are essentially different from health problems of the past or whether, like infections, they can be prevented by modifying the conditions that lead to them.

A wise man should consider that health is the greatest of human blessings, and learn how, by his own thought, to derive benefit from his illness.
—Hippocrates
460–400 BC

To answer this question, we must distinguish between genetic and chromosomal diseases determined at the moment of fertilization and all other diseases, which are attributable in greater or lesser degree to the influence of the environment. Most diseases, including the common noninfectious ones, appear to fall into the second category. Whether these diseases can be prevented is likely to be determined by the practicability of controlling the environmental influences that lead them.

The change in the character of health problems that followed the decline of infections in developed countries has not invalidated the conclusion that most diseases, both physical and mental, are associated with influences that might be controlled. Among such influences, those which the individual determines by his own behavior (smoking, eating, exercise, and the like) are now more important for his health than those that depend mainly on society's actions (provision of essential food and protection from hazards). And both behavioral and environmental influences are more significant than medical care.

The role of individual medical care in preventing sickness and premature death is secondary to that of other influences; yet society's investment in health care is based on the premise that it is the major determinant. It is assumed that we are ill and are made well, but it is nearer the truth to say that we are well and are made ill. Few people think of themselves as having the major responsibility for their own health, and the enormous resources that advanced countries assigned to the health field are used mainly to treat disease or, to a lesser extent, to prevent it by personal measures such as immunization.

The revised concept of human health cannot provide immediate solutions for the many complex problems facing society: limiting population growth and providing adequate food in developing countries, changing personal behavior, and striking a new balance between technology and care in developed nations. Instead, the enlarged understanding of health and disease should be regarded as a conceptual base with implications for services, education, and research that will take years to develop.

The most immediate requirements in the health services is to give sufficient attention to behavioral influences that are now the main determinants of health. The public believes that health depends primarily on intervention by the doctor and that the essential requirement for health is the early discovery of disease. This concept should be replaced by recognition that disease often cannot be treated effectively, and that health is determined predominantly by the way of life individuals choose to follow. Among the important influences on health are the use of tobacco, the misuse of alcohol and drugs, excessive or unbalanced diets, and lack of exercise. With research, the list of significant behavioral influences will undoubtedly increase, particularly in relation to the prevention of mental illness.

Although the influences of personal behavior are the main determinants of health in developed countries, public action can still accomplish a great deal in the environmental field. Internationally, malnutrition probably remains the most important cause of ill health, and even in affluent societies sections of the population are inadequately—as distinct from unwisely—fed. The malnourished vary in proportion and composition from one country to another, but in the developed world they are mainly the younger children of large families and elderly people who live alone. In light of the importance of food for good health, governments might use supplements and subsidies to put essential foods within the reach of everyone, and provide inducements for people to select beneficial in place of harmful foods. Of course, these aims cannot exclude other considerations such as international agreements and the solvency of farmers who have been encouraged to produce meat and dairy products rather than grains. Nevertheless, in future evaluations of agricultural and related economic policies, health implications deserve a primary place.

Perhaps the most sensitive area for consideration is the funding of health services. Although the contribution of medical intervention to prevention of sickness and premature death can be expected to remain small in relation to behavioral and environmental influences, surgery and drugs are widely regarded as the basis of health and the essence of medical care, and society invests the money it sets aside for health mainly in treatment for acute diseases and particularly in hospitals for the acutely ill. Does it follow from our appraisal that resources should be transferred from acute care to chronic care and to preventive measures?

Health signifies that one's life force is intact, and that one is sufficiently in harmony with the social, physical, and supernatural environment to enjoy what is positively valued in life, and to ward off misfortunes and evils.
—Bantu African Medical Theory

Restricting the discussion to personal medical care, I believe that neglected areas, such as mental illness, mental retardation, and geriatric care, need greatly increased attention. But to suggest that this can be achieved merely by direct transfer of resources is an oversimplification. The designation "acute care" comprises a wide range of activities that differ profoundly in their effectiveness and efficiency. Some, like surgery for accidents and the treatment of acute emergencies, are among the most important services that medicine can offer and any reduction of their support would be disastrous. Others, however, like coronary care units and iron treatment of some anemias are not shown to be effective, while still others—most tonsillectomies and routine check-ups—are quite useless and should be abandoned. A critical appraisal of medical services for acute illnesses would result in more efficient use of available resources and would free some of them for preventive measures.

What health services need in general is an adjustment in the distribution of interest and resources between prevention of disease, care of the sick who require investigation and treatment, and care of the sick who do not need active intervention. Such an adjustment must pay considerable attention to the major determinants of health: to food and the environment, which will be mainly in the hands of specialists, and to personal behavior, which should be the concern of every practicing doctor.

❖ About the Author

The late Thomas McKeown, M.D., was professor emeritus, Department of Social Medicine, University of Birmingham, England, and author of *The Role of Medicine: Dream, Mirage, or Nemesis?*

❖ Socioeconomic Inequalities in Health
No Easy Solution

NANCY E. ADLER, W. THOMAS BOYCE,
MARGARET A. CHESNEY, SUSAN FOLKMAN,
AND S. LEONARD SYME

Socioeconomic status (SES) is a strong and consistent predictor of morbidity and premature mortality. Individuals lower in the SES hierarchy suffer disproportionately from almost every disease and show higher rates of mortality than those above them.[1, 2] This association is found with each of the key components of SES: income, education, and occupational status. Various approaches have been taken to explain this association. Empirical research has mostly focused on the impact of poverty and its correlates such as poor housing and inadequate nutrition; however, the poverty-related factors have not adequately explained the SES-health association.[3–6] Policy debate has focused relatively more attention on insurance coverage as a remedy to SES-related inequalities in health; some, like Friedman,[6] argue that "although coverage is not the sole determinant of health status it is a key factor in improved health. . . . "

Each of these approaches has limited our understanding of SES influences on health. The focus on health insurance as a means to improve health may deflect attention from other factors that contribute to social inequalities in health status. In this article we argue that insurance coverage alone will have a minor impact on SES-related inequalities in health. A full understanding of health inequalities requires that we consider other factors distributed along the SES hierarchy that are likely to contribute to undue health burdens and that such factors be explored not only among the impoverished, but at all levels of the social class and health gradient.

❖ The Relationship of SES and Health

Differences in mortality by social class and occupation have been documented since the 19th century. For example, in the 1860s, only the more affluent paid taxes. The crude death rate in Providence, RI, in 1865 was 10.8 per 1000 people among the relatively small group of taxpayers vs 24.8 per 1000 people among the large population of non-taxpayers.[7] During the first half of the 20th century, the difference in life expectancy between the highest and lowest SES groups in cities in the United States, England, and Wales was about 7 years.[1]

Socioeconomic status has been associated with mortality measured both at the aggregate level (i.e., areas characterized by lower-SES indicators have higher mortality rates) and at the individual level. At the aggregate level, significant differences in mortality rates within census tracts have been associated with the median monthly rents of homes, median family income, and poverty level of the census tract.[2-11] At the individual level, SES is inversely related to all-cause mortality and to the incidence of and mortality from specific diseases including cardiovascular disease, cancer, and respiratory disease.[12-18]

Although associations between SES and health are found over time and in different countries, the mediating variables may not be identical. In earlier times (and currently in developing countries), health advantages of higher SES were likely to be associated with one's ability to avoid infection. For example, the Great Plague of London in 1665 caused a disproportionate number of deaths among the poor who were more susceptible to disease because of poor nutrition and sanitation and who, unlike the wealthy, could not flee the cities when the disease became epidemic.[18] However, in circumstances where mortality is due primarily to chronic diseases, different mechanisms must be identified. In developed countries, the majority of deaths result from chronic degenerative diseases related to life-style behaviors rather than from infection and famine.[19,20] In the remainder of this article, we examine potential pathways by which SES may now be exerting its influence on health and discuss the implications of these pathways for clinical practice and policy choices.

❖ Linear Relationship vs Threshold Effect

If SES effects are due to poverty and its correlates, one would expect to find a threshold effect above which SES would show little or no association with health outcomes. Studies at both the individual and aggregate levels challenge this expectation. An association of SES and mortality occurs throughout the SES hierarchy. While many studies have only compared those at the bottom of the SES hierarchy with those above, a number of studies that have made more fine-grained comparisons report associations of health and SES at every level of the SES hierarchy.[3-8,10,14,21] For example, using 1971 British census data, Adelstein[21] found increasing mortality as occupational status decreased. In a US sample, Kitagawa and Hauser[10] demonstrated a linear association between years of school and mortality ratios (the ratio of observed to expected deaths, and between median family incomes within neighborhoods and mortality ratios of the neighborhoods.

The association of SES and health differs by age and race. Socioeconomic status differences in health are greatest in middle age and early old age compared with both earlier and later in life. There are marked SES differences in infant mortality and in the early neonatal period.[22,23] For those who survive, SES differences are comparatively small until much later in life.[22-24] The effects of SES across racial and ethnic groups are more complex, particularly for blacks vs whites. Because blacks are disproportionately represented in lower-SES groups, race and SES are often confounded. Race is more commonly assessed than is SES, and attributions made to racial differences in health outcomes may actually be due, at least in part, to SES.

Studies examining SES and race have come to varying conclusions about their relative impact. For example, when income was taken into account, a 30% higher mortality for blacks vs whites in the Alameda County (California) Study became statistically nonsignificant.[25,35] Similarly, Dayal, et al[13] found that racial differences in incidence of and survival from cancer became nonsignificant when SES was controlled for. However, other studies have found that controlling for SES reduces but does not eliminate racial differences in disease and mortality.[17,27,28] The relationships among SES, race, and health may vary depending on the disease or condition. In addition, SES may interact with race. Kessler and Neighbors[29] reanalyzed eight epidemiologic surveys on psychological distress and found that the effects of race depended on SES level; racial differences in psychological distress were much greater among individuals with lower SES than among those with higher SES. Studies of racial differences in blood pressure have also shown different patterns of association by SES among blacks vs. whites.[14,30,31]

❖ Access to Health Care and the SES-Health Gradient

One explanation for the SES-health gradient is that individuals lower in the SES hierarchy have less access to medical care. This explanation supports the belief that universal health insurance could reduce SES differences in health in the United States. However, three sets of findings suggest that while universal health insurance may be a necessary condition, it is not likely to be sufficient to reduce substantially social inequalities in health.

First, countries that have universal health insurance show the same SES-health gradient as that found in the United States—where such insurance is not provided. In England, Townsend and Davidson[32] concluded that the establishment of the National Health Service was not followed by a reduction of SES differences in health, and that, in fact, SES differences actually widened after its initiation.[18] This may have been due to changes in social conditions that created greater disparities among individuals at different levels of the SES hierarchy. In Scandinavian countries, the SES-health gradient emerges, but it is weaker than in the United States or England.[33-35] This may reflect the more homogeneous populations in these countries, as well as social policies that have reduced social class differences in income and other social resources, in addition to universal health coverage.

Second, SES differences can be found between levels at the upper range of the SES hierarchy. At upper levels, individuals are likely to have health insurance, making lack of coverage an unlikely explanation for health effects of SES differences. A clear example of both points comes from the Whitehall studies in England. Whitehall I examined 10-year mortality rates of a group of 17,530 British civil servants first studied in 1967 through 1969.[5] Although the subject population was more homogeneous than the general population in that all were employed by the British Civil Service as well as being covered by the National Health Service, a clear gradient still emerged in 10-year mortality across four levels of employment grade. Compared with the top administrators, the executive and professional class had a relative risk (RR) of mortality of 1.6, the clerical staff had an RR of 2.2, and the unskilled laborers had an RR of 2.7.

Third, SES differences appear in a wide range of diseases, both those that are amenable to treatment and those that are not. Bunker and Gomby[26] noted that to the extent to which mortality from malignant diseases reflects differential access to care, a greater SES effect should be found in cancers most amenable to treatment. However, they concluded that "available data show either no effect, or, in fact, a greater discrepancy across social classes for those malignancies least amenable to treatment." Other evidence comes from research within a single treatment setting in which differences in care are presumably minimal and that finds an association of outcome with SES.[13] In a recent study of patients with acute myocardial infarction, patients with more education were found to have lower in-hospital mortality even when age, race, gender, and baseline severity scores were taken into account.[37] In terms of overall mortality, adequacy of care is estimated to account for about 10% of the outcome, while human biological factors and environmental factors each account for 20% and individual factors account for half.[38]

The above argument does not imply that medical care is unimportant. Rather, medical care is but one input into health status and, in some instances, will play a relatively minor role.[39–42] Further, provision of insurance does not ensure equal or adequate access, especially for primary care.[43,44] In those areas that are underserved, individuals with fewer socioeconomic resources will find it more difficult to gain access.[45] Even among individuals in the same area who technically have equal access, true access may differ for those at different SES levels. Individuals with more education and income, who may be more skilled in dealing with bureaucracies and social systems, may be more efficient in determining who provides the best care and in obtaining care when needed.

Individuals with fewer social and economic resources appear to make less use of preventive health services including screening. To some extent, this may reflect insurance-based differences in care. But Hayward et al[46] found that lower-SES women were less likely to have had Papanicolaou tests, breast examinations by a physician, or mammograms independent of age, health status, or frequency of physician visits. Harlan et al[47] found that women with less than a high school education were relatively less likely than those with more education to have been screened for cervical cancer or to have even heard of a Papanicolaou test. Research in Finland found that low-SES women were relatively less likely than those higher in SES to use cancer screening services.[48] Programs involving outreach to increase access will be more effective in reducing SES differentials. For example, Stamler et al[49] examined 5-year all-cause mortality among 11,000 hypertensive patients who were randomly referred to standard care or treatment geared to minimizing barriers to care (stepped care). The stepped-care group showed lower mortality than did the standard-care group. In the whole sample educational level was inversely related to mortality rates; in the stepped-care group, this relationship was reduced, although it still remained significant.

Because insurance alone does not guarantee equal access to and utilization of medical care, and because medical care itself has a limited association with health differences, we must consider other factors that may contribute to SES differentials in health. These must be addressed if substantial reductions in social inequalities in health outcomes are to occur.

❖ Other Factors in the SES Link

Behaviors such as smoking, diet, and lack of exercise are associated with health status.[28,50–52] Early effects of those behaviors are reflected in risk factors such as cholesterol level, obesity, and blood pressure; longer-term effects can be seen in disease and premature mortality. Both the behaviors and the risk factors show a linear relationship with SES.

Clear SES differences are shown in rates of smoking. In the Whitehall studies of the British Civil Service, smoking rates in both sexes increased as one went down the employment grade hierarchy. A significant linear trend by employment grade was also found in prevalence of exercise (the lower the employment grade, the higher the percentage reporting getting no exercise) and diet (the lower the employment grade, the lower the percentage of individuals consuming skimmed milk, wholemeal bread, and fresh fruits and vegetables).[4]

In the United States, similar patterns have been found. For example, in a community sample of 2138 women aged 42 to 50 years studied by Matthews et al.[53] the prevalence of smoking ranged from 45% of those with less than a high school education to 19% of those with advanced degrees. Intermediate rates were found for those with some college (30%) and those with a college degree (23%). Similarly, Winkleby et al[24] found a strong association of smoking with years of education among both men and women in a community sample of 3349 adults.

Risk factors also increase as SES decreases. In the community sample of women studied by Matthews et al,[53] educational level was significantly associated with cholesterol levels (higher low-density lipoprotein [LDL] and triglyceride levels, lower high-density lipoprotein [HDL], HDL2, and HDL/ LDL ratio with less education), systolic blood pressure, glucose tolerance, and body mass index. All risk factors were more adverse the less education the woman had, and the associations persisted when body mass index was taken into account. Kraus et al[14] found a linear gradient between prevalence of hypertension and six levels of SES based on education and occupation among 15,412 white males who were screened for participation in the community-based Multiple Risk Factor Intervention Trial. Smaller numbers of men from other ethnic groups were also studied; the gradient emerged for Hispanics, but not for Asians or blacks. Finally, numerous studies have shown that rates of obesity increase as SES declines, particularly among women.[55–58]

The pattern of health risk behaviors in which those with a higher SES are less likely to smoke and eat high-fat diets and are more likely to exercise has not always been true. Earlier in the 20th century, many of these behaviors (e.g., smoking, eating red meat) were not classified as health-risking behaviors but as luxuries. Epidemiological surveys documenting the prevalence of these behaviors are not available for this period. It seems likely that higher-SES individuals were relatively more likely to indulge in these activities. During this time, rates of coronary heart disease were greater in higher-SES groups.[18] However, as health promotion has become more popular, upper-SES groups have been quickest to acquire and act on information regarding health risks. Despite this seeming advantage, a few life-style differences place higher-SES individuals at relatively greater risk for specific diseases. Rates of malignant melanoma are greater in higher-SES groups, which may be due in part to differences in recreational tanning. In addition, rates of breast cancer are greater among higher-SES women, which may reflect differences in childbearing patterns. However, once breast cancer is diagnosed, survival is positively associated with SES even when stage at diagnosis is taken into account.[13]

Health behaviors represent one pathway by which SES may influence health, but they do not account for all of the association. In the Whitehall sample, for example, Marmot et al[5] found that the RR of mortality for lower employment grades was reduced but was still strong when a number of behavioral and risk factors were controlled for.

Other potential pathways by which SES may influence health are through differential exposure to physical and social contexts that are damaging to one's health. The lower an individual is in the SES hierarchy, the more likely he or she is to experience adverse environmental conditions, such as exposure to pathogens and carcinogens at home and at work, and to social conditions, such as crime.[59] As Dutton and Levin[60] note, individuals lower in the social hierarchy experience "more disruption and daily struggle as well as more simple physical hardships."

In addition to the direct health effect of exposure to adverse physical and social conditions, these experiences may trigger psychological processes that affect one's risk of disease. There is increasing evidence that stress plays a role in disease, including heart disease and susceptibility to infection.[61-63] Community studies have demonstrated that the lower one's position in the hierarchy, the greater the reported exposure to stressful life events and the greater the impact of these events on emotional adjustment.[64-66] In a study of 2320 men following a myocardial infarction, Ruberman and colleagues[67] found a strong negative association between years of education and degree of life stress and social isolation; these two variables, in turn, were strongly related to mortality following myocardial infarction. Within groups that were either low on life stress and social isolation or were high on both, education was no longer related to mortality, suggesting that the association of education and mortality was a function of the greater life stress and social isolation of those with less education.

Research on stressful life events has shown that the impact of an event on physical and mental well-being is mediated through the individual's appraisal of the event as stressful; the appraisal is a function of the individual's evaluation of the event and of the resources he or she has to handle it.[68] Appraisal of events as stressful is likely to vary by SES level. Components of SES such as education and income provide resources that can be used to address and resolve threats and may reduce the impact of the event on the body.

Socioeconomic status contributes to the development during childhood of traits and coping resources that may affect risk for disease. Rutter[69] notes that "adverse life events make it more likely that people will act in ways that create threatening situations for themselves." Exposure to greater stress in childhood reduces the likelihood that children will develop "resilience" and increases the chances that they will develop depression and helplessness, characteristics that have been linked to increased risk of disease.[70,71] Placement in the SES hierarchy is also associated with the differential ability of individuals to control their environment. A clear effect is one's ability to avoid risks of disease and injury. For example, safety features in cars (most recently air bags) have been more available in higher-priced cars. There are a myriad of ways in which higher-SES individuals can control their environment, and the experience of control itself has been linked to better health outcomes.[72-73]

❖ Implications for Policy and Clinical Practice

Public health policy is moving toward the provision of health insurance to provide universal access to health care. However, even if this goal is achieved, our review indicates that SES inequalities in health will persist. Differences related to SES in health-damaging behaviors and exposure to adverse physical and psychosocial conditions differentially place those lower in the SES hierarchy at risk of disease and premature mortality. Moreover, successful and effective utilization of care may depend on class-related contextual factors of an individual's daily life. These factors need to be addressed in clinical practice as well as in policy design.

Clinicians and policymakers should be aware that the health effects of social position occur not only at the poverty level—where even conventional wisdom acknowledges disproportionate rates of poor health—but throughout the social class hierarchy. The psychological, behavioral, and biological factors that underlie class-associated vulnerabilities remain incompletely understood, but among those that a physician should attend to involve understanding the patient's health behaviors, exposure to stressful challenges and resources to deal with such challenges, and control over important domains in his or her life that may interfere with modifying health-damaging behaviors and with obtaining adequate care.

Many providers are acutely aware of the possible influences of contextual conditions on patients' health. Yet, they may assume that these become less relevant for patients who are employed, have adequate resources for basic needs, and have access to medical care. Even above the poverty level, however, SES-related factors will affect an individual's ability to engage in health-promoting and disease-preventing behaviors, including effective use of health care services.

In many settings, job status affects the individual's control over the scheduling of his or her work: usually a manager has more flexibility than a foreman, and a foreman has more than a line worker. Control over one's work circumstances affects the individual's ability to not only obtain care, but also to follow through on prescribed regimens. For example, in a recent study of San Francisco, Calif, bus drivers, 60% of drivers with diagnosed hypertension were found to be untreated or uncontrolled despite full and complete access to primary medical care services (unpublished data, Muni Study of Stress and Hypertension, July 1991). Further exploration revealed that many drivers prescribed antihypertensive diuretics were unable to comply with treatment because bathrooms were not accessible during their tightly scheduled bus routes. This example highlights the need for physicians to consider the impact of treatment regimens on individual patient life-styles and the implications of this for their ability to adhere to treatment. In the case of hypertension, physicians may want to consider alternative treatment regimens (eg, nondiuretic antihypertensive medications, dietary changes that accommodate to the variety of foods available to the patient) that balance clinical efficacy with the likelihood that the patient will be able to accommodate the treatment into his or her life.

Our analysis underscores the importance—increasingly recognized within clinical medicine—of a strong program of preventive services accessible to populations of primary care patients. Unfortunately, preventive services may actually be offered in reverse order to the degree of need; those lower in the SES hierarchy, who have the highest rates of health-risking behaviors and risk factors, are least likely to receive information and services. Individuals at the lower ends of the SES hierarchy are more likely to use emergency departments and clinics where continuity of care is not possible and concern about prevention a luxury. Even as one ascends the SES ladder, programs to help with quitting smoking, losing weight, and learning stress management techniques are relatively more available to those at the top. At worksites with preventive health programs, for example, opportunities for exercise, smoking cessation, and stress management are often offered first to the top executives and management. Within physicians' offices, there may be a similar bias toward addressing these issues with better-educated, higher-income patients.

Health promotion programs and physician recommendations are frequently designed with upper-SES individuals in mind. For example, recommendations to increase exercise presume that patients have access to safe environments where they can swim, walk, or jog. Physicians need to recognize not only the importance of discussing risk behavior increases with patients who are lower on the SES ladder, but also that recommendations need to be tailored to the patient's life circumstances. For example, in suggesting exercise, it will be helpful to explore with patients when and where this could be accomplished, both helping them to overcome real or perceived barriers and to identify opportunities of which they may not be aware.

Beyond providing access to care and using clinical practice to reduce social inequalities in health, other inequalities associated with SES will also need to be addressed to reduce substantially the current strong association of SES and health. Vàgerö,[34] for example, attributes the fact that class differences in health are smaller in Sweden than in England to differences in income spread rather than to differences in health services. As noted earlier, Sweden's social welfare policies result in a more even distribution of income compared with England's. Other data show that in developed countries, the average life expectancy is associated with how egalitarian the income distribution is; the more egalitarian the distribution, the higher the life expectancy.[74,75] Of developed countries, the United States is among the least egalitarian nations in income distribution.[75] Thus, those concerned with the health of the nation need to be aware of social policies that increase the gap among levels in the SES hierarchy even if we enact policies that provide access to care.

In short, no single strategy will significantly reduce social inequalities in health. The problem needs to be addressed by physicians at multiple levels, from general social policy to the details of clinical practice. Expanded health care coverage and equal access to care may help reduce SES differentials in health, but attention must also be given to SES-related social, environmental, and psychological resources that influence health risk, the effective utilization of health care, and adherence to prevention and treatment regimens. Physicians have important roles to play in reducing SES inequalities in health. They can increase the likelihood that their recommendations for prevention and treatment will be effective for lower-SES as well as upper-SES patients by providing clinical care that is sensitive to SES-related influences on health and health behaviors. Physicians who are aware of the increased need for outreach to patients as SES declines can also take part in community health initiatives that increase the focus on those lower in the SES hierarchy. Finally, physicians may wish to consider advocacy for social policies to address SES inequalities that have an impact on health.

ACKNOWLEDGMENT

Preparation of this article was supported by the John D. and Catherine T. MacArthur Foundation Network on Determinants and Consequences of Health-Promoting and Disease-Preventing Behavior.

❖ About the Authors

Nancy E. Adler, M.D., is Professor and Director of the Department of Psychiatry and Professor of Pediatrics, School of Medicine, University of California, San Francisco.

W. Thomas Boyce, M.D., is Professor, Department of Pediatrics, School of Medicine, University of California, San Francisco.

Margaret Chesney, M.D., is Adjunct Professor in the Department of Medicine and Department of Epidemiology and Biostatistics, University of California, San Francisco.

Susan Folkman, M.D., is in the Department of Medicine and Center for AIDS Prevention Studies, University of California, San Francisco.

S. Leonard Syme is Emeritus Professor of Epidemiology, Department of Biomedical and Environmental Health Sciences, School of Public Health, University of California, Berkeley.

REFERENCES

1. Antonovsky A. Social class, life expectancy and overall mortality. *Milbank Q.* 1967;41:31-73.

2. Syme SL, Berkman LF. Social class, susceptibility and sickness. *Am J Epidemiol.* 1976;104:1-8.

3. Haan MN, Kaplan GA, Syme, SL. Socioeconomic states and health: old observations and new thoughts. In: Bunker JP, Gomby DS, Kehrer BH. eds. *Pathways to Health.* Menlo Park, Calif: The Henry J. Kaiser Family Foundation: 1980:76-135.

4. Marmot MG, Smith GD, Stansfeld S, et al. Health inequalities among

British civil servants: the Whitehall II study. *Lancet.* 1991;337:1387-1393.

5. Marmot MG, Shipley MJ, Rose G. Inequalities in death—specific explanations of a general pattern. *Lancet.* 1984;1:1003-1006.

6. Friedman E. The uninsured: from dilemma to crisis. *JAMA.* 1991;265:2491-2495.

7. Chapin CV. Deaths among taxpayers and nontaxpayers, income tax. Providence, 1805. *Am J Public Health.* 1924;14:647-651.

8. Coombs LC. Economic differentials in causes of death. *Med Care.* 1941;1:240-255.

9. Haan MN, Kaplan CA, Camancho T. Poverty and health: prospective evidence from the Alameda County Study. *Am J Epidemiol.* 1987;125:989-998.

10. Kitagawa FM, Hauser PM. *Differential Mortality in the United States: A Study of Socioeconomic Epidemiology.* Cambridge, Mass.: Harvard University Press, 1973.

11. Patno ME. Mortality and economic level in an urban area. *Public Health Rep.* 1960;75:841-851.

12. Berg JW, Ross R, Laitourette HR. Economic status and survival of cancer patients. *Cancer.* 1977;39:467-477.

13. Dayal HH, Power RN, Chiu C. Race and socioeconomic status in survival from breast cancer. *J Chronic Disability.* 1982;35:675-683.

14. Kraus JF, Burhani NO, Franti CE. Socioeconomic status, ethnicity, and risk of coronary heart disease. *Am J Epidemiol.* 1980;111:407-414.

15. Marmot MG, Adelstein AM, Robinson N, Rose GA. Changing social-class distribution of heart disease. *BMJ.* 1978;2:1109-1112.

16. Marmot MG, Rose G, Shipley MJ, Hamilton PJS. Employment grade and coronary heart disease in British civil servants. *J Epidermiol Community Health.* 1987;32:244-249.

17. Steinhorn SC, Myers MH, Hanky BH, Pelham VF. Factors associated with survival differences between black women and white women with cancer of the uterine corpus. *Am J Epidemiol.* 1986;124:85-93.

18. Sasser M, Watson W, Hopper K. *Sociology in Medicine.* 3rd ed. Oxford, England: Oxford University Press; 1985.

19. Caldwell JC. *Theory of Fertility Decline.* London, England: Academic Press, 1982.

20. Omran AR. The epidemiologic transition: a theory of the epidemiology of population change. *Milbank Q.* 1971;49:509-538.

21. Adelstein, AM. Life-style in occupational cancer. *J Taxicol Environ Health.* 1980;6:953-962.

22. Gould JC, LeRoy S. Socioeconomic status and low birth weight: a racial comparison. *Pediatrics.* 1988;82:896-904.

23. Wise PH, Meyers A. Poverty and child health. *Pediatr Clin North Am.* 1988;35:1169-1186.

24. House JS, Kessler RC, Herzog AR. Age, socioeconomic status, and health. *Milbank Q.* 1990;68:383-411.

25. Haan MN, Kaplan GA. The contribution of socioeconomic position to minority health. In: Heckler M, ed. *Report of the Secretary's Task Force on Black and Minority Health: Crosscutting Issues in Minority Health.* Washington DC: US Dept of Health and Human Services; 1985.

26. Kaplan GA, Haan MN. Socioeconomic position and health: prospective evidence from the Alameda County Study. Presented at the 114th annual meeting of the American Public Health Association; Las Vegas, Nev; September 29, 1986.

27. Devesa SS, Diamond EL. Association of breast cancer and cervical cancer incidences with income and education among whites and blacks. *J Natl Cancer Inst.* 1980;6:515-528.

28. Otten M, Teutsch S, Williamson, D, Marks J. The effect of known risk factors on the excess mortality

of black adults in the United States. *JAMA*. 1990;263:845-850.

29. Kessler RC, Neighbors HW. A new perspective on the relationships among race, social class, and psychological distress. *J Health Soc Behaav*. 1986;27:107-115.

30. Harburg E, Erfurt JC, Chape C, Hauenstein LS, Schull WJ, Schork MA. Socioecological stressor areas and black-white blood pressure. *J Chronic Dis*. 1973;26:595-611.

31. James AJ, Strogatz DS, Wing SB, Ramsey DL. Socioeconomic status, John Henryism, and hypertension in blacks and whites. *Am J Epidemiol*. 1987;126:664-673.

32. Townsend P, Davidson N. *Inequalities in Health: The Black Report*. Harmondsworth, England: Penguin; 1982.

33. Lundberg O. Causal explanations for class inequality in health—an empirical analysis. *Soc Sci Med*. 1991;32:385-393.

34. Vågerö D. Inequality in health—some theoretical and empirical problems. *Soc Sci Med*. 1991;32: 367-371.

35. Vågerö D, Lundberg O. Health inequalities in Britain and Sweden, *Lancet*. 1989;2:35-36.

36. Bunker JP, Gomby DS. Preface: socioeconomic states and health: an examination of underlying process. In: Bunker JP, Gomby DS, Kehrer BH. eds. *Pathways to Health*. Menlo Park, Calif: The Henry J. Kaiser Family Foundation; 1989: xv-xxiv.

37. Tofler GH, Muller JE, Stone PH, et al. Comparison of long-term outcome after acute myocardial infarction in patients never graduated from high school with that in more educated patients. *Am J Cardiol*. 1993;71:1031-1035.

38. US Dept of Health, Education and Welfare. *Healthy People: The Surgeon General's Report on Health Promotion and Disease Prevention*. Washington DC: US Dept of Health, Education and Welfare; 1979.

39. Kim K, Moody P. More resources, better health? a cross-national perspective. *Soc Sci Med*. 1992;34:837-842.

40. Doll R. Health and the environment in the 1990s. *Am J Public Health*. 1992;82:933-941.

41. Winkelstein W, Jr. Medical care is not health care. *JAMA* 1993;269-2504.

42. Diehr PK, Richardson WC, Shortell SM, LoGerfo JP. Increased access to medical care. *Med Care*. 1991;10:989-999.

43. Dalen JE, Santiago J. Insuring the uninsured is not enough. *Arch Intern Med*. 1991;151:860-862.

44. Haas JS, Udvarhelyi S, Morris CN, Epstein AM. The effect of providing health coverage to poor uninsured pregnant women in Massachusetts. *JAMA*. 1993;269:87-91.

45. Ginsberg E, Ostow M. Beyond universal health insurance to effective health care. *JAMA*. 1991;265:2559-2562.

46. Hayward RA, Shapiro MF, Freeman HE, Corey CR. Who gets screened for cervical and breast cancer? results from a new national survey. *Arch Intern Med*. 1988;148:1177-1181.

47. Harlan LC, Bernstein AB, Kessler LG. Cervical cancer screening who is not screened and why? *Am J Public Health*. 1991;81:885-890.

48. Salonen JT. Socioeconomic status and risk of cancer, cerebral stroke, and death due to coronary heart disease and any disease: a longitudinal study in eastern Finland. *J Epidemiol Community Health*. 1982; 36:294-297.

49. Stamler R, Hardy RJ, Payne GH, et al. Educational level and five-year all-cause mortality in the hypertension detection and follow-up program. *Hypertension*. 1987;9:641-646.

50. Paffenbarger RS, Hyde RT, Wing AL, Lee IM, Jung DL, Kampert JB. The association of changes in physical-activity level and other lifestyle characteristics with mor-

tality among men. *N Engl J Med.* 1993;328:538-545.

51. Wilhelmsen L. Coronary heart disease: epidemiology of smoking and intervention studies of smoking. *Am Heart J.* 1988;115:242-249.

52. Centers for Disease Control. *Smoking, Tobacco and Health: A Fact Book.* Rockville, Md: US Dept of Health and Human Services, Public Health Service, Office on Smoking and Health; 1987.

53. Matthews K, Kelsey S, Meilahn E, Kuller L, Wing R. Educational attainment and behavioral and biologic risk factors for coronary heart disease in middle-aged women. *Am J Epidemiol.* 1989;129:1132-1144.

54. Winkleby M, Fortmann S, Barrett D. Social class disparities in risk factors for disease: eight-year prevalence patterns by level of education. *Prev Med.* 1990;19:1-12.

55. Cauley JA, Donfield SM, LaPorte RF, Warhaftig NE. Physical activity by SES in two population-based cohorts. *Med Sci Sports Exercise.* 1991;23:343-352.

56. Jeffrey RW, French SA, Forester JL, Spry VM. Socioeconomic status differences in health behaviors related to obesity: the Healthy Worker Project. *Int J Obes.* 1991;15:689-696.

57. Kahn HS, Williamson DF, Stevens JA. Race and weight change in US women: the roles of socioeconomic and marital status. *Am J Public Health.* 1991;81:319-323.

58. Sobel J, Stunkard AJ. Socioeconomic status and obesity: a review of the literature. *Psychol Bull.* 1989;105:260-271.

59. Stokols D. Establishing and maintaining health environments. *Am Psychol.* 1992;47:6-22.

60. Dutton DB, Levine S. Overview, methodological critique, and reformulation. In: Bunker JP, Gomby DS, Kehrer BH. eds. *Pathways to Health.* Menlo Park, Calif: The Henry J. Kaiser Family Foundation; 1989;29-69.

61. Byrne DG, Whyte HM. Life events and myocardial infarction revisited: the role of measures of individual impact. *Psychosom Med.* 1980;42:1-10.

62. Cohen S, Tyrrell DAJ, Smith AP. Psychological stress in humans and susceptibility to the common cold. *N Engl J Med.* 1991;325:606-612.

63. Cohen S, Tyrrell DAJ, Smith AP. Negative life events, perceived stress, negative affect, and susceptibility to the common cold. *J Pers Soc Psychol.* 1993;64:131-140.

64. McLeod JD, Kessler RC. Socioeconomic status differences in vulnerability to undesirable life events. *J Health Soc Behav.* 1990;31:162-172.

65. Cohen S, Wills TA. Stress, social support and the buffering hypothesis. *Psychol Bull.* 1985;98:310-357.

66. House JS, Kessler R, Herzog AR, Mero P, Kinney A, Breslow M. Social stratification, age, and health. In: Scheie KW, Blazer D, House JS. eds. *Aging, Health Behaviors, and Health Outcomes.* Hillsdale, NJ: Lawrence Erlbaum; 1991.

67. Ruberman W, Weinblatt E, Goldberg JD, Chaudhary BS. Psychosocial influences on mortality after myocardial infarction. *N Engl J Med.* 1984;34:552-559.

68. Folkman S, Lazarus RS, Gruen RJ, DeLongis A. Appraisal, coping, health status, and psychological symptoms. *J Pers Soc Psychol.* 1986;50:571-579.

69. Rutter M. Psychosocial resilience and protective mechanisms. *Am J Orthopsychiatry.* 1987;57:316-330.

70. Carney RM, Rich MW, Freedlan KE. et al. Major depressive disorder predicts cardiac events in patients with coronary artery disease. *PsychosomMed.* 1988;50:627-633.

71. Booth-Kewley S, Friedman HS. Psychological predictors of heart disease: a quantitative review. *Psychol Bull.* 1987;101:343-362.

72. Rodin J, Langer E. Long-term effects of a control-relevant inter-

vention with the institutionalized aged. *J Pers Soc Psychol.* 1977;35: 897-902.

73. Rodin J. Aging and health: effects of the sense of control. *Science.* 1986;233:1271-1276.

74. Wilkinson RG. Income distribu-

tion and mortality a 'natural' experiment. *Social Health Illness.* 1990;12:391-412.

75. Wilkinson RC. Income distribution and life expectancy. *BMJ.* 1992;304: 165-168.

❖ Race or Class versus Race and Class: Mortality Differentials in the United States

VICENTE NAVARRO

The latest annual report of the US federal government about the health of the US population[1] has created enormous concern about the mortality differentials between whites and blacks. For example, in 1988 life expectancy at birth was 75.5 years for whites but only 69.5 years for blacks. For most causes of death, the death rate in blacks is higher than that in whites, and for many causes of death mortality differentials are increasing rather than decreasing. Alarming reports about these differences have appeared in both the lay press[2] and medical publications.[3] Consequently, it makes sense that the federal government has chosen the reduction of these differentials as one of its top objectives and has called for a "decrease [of the] disparity in life expectancy between white and minority populations to no more than four years."[4]

Although this emphasis on reducing race differentials is undoubtedly very important, another component of the nation's health that is highly relevant to race differentials in mortality has passed unnoticed. The stark fact is that these differentials cannot be explained merely by looking at race. After all, some blacks have better health indicators (including mortality rates) than some whites, and not all whites have similar mortality indicators. Thus we must look at class differentials in mortality in the US, which are also increasing rather than declining. Class is harder to define than race, but the most frequent indicators of social class used for morbidity and mortality statistics in the western industrialised world are occupation, education, and income.[5]

❖ Importance of Class Differentials

The US is the only western developed nation whose government does not collect mortality statistics by class. The federal report[1] on health indicators in the US—*Health, United States, 1989*—tabulates mortality statistics by age, sex, and race but not by class indicators such as income, education, or occupation. With the active encouragement of the European office of the World Health Organisation, most European countries have chosen as the top target in their health policies a reduction, by the year 2000, of the differentials in health status among classes.[6] By contrast, the US is alone among major industrialised nations in not aiming for this goal—in the US, race is used as a *substitute* for class. What the US government seems to ignore is that even if there were no race differentials in mortality, most blacks would still have higher mortality rates than the median or the mean rate in the US population. To understand this point, one has to appreciate that the US has classes as well as races.

How people live, die, and get sick depends not only on their race, gender, and age but also on the class to which they belong. There is empirical information to sustain this position. On one of the few occasions (in 1986) that the US government collected information on mortality rates (for heart and cerebrovascular disease) by class, the results showed that, by whatever indicators of class one might choose (level of education, income, or occupation), mortality rates are related to social class. People with less formal education, with lower income, and belonging to the working class (eg, labourers in the US Census categories of operator and services) are more likely to die of heart disease than are people with more formal education, with higher income, and belonging to the upper classes (eg, managerial and professional).[7]

Mortality Differentials

Managerial and professional groups had lower mortality rates for heart disease than did major components of the working class, such as operators and service workers.

Data from the same survey (1986 National Mortality Followback Survey) also show that most of those who died of cerebrovascular disease and all other causes had family incomes of less than $25,000 in 1985 and less than a high school education; the largest proportion of the deceased had worked in technical, sales, and operator occupations—the main occupational groups in the working class.[8] Similar class mortality differentials have been found for breast cancer and for all causes of death.[9,10]

For both causes of mortality—heart disease and cerebrovascular disease—the class differentials in mortality were larger than the race differentials. The mortality rate for heart disease in blue-collar workers (operators) was 2.3 times higher than the rate in managers and professionals.

For 1986, the heart disease mortality rate for black males was 1.2 times higher than for white males, and for black females was 1.5 times higher than for white females.[11]

Morbidity Differentials

Although there are no published data to show mortality rates by class and race, it is likely that the mortality rates for white service workers, for example, are closer to those of black service workers than to those of white professionals. Since there are no data to establish this point, we can look instead at data on morbidity. Morbidity differentials by class are much larger than differentials by race. In 1986, those making $10,000 or less per year reported 4.6 times more morbidity than those making over

$35,000, while blacks reported 1.9 times more morbidity than whites.[12] The race differentials were less than half the class differentials. The same report shows that race differentials within each income group are less pronounced than those between income groups. Morbidity rates for blacks making less than $20,000 were much closer to those for whites in the same income group than to those for blacks in income groups greater than $20,000. Similarly, morbidity rates for whites with incomes below $20,000 were closer to those of blacks in the same income group than to those of whites in income groups over $20,000. Whites making under $20,000 had higher morbidity rates than blacks earning over $20,000.

A similar pattern is observed when occupation is used rather than income. Thus blue-collar workers (operators) reported a morbidity rate (9.5%) that was 2.9 times higher than that of professionals (3.2%), while blacks reported a morbidity rate 1.9 times higher than that of whites.[13]

Consideration of the annual percentage of persons with limited activity due to chronic conditions rather than self-reported morbidity provides further confirmation. Class differentials (measured by income differentials) are larger than race differentials.[14] Moreover, these class differentials have grown larger during the 1980s—even larger than race differentials.

❖ Disparity of Wealth and Income by Class

Within each class (measured by education, income, or occupation), blacks often have worse health indicators than whites. These are the differentials that the US government is targeting for reduction, an important and much-needed task. But the overwhelming majority of blacks (and other minorities) are members of the low-paid, poorly educated working class that have higher morbidity and mortality rates than high-earning, better educated people. The growing mortality differentials between whites and blacks cannot be understood by looking only at race; they are part and parcel of larger mortality differentials—class differentials. In the 1980s, the US witnessed an increased class polarisation of the population, with a reduction of the middle class, and a rapid growth of the low-paid, unskilled working class. Members of the working class are increasingly non-unionised, poorly paid, and part-time, and with a preponderance of minorities and women. The low-earners comprise a heterogeneous group—blacks, Hispanics, whites, men, and women—whose standards of living are rapidly deteriorating because of the growing wealth and income differentials between the upper and lower classes. These social groups belong to the 40% of the population who received only 15.7% of the total income in 1984, the lowest figure since data collection was initiated in 1947. By contrast, the wealthiest 20% received 42.9% of total income, the highest ever.[15] This growing disparity of wealth and income by class mainly, but not exclusively, explains the race differentials in morbidity and mortality.

The growing class differential in mortality rates is not unique to the

US. Other countries have noticed that these differentials are not only persistent but growing,[16] and a large national and international debate about the reasons for these class differentials has been initiated.[17] However, in the US there is a deafening silence on this topic. If a prerequisite for finding the right answer is to ask the right question, then it is unlikely that by concentrating solely on race differentials we will ever be able to understand why the health indicators of our minorities are getting worse.

❖ About the Author

Vicente Navarro, Ph.D., is Professor of Public Policy, Sociology and Policy Studies, Department of Health Policy and Management, School of Hygiene and Public Health at Johns Hopkins University in Baltimore, Maryland.

REFERENCES

1. Health, United States, 1989. Washington, DC: US Department of Health and Human Services, 1990.
2. US health gap is widening between whites and blacks. *New York Times*, March 23, 1990: A17.
3. Greenberg DS. Black health: grim statistics. *Lancet*. 1990;335:780–81.
4. Goals for the nation for the year 2000. Washington, DC: Public Health Service, US Department of Health and Human Services, 1989.
5. Liberatos P, Link GB, Kelsey LJ. The measurement of social class in epidemiology. *Epidemiol Rev*. 1988; 10:87–121.
6. Targets for health for all: targets in support of the European regional strategy for health for all. Copenhagen: World Health Organisation, Regional Office for Europe, 1980:24–25.
7. Kapantais G, Powell-Griner E. Characteristics of persons dying of diseases of the heart. Preliminary data from the 1986 national mortality follow-back survey. Washington, DC: National Center for Health Statistics. Advance data from vital and health statistics. No. 172, Aug. 24, 1989: 7, 9, 12 (tables 3, 4, 5).
8. Powell-Griner E. Characteristics of persons dying from cerebrovascular diseases. Washington, DC: National Center for Health Statistics. Preliminary data from vital and health statistics, No. 180, Feb. 8, 1990: 2–3.
9. Krieger N. Social class and the black white crossover in the age-specific incidence of breast cancer: a study linking census derived data to population-based registry records. *Am J Epidemiol* 1990;131: 804–14.
10. Marmot MG, Kogevinas M, Elston MA. Social economic status and disease. *Annu Rev Publ Health*. 1987;8:111–13.
11. Age adjusted death rates for selected causes of death, according to sex and race: United States, selected years, 1950–87. Table 23 in Health, United States, 1989. Washington, DC: US Department of Health and Human Services, 1990: 121–22.
12. Self assessment of health according to race and income. Table 45 in Health, United States, 1987. Washington, DC: US Department of Health and Human Services, 1988:91.

13. Percent of persons 18 years of age and over in the labor force with respondent-assessed health status of either fair or poor, by employment status and by occupation: US, 1983–85. Table D in Health Characteristics by Occupation and Industry: US, 1983–85. Washington, DC: US Department of Health and Human Services, 1989:11.

14. Average annual percent of persons with limitation of activity due to chronic conditions by race, age, and family income: US, 1985–87. Fig. 4 in Health of black and white Americans, 1985–87. Vital and health statistics. Washington, DC: National Center for Health Statistics, 1990; ser 10, no 171:12.

15. Harrison B, Bluestone B. The great U-turn: corporate restructuring and the polarization of America. New York: Basic Books, 1988:128.

16. Vagerö, D, Lundberg O. Health inequalities in Britain and Sweden. *Lancet.* 1989;ii:35–36,

17. Townsend P. Widening inequalities of health: a rejoinder to Rudolph Klein. *Int J Health Serv.* 1990; 20:363–72.

❖ Chapter 2
The Health of
the Nation

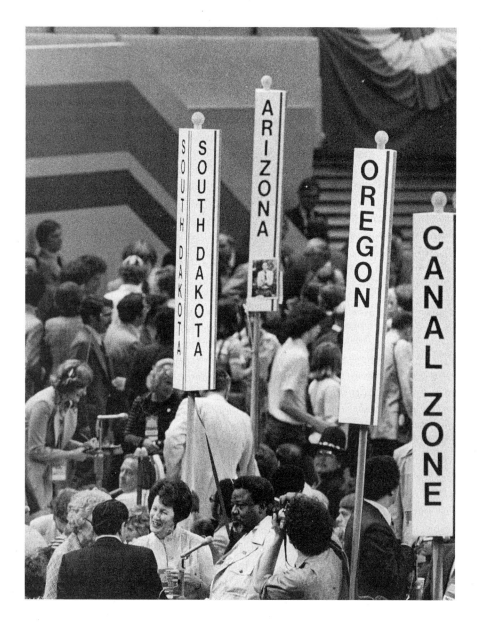

The dramatic improvements in the health of the population of the United States during the past 200 years have been reviewed by Duffy (1990), Fee (1991), and Breslow (1990). In the early years of the republic, before the sanitary revolution which began in the 1850s, mortality rates from infectious diseases were high. Although the recurrent epidemics of cholera, yellow fever, and small pox attracted the most public attention, mortality was also high for tuberculosis, pneumonia, and influenza.

The sanitary revolution began in the 1850s with the beginnings of organized community efforts to deal with the unsanitary conditions in the environment, contamination of water supplies, human and animal wastes, and miserable, overcrowded housing. The initial focus on environmental sanitation produced dramatic benefits for the health of the population, particularly with a reduction in mortality from the recurrent yellow fever and cholera epidemics. Although small pox vaccination was begun by Jenner in the late 18th century, it did not become widespread until almost a century later. Tuberculosis began to decline even before the pioneering studies by Koch in the late 1900s, but tuberculosis was still the nation's leading cause of death in 1900.

The application of Pasteur's research began to bear fruit after the turn of the 20th century with the pasteurization of milk. The New York City Health Department lead the nation in its development of milk stations to distribute safe milk to poor infants. These efforts, as well as the chlorination of water supplies, were to dramatically reduce mortality from communicable diseases prior to the influenza pandemic of 1918–1919.

By the 1920s, the great killers had become heart disease, cancer and stroke. These three chronic diseases remain at the top of the list of killer diseases, but mortality rates for heart disease and stroke began to fall in the 1960s, with the advent of the second public health revolution (Breslow, 1990). Recently, mortality rates from cancer have also begun to decline. The dramatic decline in cardiovascular death rates has been the result of the combined effect of public health (e.g., smoking control) and medical care (e.g., improved treatment of hypertension).

In the late 1970s, a national focus began to be placed on achieving broader national health objectives as noted by McGinnis and Lee (1994) and Lee (1995). It began with Surgeon General Julius Richmond's 1977 report on Disease Prevention and Health Promotion (1977). A process to establish national health objectives for 1990 was initiated that included state governments and many private sector organizations, including both commercial and voluntary organizations.

Based on the experience in the 1980s with the health objectives for 1990, the health objectives for the year 2000, *Healthy People 2000 National Health Promotion and Disease Prevention Objectives*, were launched in 1990 as described in the article by McGinnis and Lee included in this chapter. Healthy People 2000 has three goals: (1) increase the span of healthy life for all Americans, (2) reduce health disparities among Americans, and (3) achieve access to preventive health care services for all Americans.

To accomplish the goals, Healthy People 2000 sets forth 300 objectives in 22 priority areas, grouped into four categories: (1) health promotion, (2) health protection, (3) clinical preventive services, and (4) surveillance and data systems. The health promotion category addresses the social context, personal attitudes, and behaviors that affect health. The health protection priority emphasizes population-wide interventions that can confer protection for entire communities (e.g., safe water, food safety, automobile safety). Clinical preventive services include counseling, screening, immunization, and chemoprophylaxis that are often provided through personal health services. Finally, surveillance and data systems include both public health data systems such as vital statistics and surveys (Behavioral Risk Factor Survey, National Health Intervention Survey), as well as administrative data often collected for other purposes (e.g., medical care encounter, billing data).

In their article, McGinnis and Lee describe the progress at mid-decade in achieving the Healthy People 2000 Objectives. In health promotion, 10 of 17 sentinel targets are moving in the right direction, four in the wrong direction, two are without change, and two have no data available upon which to assess progress. In the health promotion category, 8 of 10 sentinel targets are moving in the right direction, one in the wrong direction, and one has insufficient data available to assess progress. In the clinical preventive services category, only 11 of 19 sentinel objectives are moving in the right direction, four are moving in the wrong direction, two show no change, and two have insufficient data upon which to draw conclusions. This midcourse review did not address progress on surveillance and data systems.

❖ *Healthy People 2000* at Mid Decade

J. MICHAEL MCGINNIS, PHILIP R. LEE

The nation's health goals for the year 2000 were set forth with the 1990 release of *Healthy People 2000*,[1] which reviewed the principal health challenges for Americans and identified in measurable terms the opportunities for health gains during the 1990s. The arrival of the decade's midpoint prompts an assessment of progress to date.

Healthy People 2000 was based on the previous experience with setting national health targets for the year 1990,[2,3] the results for which have been described elsewhere.[4] The targets contained in *Healthy People 2000* were developed between 1987 and 1990 through an extensive consultative and hearings process conducted and managed by the US Public Health Service (PHS) in partnership with the National Academy of Sciences' Institute of Medicine.[5] To provide guidance to the effort, a national consortium was formed that included the principal health officials of the 50 states and representatives of more than 300 professional and voluntary national membership organizations. The final document was issued in September 1990.

Healthy People 2000 presents three broad goals for the health of the nation: (1) to increase the span of healthy life for Americans, (2) to reduce health disparities among Americans, and (3) to achieve access to preventive services for all Americans.

To foster accomplishment of these goals, *Healthy People 2000* also set forth 300 measurable objectives to be accomplished by the year 2000 in 22 areas of priority for health promotion, health protection, and clinical preventive services (Table 1). The health promotion priorities are those with a prominent behavioral component, requiring strategies that address the social context that gives shape to personal attitudes and choices. The health protection priorities feature those strategies with special emphasis on population-wide interventions that can confer protection on entire communities. Clinical preventive services priorities represent those counseling, screening, immunization, and chemoprophylaxis interventions that are often best provided through clinical settings. Objectives specific to people in certain age, ethnic, or socioeconomic groups are found in each of the priority areas. In addition, objectives were established for improving surveillance and data systems at national, state, and local levels to target interventions more strategically to areas of greatest need.

❖ Implementation

A central principle of the *Healthy People 2000* process has been the national (as distinct from federal) character of the effort. Because

TABLE 1   Priority Areas for 2000

Health promotion
  Physical activity and fitness
  Nutrition
  Tobacco
  Alcohol and other drugs
  Family planning
  Mental health and mental disorders
  Violent and abusive behavior
  Educational and community-based programs
Health protection
  Unintentional injuries
  Occupational safety and health
  Environmental health
  Food and drug safety
  Oral health
Preventive services
  Maternal and infant health
  Heart disease and stroke
  Cancer
  Diabetes and chronic disabling conditions
  Human immunodeficiency virus infection
  Sexually transmitted diseases
  Immunization and infectious diseases
  Clinical preventive services
Surveillance and data systems

the strategies prompted by the objectives in the priority areas depend on the involvement of many sectors of US society, the participatory nature of the process of establishing the objectives was designed to yield a product that to the extent possible reflects the full spectrum of national opinion, not merely that of the federal policy apparatus. Accordingly, implementation efforts have focused simultaneously on stimulating the contributions of (1) federal agencies, (2) state agencies, (3) local agencies, and (4) private, voluntary, and other community-based organizations.

Federal Action

Several steps have been taken to enhance the federal contribution to achievement of the *Healthy People 2000* objectives.[6] Lead responsibility has been assigned among agencies of the PHS for each of the 22 priority areas. Those agencies have been charged with leading federal action engaging multiple agencies in efforts to attain the objectives, forging partnerships with states and the private and voluntary sectors important to the task, and monitoring progress by ensuring collection of the necessary data. In addition, PHS agencies have been asked to take account of the *Healthy People 2000* objectives when they prepare their annual agency budget requests, and since 1992, all relevant grant announcements of PHS agencies require that applicants address ways that proposals can help achieve the *Healthy People 2000* targets.

Monthly progress reviews have been scheduled as a means of holding PHS agencies accountable. These sessions are chaired by the assistant secretary for health (P.R.L.) to assess the status of objectives and to engage various state, local, and private sector partners in a discussion of policy issues, implementation efforts to reach the year 2000 targets, barriers to attaining the targets, and strategies to overcome those barriers. Another mechanism for reporting both the successes and remaining challenges is *Healthy People 2000 Review,*[7] an annual statistical abstract produced by the National Center for Health Statistics of the Centers for Disease Control and Prevention (CDC), to provide the current data on the national health status indicators and the full set of objectives.

Federal action is not limited to the executive branch. Congress has enacted three laws that incorporate *Healthy People 2000* objectives. The first was the 1989 authorization of the maternal and child health block grant, which requires reporting on the national objectives for maternal and infant health. Second was the 1992 Indian Health Care Improvement Act, directing the Indian Health Service to report annually the allocation of resources to 61 *Healthy People 2000* objectives related to American Indians. Third was the 1993 authorization of the Preventive Health and Health Services Block Grant.

State Action

Particularly important are the *Healthy People 2000* initiatives at the state and local levels.[8] All states have been encouraged to develop state-specific goals and objectives tailored to their individual needs and conditions. To date, 41 of the 50 states and the District of Columbia have issued their own *Healthy People 2000* plans, another three have completed health status assessments based on the year 2000 framework, and the remaining states and Puerto Rico are each pursuing a variety of activities based on the year 2000 framework. Some states have drafted documents that parallel the 22 priority areas; others have adopted only selected priority areas and objectives. Most states have set their own targets, more or less ambitious than in *Healthy People 2000*, depending on circumstances. These state-specific plans are used to marshal participation of multiple sectors around activity important to public health priorities, as well as to help improve their data systems and monitor the health status of state residents.

Local Action

At the community level, *Healthy People 2000* has provided a framework for local health initiatives. To assist communities in planning and implementing prevention agendas, the American Public Health Association and the CDC jointly developed *Healthy Communities 2000: Model Standards, Guidelines for Community Attainment of Year 2000 National Health Objectives.*[9] Linked to *Healthy People 2000* objectives, model standards provide public health agencies with a tool to use in determining a community's priority health issues. A 1993 survey of 2072 local health departments found that 70% used *Healthy People 2000* and 47% used *Healthy Communities 2000* for program or organizational planning.[10]

The National Association of County Health Officials developed the Assessment Protocol for Excellence in Public Health[11] in collaboration with the American Public Health Association, the Association of Schools of Public Health, the Association of State and Territorial Health Officials, and the US Conference of Local Health Officers, with the support of the CDC. This protocol provides public health agencies with a tool for assessing their organizational capacity to meet community needs, assessing community health status, setting priorities for action, and monitoring progress toward achieving established objectives. The CDC also promotes use of the Planned Approach to Community Health model,[12] which, with its strong health education framework, helps communities establish programs that rely on local health data and goals, broad participation, and proven intervention models.

Private and Voluntary Action

The *Healthy People 2000* Consortium was formed in 1987 to facilitate broad participation in the process of developing the national prevention agenda and to engage local chapters and their members in the provision of community and neighborhood leadership for *Healthy People 2000.*[13] The American Dietetic Association, the American Academy of Pediatrics, the National Recreation and Park Association, and the National Medical Association are examples of consortium members using their expertise, contacts, and resources to achieve the national health objectives. The Wellness Councils of America, with 26 locally affiliated wellness councils in 20 states and 2500 company members, has adopted the *Healthy People 2000* work-site objectives as their agenda for the decade; the American Hospital Association, which represents nearly 5500 institutional members, has developed a resource kit, *Healthy People 2000:* America's Hospitals Respond,[14] for hospital administrators to help mobilize health promotion initiatives at the community level; and the American Medical Association and its National Adolescent Health Coalition have used the *Healthy People 2000* objectives for adolescents as a framework to address adolescent health issues through the project Healthy Youth 2000.[15]

❖ Results To Date

Broad multisector involvement in efforts to achieve better health for Americans has been a primary purpose of the *Healthy People 2000* process from the outset. Ultimately, the most important result relates to progress with respect to the health of the nation. Data are now being compiled from more than 200 sources on the mid-decade status for the goals and each of the 300 objectives (and their related subobjectives) of *Healthy People 2000*. Most of these data sources provide information for one or two of the objectives; a few provide data for multiple objectives. The most frequently used data sources are the National Vital Statistics System, National Health Interview Survey, and National Health and Nutrition Examination Survey, all the responsibility of the National Center for Health Statistics. Because of lag times in the compilation and analysis of data, it will be at most another 3 years before information will be available from data collected in 1995. However, a preliminary indication of the general trends may be obtained by examining the developments since the baseline years, with respect to a subset of 47 objectives identified in *Healthy People 2000* as representative or "sentinel" indicators of general progress for each of the 22 priority area categories, and assessing how those developments have affected progress on the broad goals of *Healthy People 2000*.

Health Promotion Priorities

In the health promotion priority areas, 10 of the 17 sentinel targets are proceeding in the right direction, four are proceeding in the wrong direction, one is without change, and two have no data available on which to make comments. Particularly good progress continues for reductions in adult use of tobacco products and in alcohol-related automobile deaths. Positive but less striking gains are recorded for the proportion of adults exercising regularly, eating less fatty diets, and reporting stress-related problems. Perhaps contributing to some of the favorable trends among adults is the increase in the proportion of workplaces with health promotion programs accessible to workers. On the other hand, there has been no decline in the proportion of people who lead essentially sedentary lifestyles, and there have been increases in the share of the population that is overweight.

For youth, the trend has also been mixed for patterns of behavior with health consequences. Data from early in the decade indicate improvements with respect to the proportion of youth using tobacco, alcohol, or marijuana, although surveys reported in the last 12 months suggest the possibility of setbacks for substance abuse among youth.[16] Especially alarming are the increases seen among young people with respect to homicides, other violence, and pregnancies.

Health Protection Priorities

In the health protection priority areas, 8 of the 10 sentinel objectives are progressing in the right direction, one is progressing in the wrong direction, and one has insufficient data available on which to base a conclusion. The reduction in unintentional injury deaths is in large part attributable to the declining number of motor vehicle deaths. Greater attention to reducing the occurrence of drunk driving and laws requiring use of child safety seats, seat belt use, 55-mph speed limits, and air bags in new vehicles have all advanced highway safety and saved lives.

In the area of environmental health, notable successes have occurred in improving air quality and in reducing blood lead levels among children. However, as evidenced in part by increased asthma hospitalizations, substantial challenges remain for the improvement of indoor air quality. In the area of occupational safety and health, work-related deaths have declined, but there has been a slight increase in work-related injuries.

There is continued progress in food safety as measured by the decline in salmonella outbreaks, although the occurrence of at least one widespread outbreak of food poisoning by *Escherichia coli* indicates the need for public health vigilance in this area.[17] In oral health, more older people are keeping their teeth and avoiding complete tooth loss. For children, no new data are available on occurrence of dental caries, but some concerns exist about a declining percentage of children visiting the dentist and receiving protective sealants. The percentage of the population served by fluoridated water has not changed.

Clinical Preventive Service Priorities

In the priority areas for clinical preventive services, 13 of the 19 sentinel objectives are progressing in the right direction, four are progressing in the wrong direction, one shows no change, and one has insufficient data available on which to draw a conclusion. Significant progress has been made in reducing cholesterol levels and controlling hypertension. The results are measured by steady declines in coronary heart disease deaths and reductions in stroke deaths, which by 1992 had declined from the 1987 baseline rates by approximately 16% and 13%, respectively.[18]

Cancer death rates have shown slight improvement as yet, but people are increasingly using recommended cancer screening services. The percentage of women older than 50 years who received a recent mammogram has increased from 25% in 1987 to 55% in 1993.[19] Approximately 95% of all women older than 18 years surveyed in 1993 have had a Papanicalaou test, and 75% had a cervical cancer screening within the preceding 3 years.[19] Rates of fecal occult blood screening tests have shown a slight increase.

More pregnant women are seeking prenatal care during the first trimester, with greater improvements noted among blacks, American Indians, and Hispanics than in the general population. On the infectious disease front, solid progress has been made toward the targets for fewer cases of gonorrhea and syphilis. The number of children (aged 19 to 35 months) receiving immunizations is increasing,[19] and the number of cases of vaccine-preventable diseases (ie, measles, mumps, and rubella) has declined.[20] The number of pertussis cases, however, has been increasing.[20]

Particular problems remain for the most vulnerable populations. As measured by the proportion of Americans who lack health insurance, financial barriers to medical care and preventive services have increased for many. Some of the more tangible consequences are apparent in population-wide data and include reverses with respect to the targets for achieving fewer pneumonia and influenza deaths through enhanced immunization rates, achieving fewer newborns with low birth weight through better prenatal care, and achieving fewer people disabled by complications of chronic conditions such as diabetes. Diabetes-related death rates are unchanged for the white population but have increased among blacks, American Indians, and Hispanics. Finally, in one of the most difficult challenges to public health policies and programs, progress is difficult to discern for the national prevalence of infection with the human immunodeficiency virus (HIV). Because of difficulties in estimating rates of HIV infection, no update is yet available on the rate of HIV infection nationwide, but the level of concern about the ability to control this problem is manifest in the fact that the work group establishing this target felt that the nation would be doing well to limit the spread of the virus to twice the 1989 levels of approximately 400 per 100,000 people.[21]

Progress on Objectives for Ethnic Minorities

Experience with the 1990 objectives indicates the importance of looking beyond the aggregate data and examining the data for special population groups. Given the mixed results for these groups with respect to sentinel objectives, in many cases their situation is compromised in comparison with the aggregate national results. Preliminary analysis for the full set of 300 *Healthy People 2000* objectives indicates that overall 48% are proceeding in the right direction, 19% are proceeding in the wrong direction, 3% are unchanged, and 30% lack sufficient data to determine progress. Although approximately the same proportion of all special population targets established are known to be proceeding in the right direction, the proportion proceeding in the wrong direction is considerably greater for minorities.

For blacks, there is progress on prenatal care, breast-feeding, infant deaths, and neonatal and postneonatal mortality. Death rates from coronary heart disease, stroke, cirrhosis, and unintentional injuries are also showing improvement. On the other hand, asthma hospitalizations, adolescent pregnancies, acquired immunodeficiency syndrome (AIDS) incidence, and homicides are increasing and moving away from the year 2000 targets. For Hispanics, there have been increases in the number of women being screened for breast and cervical cancers, and increased rates of breastfeeding. There has been progress in declining teen pregnancy rates, infant mortality, and cigarette smoking. Access to primary care, however, has declined because of lack of health insurance coverage among Hispanics. Furthermore, AIDS cases, homicides, tuberculosis, and overweight prevalence among Hispanic women are all headed away from the year 2000 targets. For American Indians and Alaska Natives, progress has been made on increasing breast-feeding and decreasing the use of smokeless tobacco, alcohol-related motor vehicle deaths, and cirrhosis deaths. Progressing in the wrong direction are untreated dental caries, diabetes-related complications and deaths, overweight prevalence, and homicides. For Asian and Pacific Islander Americans, the number of tuberculosis cases is increasing, but improvements are evident in reduced cigarette smoking, reduced rates of hepatitis B infection among Asian children, and declines in growth retardation in low-income children younger than 1 year and among 2- to 4-year-olds.

Progress on the Goals

Progress on the *Healthy People 2000* objectives is intended to facilitate progress toward its broad goals. Here, too, the results are varied. The first goal of *Healthy People 2000* targets increasing the span of healthy life. Life expectancy for Americans is now at a record 75.8 years. The overall decline in mortality rates is advancing the nation toward the life-stage goals for reduced death rates, continuing the gains achieved in the last decade for the 1990 objectives. Infant deaths (younger than 1 year) were at a record low level in 1992, with 850 deaths per 100,000 infants. For children (aged 1 to 14 years), the 1992 death rate is already close to the year 2000 target. Although the 1992 death rate for young people (aged 15 to 24 years) has declined from the 1987 baseline, it had actually increased in the years between 1987 and 1990 because of an increase in violent deaths among this age group. The adult death rate continues to decline toward the established target.

The *Healthy People 2000* goal, however, emphasizes the quality of life—not just its quantity—as measured through the use of quality-adjusted life expectancy (years of healthy life). Although there are unresolved issues related to the measurement of years of healthy life, an interim measure has been developed and will be used to track progress toward this goal. Current data show that on average people can expect to experience about 64 years of healthy life—a level that has been essentially static or may have even slightly declined in the last several years.[7] In part, the lack of progress in improved quality of life is related to disparities among population groups. The mortality differences among racial and ethnic groups offer a notion of how the nation is faring on the second *Healthy People 2000* goal of reducing health disparities among Americans. This goal addresses the higher rates of preventable death, morbidity, and disability among people with low incomes, people with disabilities, and people of certain racial and ethnic minority groups. It recognizes that the health and productive capacity of the nation is undermined by the continuing high incidence among those population groups of infant mortality, low birth weight, teen pregnancies, and homicides. Real progress in public health demands special attention to those who are at highest risk, but the nation has not made enough progress eliminating the disparities that exist for certain groups.

The 7-year gap between the life expectancy at birth of 69.6 years for blacks and that of 76.5 years for whites has persisted for more than a decade. Among males, the gap has actually widened, with life expectancy for blacks increasing by only 1.2 years since 1980, in contrast to the 2.5-year gain for whites.[18] One of the most intractable gaps is that between whites and blacks for infant deaths. Although the death rate has declined for black infants, progress has been even greater for white infants, with the result that the gap has widened and the rate for blacks is nearly double the rate for whites.[18] The disparities in health status are also evident for some of the leading causes of mortality among adults. Age-adjusted death rates for coronary heart disease were more than 35% greater for blacks than whites in 1992, and stroke deaths were 86% greater.[18] Cancer death rates were 37% greater for blacks than whites in 1992.[18]

American Indians and Alaska Natives, Asians and Pacific Islanders, and Hispanics all had lower death rates than whites for coronary heart disease, stroke, and cancer. American Indians and Alaska Natives had considerably higher death rates from unintentional injuries, 99% greater than whites in 1992.[18] Deaths from HIV infection have disproportionately affected the lives of minorities. In 1990, approximately 30% of the deaths due to HIV infection occurred among blacks, yet their proportion of the total population is less than 12%. Similarly, 17% of the deaths due to HIV infection occurred among Hispanics, in contrast to their 9% proportion of the total population.[18]

Another example of a national shortfall in closing the gap in health disparities is found in the experience with respect to the third *Healthy People 2000* goal—to achieve access to preventive services for all Americans. This goal put the nation on record in 1990 as being committed to universal access to preventive and primary care health services. But without health system reform legislation ensuring all Americans coverage for medical care, including basic clinical preventive services recommended by the US Preventive Services Task Force,[22] this will be an elusive goal, and minority groups continue to be affected disproportionately. In 1990, when *Healthy People 2000* was released, approximately 35 million Americans or 14% of the population had no health insurance.[23] As of 1992, the proportion of Americans without health insurance had increased to more than 15% for the nation as a whole and 21% for blacks and 32% for Hispanics.[23]

❖ Midcourse Corrections

The variable results, especially among certain populations, for *Healthy People 2000* goals and objectives at mid decade suggest the need for a number of course corrections. In part, corrections are required for some of the targets. The PHS agencies have been carefully reviewing the existing targets for their appropriateness, given changes that have occurred with respect to scientific developments, data availability, and understanding about the importance of issues. As a result of this review, changes have been proposed related to language revisions to encompass current issues and data reporting systems; new special population targets to focus on groups that are at highest risk of premature death, disease, or disability; revisions where the baseline had changed; or, in some cases, new objectives. The original criteria for developing year 2000 objectives—credibility, freedom from data constraints, and measurability—continue to pertain. Proposed revisions were published for public review and comment in October 1994.[24] Although targets have not been proposed that are less ambitious than the original objectives, some, such as several related to injury control that have already been nearly achieved, have had more challenging targets proposed. Because of the continued need for efforts to reduce disparities among population groups, more than 100 special population targets have been proposed to sharpen the focus on closing gaps that may exist. Based on comments received from consortium members and the public, the PHS lead agencies will submit final revisions for release in mid 1995.

More important than corrections in the targets themselves are corrections in the strategies to achieve them. From the nature of those areas in which our national failures are most prominent, such as violence, teen pregnancy, and overweight prevalence, it is evident that many strategies currently in place are not working. Clearly, the nation needs stronger education and incentives targeted to behavioral factors that shape personal health prospects and to strengthen the state and local public health infrastructures that are important to protecting the health of entire populations. Our inability to narrow the gaps experienced by some groups suggests that social factors may also be playing a prominent role for several of these problems, with progress shaped by developments with respect to education, employment, public assistance, and other factors outside the health arena. It also calls into question the effectiveness of strategies that compartmentalize elements of the problems. Because of concerns that the nature of many categorical public health programs may even detract from the citizen participation and responsibility necessary to the revitalization of communities at greatest risk, a change in approach may be warranted. As a result, the PHS budget proposal offered this year for the consideration of Congress calls for consolidation of many of the categorical grant programs into larger partnership grants characterized by a greater degree of flexibility in the way they are administered and by accountability provisions that are focused not on the processes of program management, but on outcomes of the sort embodied in *Healthy People 2000*. This concept seeks to enhance the role of local leadership in shaping programs and the level of communication and cooperation among principals at the federal, state, and local levels concerning agreed-on outcomes. Such a change in program philosophy holds the prospect of advancing two of the major aims of *Healthy People 2000*: broad participation in the development of a shared vision of issues, approaches, and opportunities and promotion of measurable indexes on which to assess results.

Also of great importance to the accomplishment of the targets of *Healthy People 2000* is what happens in efforts related to medical care access and health financing reform around the country. Even though access to medical services has limited potential by itself to change the overall health status of a population, the structure and incentives for institutions that deliver those services can do much to shape their involvement in the broader issues that determine the health profile of a community and its citizens. Full accomplishment of the goals of *Healthy People 2000* is dependent on success in reaching all Americans through a comprehensive health system that integrates personal health care and population-based public health.[25] With the growth in managed care throughout the nation—and the extensive use in managed care of a Health Plan Employer Data and Information Set performance evaluation instrument based in part on the *Healthy People 2000* objectives[26]—a medical care financing and payment system is developing that has the potential to reward providers and health plans for keeping populations healthy. That potential will, however, only be reached if the financing system extends to all the nation's citizens and if it does so in a fashion that fosters true accountability for keeping people healthy.

Healthy People 2000 at mid decade offers both promise and challenge. The challenge is evident in the magnitude of our shortfalls with respect to our aspirations and of the changes necessary to rebuild the eroding infrastructures of many of our communities. However, *Healthy People 2000* also offers the opportunity to celebrate what has been accomplished, and what is yet feasible, for the health status of Americans.

ACKNOWLEDGMENTS

We gratefully acknowledge the important contribution to the preparation of the manuscript made by Deborah Maiese, MPA, of the Office of Disease Prevention and Health Promotion, US Department of Health and Human Services, Washington, DC. We would also like to thank Richard Klein, MPH, Kathleen Turezyn, MPH, Fred Seitz, PhD, Susan Schober, PhD, and Christine Plepys, MS, of the Division of Health Promotion Statistics at the Centers for Disease Control and Prevention's National Center for Health Statistics, and Ashley Files, MA, Marthe Gold, MD, MPH, James Harrell, MA, Kristine McCoy, MPH, Debbie Rothstein, Phd, and Nicole Walls of the Office of Disease Prevention and Health Promotion for their helpful comments on the manuscript.

❖ About the Authors

J. Michael McGinnis, M.D., J.D., is Director of the National Academy of Sciences and Former Assistant Surgeon General, Deputy Assistant Secretary for Health, and Director of the Office of Disease Prevention and Health Promotion in the U.S. Department of Health and Human Services.

Philip R. Lee, M. D., is Emeritus Professor of Social Medicine and former Assistant Secretary for Health, Department of Health and Human Services (1993-1997)

REFERENCES

1. US Public Health Service. *Healthy People 2000: National Health Promotion and Disease Prevention Objectives.* Washington, DC: US Dept of Health and Human Services; 1991. Publication PHS 91-50212.

2. US Public Health Service. *Healthy People: Surgeon General's Report on Health Promotion and Disease Prevention.* Washington, DC: US Dept of Health, Education, and Welfare; 1979. Publication PHS 79-55071.

3. US Public Health Service, *Promoting Health/Preventing Disease: Objectives for the Nation.* Washington, DC: US Dept of Health and Human Services; 1980.

4. McGinnis JM, Richmond JB, Brandt EN, Windom RE, Mason JO. Health progress in the United States: results of the 1990 objectives for the nation. *JAMA.* 1992; 268:2545-2552.

5. Institute of Medicine, National Academy of Sciences. *Healthy People 2000: Citizens Chart the Course.* Washington, DC: National Academy Press; 1990.

6. US Public Health Service. *Healthy People 2000: Public Health Service Action.* Washington, DC: US Dept of Health and Human Services; 1992.

7. National Center for Health Statistics. *Healthy People 2000 Review, 1993.* Hyattsville, Md: US Dept of Health and Human Services; 1994. PHS 94-1232-1.

8. US Public Health Service. *Healthy People 2000: State Action.* Washington, DC: US Dept of Health and Human Services; 1992.

9. American Public Health Association. *Healthy Communities 2000: Model Standards, Guidelines for Community Attainment of Year 2000 National Health Objectives.* 3rd ed. Washington, DC: American Public Health Association; 1991.

10. National Association of County and City Health Officials and the Centers for Disease Control and Prevention. *1992-1993 National Profile of Local Health Departments.* Washington, DC: National Association of County and City Health Departments and the Centers for Disease Control and Prevention. In press.

11. American Public Health Association, the Association of Schools of Public Health, the Association of State and Territorial Health Officials, the Centers for Disease Control, the National Association of County Health Officials, the US Conference of Local Health Officers. *Assessment Protocol for Excellence in Public Health (APEX-PH).* Washington, DC: National Association of County Health Officials; 1990.

12. Kreuter MW. PATCH: its origin, basic concepts, and links to contemporary public health policy. *J Health Educ.* 1992;23:135-139.

13. US Public Health Service. *Healthy People 2000: Consortium Action.* Washington, DC: US Dept of Health and Human Services; 1992.

14. American Hospital Association. *Healthy People 2000: America's Hospitals Respond.* Chicago, Ill: American Hospital Association; 1990.

15. American Medical Association. *Healthy Youth 2000.* Chicago, Ill: American Medical Association; 1990.

16. Substance Abuse and Mental Health Administration. *National Household Survey on Drug Abuse.* Rockville, Md: US Dept of Health and Human Services; 1988, 1990-1993.

17. Centers for Disease Control and Prevention. Update: multistate outbreak of *Escherichia coli* O157: H7 infections from hamburgers: Western United States, 1992-1993. *MMWR Morb Mortal Wkly Rep.* 1993;42:258–263.

18. Centers for Disease Control and Prevention, National Center for Health Statistics. *Vital Statistics of the United States, Vol II, Mortality Part A,* published annually and unpublished data, 1987-1992, Washington, DC, National Center for Health Statistics.

19. Centers for Disease Control and Prevention. Vaccination coverage of 2-year-old children: United States, January-March 1994. *MMWR Morb Mortal Wkly Rep.* 1995;44:142-150.

20. Centers for Disease Control and Prevention, Epidemiology Program Office. National Notifiable Disease System, published weekly in *MMWR Morb Mortal Wkly Rep.*

21. Centers for Disease Control and Prevention. HIV prevalence estimates and AIDS case projections for the United States: report based upon a workshop. *MMWR Morb Mortal Wkly Rep.* 1990;39(No. RR-16):1-31.

22. US Preventive Services Task Force. *Guide to Clinical Preventive Services: An Assessment of the Effectiveness of 169 Interventions.* Baltimore, Md: Williams & Wilkins; 1989.

23. US Bureau of the Census. *March 1993 Supplement to the Current Population Survey.* Washington, DC: US Bureau of the Census; 1993.

24. US Public Health Service. Availability and request for comment on the *Healthy People 2000* midcourse revisions. *Federal Register.* October 3, 1994;59:50253.

25. Lasker RD, Lee PL. Improving health through health system reform. *JAMA.* 1994;272:1297-1298.

26. National Committee for Quality Assurance. *Health Plan Employer Data and Information Set.* Washington, DC: National Committee for Quality Assurance; 1993.

❖ PART II

Public Health in the '90s

❖ Chapter 3
Foundations of
Public Health

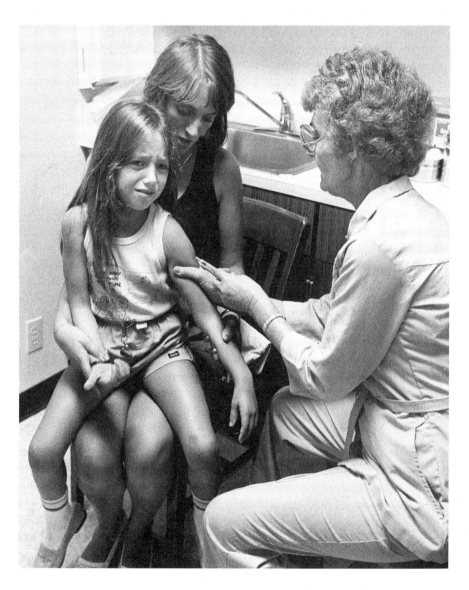

In 1988, the Institute of Medicine (IOM) issued a critically important report, *The Future of Public Health* (a portion is included in Chapter 3), that reviewed the health problems facing the nation and proposed a conceptual framework for public health. They defined public health broadly:

> Public health is what we, as a society, do collectively to assure the conditions in which people can be healthy. This requires that continuing and emerging threats to the health of the public be successfully countered. These threats include immediate crises, such as the AIDS epidemic; enduring problems, such as injuries and chronic illness; impending crises, foreshadowed by such developments as the toxic by-products of a modern economy (IOM, 1988, p. 2).

The IOM proposed that the three broad functions of public health include assessment, policy development, and assurance. These functions are described more fully in the IOM Report and by Afifi and Breslow, who define the core disciplines of public health as epidemiology and biostatistics (composing the "diagnostic tools") and health behaviors, environmental health and personal health services (the "treatment tools" of public health). They note that public health practice "embraces all those activities that are directed to assessment of health and disease problems or the population; the formulation of policies for dealing with such problems; and the assurance of environmental, behavioral and medical services designed to accelerate favorable health trends and reduce the unfavorable" (Affifi and Breslow, 1994, p. 232).

Three papers published in the *Annual Review of Public Health,* Breslow (1990), Affifi and Breslow (1994), and Lee and Paxman (1997), update developments in public health since the 1988 IOM Report.

Breslow (1990) identified five major issues facing public health in the final decade of the 20th century: (1) the reconstitution of public health, (2) setting objectives for public health, (3) refocus from disease control to health promotion; (4) redress continuing social inequities and their impacts on health; and (5) the health implications of accelerating developments in technology. Developments in these areas were updated by Lee and Paxman (1997).

Breslow also noted that the 1990s would bring discussions that were critical to public health. This prediction proved quite accurate as Lee and Paxman noted in their 1997 review. After the 1988 IOM Report, discussions about the role and future of public health took place in many settings. The IOM established a public health roundtable funded by the U.S. Public Health Service and several major private foundations, and it carried out major studies of public health problems. In addition, the Robert Wood Johnson and the Kellogg Foundations launched a major public health initiative to strengthen state and local public health departments. The U.S. Public Health Service in 1993, under the leadership of the Assistant Secretary for Health, established a working group of federal, state, and local public health leaders to develop a clearer definition of public health functions, organizations, and expenditures. The working group identified ten core services that support public health agencies in order to: prevent epidemics and the spread of disease; protect against environmental threats; prevent injuries; promote and encourage healthy behaviors; respond to disasters and assist communities in recovery; and assure the quality and accessibility of health services (see Lee and Paxman reference in Recommended Reading).

While the concept of core public health functions is useful at a very broad level, it does not translate easily into population-based services actually provided in the community. A study is currently under way that should help to better describe the core services at the local level and how these can be characterized after 60 years of federal categorical grants (e.g., tuberculosis, immunizations, STDs, HIV/AIDS, maternal and child health). The proliferation of categorical grants, particularly since the 1960s, has made it increasingly difficult for states and local health departments to set priorities and allocate resources in relation to needs as identified at the local level.

Two recent reports—"For a Healthy Nation: Returns on Investments in Public Health" (DHHS, 1995) and the 1992–1993 National Profile of Local Health Departments (DHHS, 1995)—give the most up-to-date picture of public health programs such as polio immunization, fluoridation of water supplies, elimination of lead in gasoline. These references are included in the Recommended Reading list.

The public health system is, of necessity, large and complex because of the multiplicity of responsibilities thrust upon public health agencies. Some of these are in traditional health departments. Others, such as occupational health and safety, are in the federal Department of Labor and comparable state agencies. In many states, air and water pollution are in an environmental protection agency, as they are at the federal level. Mental health and substance abuse prevention and treatment services may be in separate agencies at the state and local level. In addition, medical care for indigent populations may be provided by local health departments or by separate counties or municipal public hospital systems.

The organizational fragmentation makes it very difficult to determine how much of the one trillion dollars in health expenditures actually supports population health services (Lee, 1995). In 1993, only 2.8 percent ($24.7 billion) was for government public health activities, including $11.4 billion (1.4 percent of the total) for population-based health promotion, health protection, and disease prevention programs (Lee, Benjamin, and Weber, 1997; HCFA Review, 1996). Spending by state and local governments for essential public health functions in 1993 was estimated to be $6.4 billion, a little more than half of the total. By contrast, Medicaid expenditures (federal, state, and local) were $101 billion for acute and long-term care, and Medicare expenditures were $150 billion. Expenditures for these two publicly funded medical care programs were ten times those for government public health programs and twenty-five times those for essential public health services.

The foundations of public health remain in a precarious state on the eve of the 21st century, as they were when the IOM Report (1988) described them as in "disarray." The current national attention that is being focused on the critical role of population based public health functions may, or may not, result in a stabilization, or even strengthening of the public health infrastructure. While managed care, both in the private sector and in the Medicaid and Medicare programs, provides an opportunity to achieve population based public health objectives, it may divert resources from public health, increase the number of uninsured, and increase the burden on local public health departments without commensurate increases in resources.

❖ The Future of Public Health
Summary and Recommendations
INSTITUTE OF MEDICINE

❖ The State of U.S. Public Health

Throughout the history of public health, two major factors have determined how problems were solved: the level of scientific and technical knowledge, and the content of public values and popular opinions. Over time, public health measures have changed with important advances in understanding the causes and control of disease. In addition, practice was affected by popular beliefs about illness and by public views on appropriate governmental action. As poverty and disease came to be seen as societal as well as personal problems, and as governmental involvement in societal concerns increased, collective action against disease was gradually accepted. Health became a social as well as individual responsibility. At the same time, advances such as the discovery of bacteria and identification of better ways to control and prevent communicable disease made possible effective community action under the auspices of increasingly professional public health agencies.

The Public Health Mission

Knowledge and values today remain decisive elements in the shaping of public health practice. But they blend less harmoniously than they once did. On the surface there appears to be widespread agreement on the overall mission of public health, as reflected in such comments to the committee as "public health does things that benefit everybody," or "public health prevents illness and educates the population." But when it comes to translating broad statements into effective action, little consensus can be found. Neither among the providers nor the beneficiaries of public health programs is there a shared sense of what the citizenry should expect in the way of services, and both the mix and the intensity of services vary widely from place to place.

In one state the committee visited, the state health department was a major provider of prenatal care for poor women; in other places, women who could not pay got no care. Some state health departments are active and well equipped, while others perform fewer functions and get by on relatively meager resources. Localities vary even more widely: in some places, the local health departments are larger and more sophisticated technically than many state health departments. But in too many localities, there is no health department. Perhaps the area is visited occasionally by a "circuit-riding" public health nurse—and perhaps not.

Lack of agreement about the public health mission is also reflected in the diversion in some states of traditional public health functions, such as water and air pollution control, to separate departments of environmental services, where the health effects of pollutants often receive less notice.

In some states, mental health is seen as a public health responsibility, but in many the two are organizationally distinct, making it difficult to coordinate services to multiproblem clients. Some health departments are part of larger deportments of "social and health services," where public health scientists find their approaches, which benefit society as a whole, stamped with a negative welfare label.

Such extreme variety of available services and organizational arrangements suggests that contemporary public health is defined less by what public health professionals know how to do than by what the political system in a given area decides is appropriate or feasible.

Professional Expertise and the Political Process

Tension between professional expertise and politics can be observed throughout the nation's public health system. Public health professionals rely on expert knowledge derived from such areas as epidemiology and biostatistics to identify and deal with the health needs of whole populations. A central tenet of their professional ethic is commitment to use this knowledge to fulfill the public interest in reducing human suffering and enhancing the quality of life. Thus their aim is to maximize the influence of accurate data and professional judgment on decision-making—to make decisions as comprehensive and objective as possible.

The dynamics of American politics, however, make it difficult to fulfill this commitment. Decision-making in public health, as in other areas, is driven by crises, hot issues, and the concerns of organized interest groups. Decisions are made largely on the basis of competition, bargaining, and influence rather than comprehensive analysis. The idea that politics can be restricted to the legislative arena, while the work of public agencies remains neutral and expert, has been discredited. Professional analysis and judgment must compete with other perspectives for policy attention and support.

Public health has had great difficulty accommodating itself to these political dynamics. Technical knowledge in fact plays a much more restricted role in public health decision-making than it once did, despite the fact that we now know more. The impact of politics is clearly evident in the rapid turnover among public health officials (the average tenure of a state health officer is now only 2 years); in a marked shift toward political appointees as opposed to career professionals in the top ranks of health agencies; and in the gradual disappearance of state boards of health, which have dwindled by half (from nearly all states to 24) in only 25 years. Too frequently during its investigations, the committee heard legislators and members of the general public castigate public health professionals as paper-shufflers, out of touch with reality, and caught up in red tape. There is a sharp tendency to take what are perceived as "important" programs (for example, Medicaid and environmental programs) away from health departments. The growing perception of health as big business has led to attempts to take public health "out of the hands of the doctors" by interposing a nonmedical administrator between the health officer and elected officials.

Perhaps because they view their professional knowledge and skills as effective and therefore obviously valuable, public health professionals appear to have been slow in developing strategies to demonstrate the worth of their efforts to legislators and the public. Public health crises, not public health successes, make headlines. A number of well-informed members of the public had only vague ideas about what their local health department did. Without broad support, public health officials appear defensive and self-serving when they attempt to answer the criticisms of legislators or mobilize needed resources. Yet many public health professionals who talked with us seemed to regard politics as a contaminant of an ideally rational decision-making process rather than as an essential element of democratic governance. We saw much evidence of isolation and little evidence of constituency building, citizen participation, or continuing (as opposed to crisis-driven) communications with elected officials or with the community at large.

Public Health and the Medical Profession

The political difficulties of public health are reflected in an especially vivid way in its associations with private medicine. Historically, this has been an uneasy relationship. The discovery of bacteria, which proved such a boon to public health's disease control efforts, also brought it into competition with physicians, inasmuch as control measures such as immunizations were carried out not in the environment but on individual patients, who were the purview of the private doctor. Today, while numerous examples can be found of medical community support for public health activities (witness the American Medical Association's stance on AIDS), too often confrontation and suspicion are evident on both sides. For example, the director of one state medical association characterized the health department as distrustful of physicians and cited the director's effort to push a mandatory data-reporting system through the legislature without consulting the society. The committee found medical leaders who were unaware of public health activities in their communities; yet these same leaders are crucial to the implementation of many public health measures and vital in building political support.

The Knowledge Base and Its Application

This summary of the state of U.S. public health began with the observation that both technical knowledge and public values determine how public health is practiced. Clearly, the current impact of public values is troublesome, as political dilemmas attest. But there are also problems on the knowledge front.

Effective public health action must be based on accurate knowledge of the causes and distribution of health problems and of effective interventions. Despite much progress, there are still significant knowledge gaps for many public health problems, for example, the health risks of long-term exposure to certain toxic chemicals or the role of stress in disease.

Because public health is an applied activity, operating under fiscal constraints, it is often difficult to mobilize and sustain necessary research. In our site visits, we found that only one of six states had made a substantial investment in research. Similarly, technical expertise is unevenly distributed: public health employees in some larger states have a considerable skill level, but many others do not. The problem is exacerbated by a shortage of epidemiologists and other trained experts. In many jurisdictions low salary structures and unrewarding professional environments may further inhibit the acquisition of expertise.

In addition, there has been little attention in public health to management as a technical skill in its own right. Management of a public health agency is a demanding, high-visibility assignment requiring, in addition to technical and political acumen, the ability to motivate and lead personnel, to plan and allocate agency resources, and to sense and deal with changes in the agency's environment and to relate the agency to the larger community. Progress in public health in the United States has been greatly advanced throughout its history by outstanding individuals who fortuitously combined all these qualities. Today, the need for leaders is too great to leave their emergence to chance. Yet there is little specific focus in public health education on leadership development, and low salaries and a low public image make it difficult to attract outstanding people into the profession and to retain them until they are ready for top posts.

❖ The Future of Public Health: Recommendations

In conducting this study, the committee has sought to take a fresh look at public health—its mission, its current state, and the barriers to improvement. The committee has concluded that effective public health activities are essential to the health and well-being of the American people, now and in the future. But public health is currently in disarray. Some of the frequently heard criticisms of public health are deserved, but this society has contributed to the disarray by lack of clarity and agreement about the mission of public health, the role of government, and the specific means necessary to accomplish public health objectives. To provide a set of directions for public health that can attract the support of the total society, the committee has made three basic recommendations dealing with:

- ❖ the mission of public health,
- ❖ the governmental role in fulfilling the mission, and
- ❖ the responsibilities unique to each level of government.

The rest of the recommendations are instrumental in implementing the basic recommendations for the future of public health. These instrumental recommendations fall into the following categories: statutory framework; structural and organizational steps; strategies to build the fundamental capacities of public health agencies—technical, political, managerial, programmatic, and fiscal; and education for public health.

❖ The Public Health Mission, Governmental Role, and Levels of Responsibility

Mission

The committee defines the mission of public health as fulfilling society's interest in assuring conditions in which people can be healthy. Its aim is to generate organized community effort to address the public interest in health by applying scientific and technical knowledge to prevent disease and promote health. The mission of public health is addressed by private organizations and individuals as well as by public agencies. But the governmental public health agency has a unique function: to see to it that vital elements are in place and that the mission is adequately addressed.

The Governmental Role in Public Health

The committee finds that the core functions of public health agencies at all levels of government are assessment, policy development, and assurance.

Assessment

The committee recommends that every public health agency regularly and systematically collect, assemble, analyze, and make available information on the health of the community, including statistics on health status, community health needs, and epidemiologic and other studies of health problems. Not every agency is large enough to conduct these activities directly; intergovernmental and interagency cooperation is essential. Nevertheless each agency bears the responsibility for seeing that the assessment function is fulfilled. This basic function of public health cannot be delegated.

Policy Development

The committee recommends that every public health agency exercise its responsibility to serve the public interest in the development of comprehensive public health policies by promoting use of the scientific knowledge base in decision-making about public health and by leading in developing public health policy. Agencies must take a strategic approach, developed on the basis of a positive appreciation for the democratic political process.

Assurance

The committee recommends that public health agencies assure their constituents that services necessary to achieve agreed upon goals are provided, either by encouraging actions by other entities (private or public sector), by requiring such action through regulation, or by providing services directly.

The committee recommends that each public health agency involve key policymakers and the general public in determining a set of high-priority personal and communitywide health services that governments will guarantee to every member of the community. This guarantee should include subsidization or direct provision of high-priority personal health services for those unable to afford them.

Levels of Responsibility

In addition to these functions, which are common to federal, state, and local governments, each level of government has unique responsibilities.

States

The committee believes that states are and must be the central force in public health. They bear primary public sector responsibility for health.

The committee recommends that the public health duties of states should include the following:

❖ assessment of health needs in the state based on statewide data collection;

❖ assurance of an adequate statutory base for health activities in the state;

❖ establishment of statewide health objectives, delegating power to localities as appropriate and holding them accountable;

❖ assurance of appropriate organized statewide effort to develop and maintain essential personal, educational, and environmental health services; provision of access to necessary services; and solution of problems inimical to health;

❖ guarantee of a minimum set of essential health services; and

❖ support of local service capacity, especially when disparities in local ability to raise revenue and/or administer programs require subsidies, technical assistance, or direct action by the state to achieve adequate service levels.

Federal

The committee recommends the following as federal public health obligations:

❖ support of knowledge development and dissemination through data gathering, research, and information exchange;

❖ establishment of nationwide health objectives and priorities, and stimulation of debate on interstate and national public health issues;

❖ provision of technical assistance to help states and localities determine their own objectives and to carry out action on national and regional objectives;

❖ provision of funds to states to strengthen state capacity for services, especially to achieve an adequate minimum capacity, and to achieve national objectives; and

❖ assurance of actions and services that are in the public interest of the entire nation such as control of AIDS and similar communicable diseases, interstate environmental actions, and food and drug inspection.

Localities

Because of great diversity in size, powers, and capacities of local governments, generalizations must be made with caution. Nevertheless, no citizen from any community, no matter how small or remote, should be without identifiable and realistic access to the benefits of public health protection, which is possible only through a local component of the public health delivery system.

The committee recommends the following functions for local public health units:

❖ assessment, monitoring, and surveillance of local health problems and needs and of resources for dealing with them;

❖ policy development and leadership that foster local involvement and a sense of ownership, that emphasize local needs, and that advocate equitable distribution of public resources and complementary private activities commensurate with community needs; and

❖ assurance that high-quality services, including personal health services, needed for the protection of public health in the community are available and accessible to all persons; that the community receives proper consideration in the allocation of federal and state as well as local resources for public health; and that the community is informed about how to obtain public health, including personal health, services, or how to comply with public health requirements.

❖ Concluding Remarks

This report conveys an urgent message to the American people. Public health is a vital function that is in trouble. Immediate public concern and support are called for in order to fulfill society's interest in assuring the conditions in which people can be healthy. History teaches us that an organized community effort to prevent disease and promote health is both valuable and effective. Yet public health in the United States has been taken for granted, many public health issues have become inappropriately politicized, and public health responsibilities have become so fragmented that deliberate action is often difficult if not impossible.

Restoring an effective public health system neither can nor should be achieved by public health professionals alone. Americans must be concerned that there are adequate public health services in their communities, and must let their elected representatives know of their concern. The specific actions appropriate to strengthen public health will vary from area to area and must blend professional knowledge with community values. The committee intends not to prescribe one best way of rescuing public health, but to admonish the readers to get involved in their own communities in order to address present dangers, now and for the sake of future generations.

❖ About the Author

The Institute of Medicine (IOM) was chartered in 1970 as a component of the National Academy of Sciences to enlist distinguished members of the appropriate professions in the examination of policy matters pertaining to the health of the public. The mission of the Institute of Medicine is to advance scientific knowledge and the health and well-being of all people of this nation and the world.

❖ Chapter 4
Policy Issues: Behavior, Environment, and Human Biology

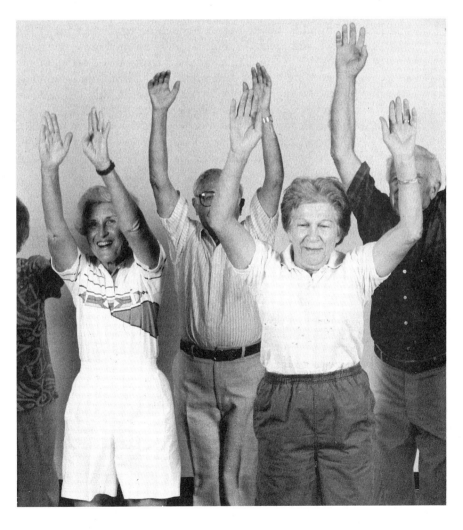

The problems facing public health on the eve of the 21st century are much the same as those identified in the IOM (1988) report and reviewed by Breslow in 1990. Included in the list of major public health problems are tobacco use; HIV/AIDS and other newly emerging or re-emerging infections; current dietary patterns and sedentary life styles; alcohol and illicit drug abuse; injuries (including those due to violence); adolescent health, including unintended pregnancies; vaccine preventable illnesses in children (e.g., poliomyelitis, measles, pertussis) and adults (e.g., pneumonias, influenza); chronic diseases including heart disease, cancer, cerebrovascular disease, diabetes mellitus, and obesity; and a growing list of environmental hazards. The public health and medical care response to terrorism, or the threat of terrorism, whether nuclear, chemical, biological or conventional weapons (e.g., bomb), must be added to the response to natural disasters as public health responsibilities.

In this section on public health issues we include articles on only a few of these issues, but we will touch on more in this introduction. Rather than dealing with these health problems facing communities as a series of categorical problems requiring federal categorical public health programs, we will group them into the four broad determinants of health: (1) personal behavior; (2) environment; (3) human biology (genetics); and (4) health care. We do not include socioeconomic status as a separate determinant of health, but note that it affects all others, except human biology. The fourth broad determinant of health, health care, is covered extensively in Parts III and IV of this volume.

❖ Personal Behavior

The importance of personal behavior in health began to attract serious attention 33 years ago with the release of the first *Surgeon General's Report on Smoking and Health* (1964). Since that time, a number of critically important Surgeon General's Reports on smoking have been released, including the 1988 report that identified nicotine as an addicting substance and the 1994 report that stressed the role of smoking and adolescents (U. S. Department of Health and Human Services).

Two other areas of human behavior, dietary patterns and physical activity, were the subjects of major Surgeon General's Reports in 1988 (nutrition) and 1996 (physical activity).

In addition to smoking, eating, and physical activity, other behavioral determinants include substance abuse, violence, alcohol abuse (including driving under the influence of alcohol) and sexual activity. Behavioral determinants exert a profound influence on whether or not an individual dies prematurely of lung cancer, colon cancer, coronary artery disease, chronic obstructive pulmonary disease, diabetes mellitus, liver cirrhosis, and HIV/AIDS or from injuries resulting from a variety of high risk behaviors.

We will first address the topic of personal behavior, including the Surgeon General's Reports on smoking, nutrition, and physical activity; we will then turn to the environment and human biology. Because of the magnitude of the expenditures on Medicare and Medicaid and the potential role of health care in contributing to population health, health care will be dealt with separately in the chapter on health care and health care reform.

Tobacco Use

The release of the first Surgeon General's Report on smoking and health was among the most important public health actions in this century because it signaled the beginning of a broad-based public health approach to the health problems caused by tobacco use. Since the first Surgeon General's Report on smoking, there have been 23 Surgeon General's Reports dealing with a wide range of topics. Two reports are particularly important to the current federal strategy. The 1988 Report identified nicotine as an addicting substance and the 1994 Report, *Preventing Tobacco Use Among Young People,* described the magnitude of the problem among youth and the fact that over two thirds of adult smokers began smoking before the age of 18 years. The topic of tobacco use has long been a priority because of the magnitude of the health problems associated with tobacco. Tobacco use has long been the leading cause of death in the United States, contributing to more than 400,000 deaths per year, primarily due to cancer, cardiovascular disease, and chronic obstructive pulmonary disease.

The most significant developments in tobacco control in recent years have been at both the state and federal level. Important developments include: (1) a series of state initiatives (e.g., California, Washington, Michigan, Massachusetts, Arizona) that raised taxes on tobacco products, provided funds for education campaigns to counter tobacco industry promotion and advertising, and provided funds to pay for medical care for the uninsured; (2) the new federal initiatives to reduce tobacco use among children, including the Synar regulations, the FDA regulations regulating tobacco products issued in August 1996, and support to state/local tobacco control programs by the CDC and the National Cancer Institute; (3) a major private sector initiative involving foundations, voluntary organizations (e.g., American Cancer Society, American Lung Association, PTA, Girl Scouts, Oral Health); and (4) a series of law suits filed by state governments against tobacco companies to recover Medicaid costs related to tobacco use.

While we include only one paper on tobacco use in this section because of space limitations, it does not diminish the importance of the issue and the rapid developments in tobacco control in the past five years. The paper by Max and Rice (1993), which we have included in the recommended reading list, is important because it details the cost of smoking related illness in California and it has been used by a number of states in their suits against tobacco companies. The article by Kessler (1995) was the first to define cigarette smoking as a "pediatric disease." This approach became the basis for the FDA regulations that focus on children's access to cigarettes (e.g., it would ban cigarette vending machines in all locations easily accessible to children under age 18 years) and reduce the appeal of cigarettes and spit tobacco through advertising and promotion directed at children by tobacco companies. The FDA regulation of tobacco products described by Kessler et al. (1996) that we have included in chapter 4, is strongly supported by the Secretary of Health and Human Services, the Vice President and the President. The 1996 FDA regulation of tobacco products represents a new strategy and a different focus for federal tobacco control efforts.

Ronald M. Davis' (1996) recent paper "The Ledger of Tobacco Control: Is the Cup Half Empty or Half Full?" "takes stock of our balance sheet in tobacco control," and presents a timely, cogent, and thorough accounting of the accomplishments to date and the continuing and new obstacles hindering progress.

While the emphasis during the past year has been on the FDA initiative to regulate tobacco products as medical devices, there has been a three-pronged federal strategy to limit children's access to tobacco products. The first of these was the Synar Amendment to the federal authority to grant substance abuse prevention and treatment dollars to states. The regulations implementing the Synar Amendment require the states to enforce their laws related to the purchase of tobacco products by minors. Failure to achieve federally established goals can result in the loss of federal block grant funds for substance abuse prevention and treatment.

The Centers for Disease Control and Prevention administer a grant-in-aid program (Project IMPACT) that provides funds and assists states with the establishment of state tobacco control programs. Currently, 35 states receive federal assistance.

The National Cancer Institute is in the fifth year of a major demonstration program to evaluate the effectiveness of state/local tobacco control programs. Projects are funded in seven states and preliminary evidence suggests that these comprehensive efforts have been effective in reducing smoking prevalence.

Dietary Habits and Physical Activity

Ranking second only to tobacco use in contributing to premature mortality, dietary patterns (eating habits) and the sedentary lifestyle of most Americans have not received the attention of public health authorities that has been accorded to tobacco. While public health authorities throughout the world had long been concerned about the relationship of poverty to undernutrition, the relationship of diet to chronic illness in the United States did not attract much attention outside a select group of investigators until the past 20 years. It is now widely recognized that the major nutritional problem is overnutrition, particularly the excess consumption of fat. The foods that Americans choose to eat play a major role in cardiovascular disease, diabetes mellitus, and cancer. It has been established that 40–60 percent of all cancers, and as many as 35 percent of all cancer deaths, are linked to current diets in the United States.

Although a series of publications by the federal government, including dietary guidelines and the Food Guide Pyramid published by the Department of Agriculture, pointed out problems and possible strategies, it was not until the 1988 Surgeon General's Report on nutrition that there was a comprehensive review by the federal government of the link between diet and chronic illness.

A number of barriers prevent Americans from following the recommendations of the Surgeon General's Report on nutrition and those of the dietary guidelines issued every five years by the Department of Agriculture/Department of Health and Human Services. Among these are the misunderstanding and confusion of a number of terms used in the Guidelines and strong political pressures from food lobbies to weaken the language that might decrease consumer demand for their products (Nestle, 1993).

Despite inadequacies in the diets of most Americans, low income populations, African Americans, Hispanics, American Indians, and Alaska Natives, bear a disproportionate burden of chronic illness associated with poor diets. Nutrition educators are encouraged to target multicultural populations and focus on dietary change as a key area of intervention to reduce the burden of chronic illness (Nestle & Cowell, 1993).

Few have done more since the publication of the Surgeon General's Report to point out the multiplicity of issues related to diet, human nutrition, and chronic illness than the editor of that report, Professor Marion Nestle of New York University. In a series of articles and book chapters (1993a, 1993b, 1995) she has documented the problems and proposed solutions. In one of her recent papers, she addresses the needs for the 21st century. We have included this paper in this section.

Physical inactivity has increasingly been recognized as a major risk factor for chronic disease, particularly cardiovascular disease and cancer. *The Surgeon General's Report on Physical Activity and Health* (1996), like the previous reports on smoking and nutrition, is a landmark in public health. The report summarizes the evidence from the literature, particularly over the past 20 years, on the role of physical activity and health. It demonstrates the extent and strength of the evidence from the fields of epidemiology, exercise physiology, medicine, and behavioral sciences linking physical activity and the risk of cardiovascular disease, cancer, and diabetes mellitus. Regular activity in moderate physical activity of 30 minutes per day can reduce the risk of premature mortality from these killer diseases. Greater levels of aerobic physical activity can increase the protection benefits of exercise.

The article, "How Fast Do We Age: Exercise Performance Over Time as a Biomarker," by Walter M. Boortz, IV, and Walter M. Boortz, II, is a significant recent example of the rigor with which physical activity may both be investigated as a tool for assessing biological aging as well as a mechanism for promoting healthy aging. We have included it in chapter 4.

While including only a portion of the Executive Summary of the Surgeon General's Report and the Boortz and Boortz article in Chapter Four, we recommend also reading recent articles by three other leaders in the field (Blair, Paffenbarger, and Stewart) and their associates that illustrate the growing evidence from different disciplines related to physical activity and health. Recent studies of interest are included in the Recommended Reading list.

Sexual Activity

While the literature on HIV/AIDS is huge, we include only one article because it focuses on the global nature of the HIV/AIDS epidemic. The article by Kimball et al. (1996) reviews the current status of the global epidemic of HIV/AIDS and makes clear why the possible solution is a public health approach. While some of the behavioral interventions (e.g., condom use) have proved feasible in limited demonstration projects, they have not been widely adopted in countries in Africa or in India, where the epidemic is raging. Although the recent introduction of protease inhibitors in the United States will greatly enhance the combined medical care/ public health approach to HIV prevention and care in the US they are too costly to be practically used in many developing nations. The only long-term solution is the development of an effective vaccine or vaccines.

Even after more than a decade of experience with one of the foundations of the public health approach, HIV testing and counseling, a number of problems remain as described by Phillips and Coates (1995). They pose a clear challenge to public health in their very thorough review of these issues and we have included this article in the Recommended Reading list.

We also highly recommend Claire Brindis' article on "Promising Approaches for Adolescent Reproductive Health Service Delivery: The Role of School-Based Health Centers in a Managed Care Environment," which highlights a system level public health intervention that addresses two very serious threats to adolescent health—unwanted pregnancy and HIV/ AIDS—and does so under a contemporary managed care model. Coordination of services between managed care providers and school based health centers can work effectively to provide comprehensive, potentially cost-effective, and accessible reproductive health services to adolescents. As the most critical service delivery issue in adolescent health, access to care is enhanced by this type of cooperative venture

❖ Environment

The environment is of critical importance to the public health. The sanitary revolution produced the most dramatic improvements in health in human history, largely dealing with assuring proper waste disposal and safe water and food. The great killers had been water-borne and airborne bacterial and viral infections. The decline in tuberculosis that occurred during this period appeared related primarily to improved socioeconomic conditions, including improved nutrition and less crowded housing, rather than public health measures per se.

Today, infection—newly emerging and re-emerging (e.g., tuberculosis) continue to pose a major threat. The HIV/AIDS epidemic throughout the world (see Kimball) illustrates the power of a newly emerging infectious disease. Malaria continues to kill and disable millions throughout the world, as do the diarrheal and respiratory infections that kill millions of children annually. In the United States, newly emerging diseases, in addition to HIV/AIDS, have included toxic shock syndrome, Legionnaire's disease, Lyme disease and Hanta virus infection. Food borne infections, such as those caused by E. coli 157, continue to pose a threat in the United States. The overuse and misuse of antibiotics throughout the world has created a worldwide problem of antibiotic resistant organisms.

Environmental threats have increasingly become associated with exposure to man-made chemical and physical agents and hazards in the workplace, including silicosis in miners and scrotal cancers in chimney sweeps which were recognized early. Later the relationship between asbestos and pulmonary disease was clarified (OTA, 1994).

In the past 30 years, issues arose related to the use of pesticides, both the acute effects on workers exposed during spraying and the latent effects on people who ate food with pesticide residues (Dunlop, 1988). In 1958, Congress enacted legislation that prohibited the use of any food additive that had been shown to induce cancer in humans or animals (Delaney Clause). This law remained in effect until 1996, when a more scientifically based law, the Food Quality Protection Act, was signed into law. Policies regulating potentially toxic agents have classified these agents into carcinogens and non-carcinogens (OTA 1989, EPA 1986). The problem with the Delaney Clause was that chemicals causing cancer in some experimental animals did not have a carcinogenic effect in humans because the biologic pathway did not exist in humans, but the additives could not be used.

The great strides in biomedical research in the past decade have begun to reveal the cellular and molecular mechanisms by which environmental agents can cause disease. One result has been the shift from a focus on cancer to a study of the immunologic, neurologic, respiratory, and developmental effects of chemical and physical agents in the environment (OTA, 1994). Among the recent studies are those that suggest some environmental agents may be disrupting the human endocrine system. For instance, Davis and Bradlow (1995) discuss the role of "endocrine disrupters" in breast cancer.

Because people are exposed daily to many environmental hazards, more data is needed about the exposure to chemical mixtures of all kinds, as well as in combinations of chemical, physical, and biologic agents (Commission on Risk Assessment and Risk Management, 1995). In their paper included in chapter 4, Thacker, Stromp, Parrish, and Anderson (1996) provide a review of the requirements for an environmental health surveillance system.

Nuclear wastes continue to pose a long-term threat to public health and the failure to deal effectively with the nuclear wastes as well as the continual threat of nuclear disasters such as Chernobyl have undermined public confidence in nuclear power in the United States.

The increasing complexity and often hazard-specific nature of federal statutes and regulatory requirements has resulted in a greater reliance on regulatory approaches rather than a broader public health approach to environmental hazards (Burke, Shalavta, and Tran, 1994, USPHS). The primary functions of regulatory agencies include activities relating to permitting, enforcement, record keeping, remediation, and standard setting. The broader public health functions that relate to health surveillance, environmental epidemiology, applied and basic research, toxicology, communication, education, and training, and community-based interventions (e.g., smoke-free workplace, public building) have had less emphasis. Future progress will require a return to a broader public health approach that includes regulation but is not so dependent upon it.

❖ Human Biology

The Human Genome Project, initiated by the National Institutes on Health (NIH) and the Department of Energy in 1988, is rapidly advancing the understanding of human genetics. The project has a goal to establish the location of the estimated 100,000 human genes and read the entire set of genetic instructions encoded in human DNA. The specific goals of the project are the construction of a set of useful maps of the human genomes; the determination of the complete sequence of DNA; the parallel analysis of the genomes of a small number of well characterized nonhuman organisms; and, the development of the new technology needed to accomplish these goals (Guyer and Collins, 1993, 1995).

The initial phases of the human genome project have been remarkably successful (Collins, 1995, 1996; Guyer and Collins, 1995). The contributions to advancing the study of inherited diseases and other biologic phenomena are widely recognized within the scientific community.

Genetic errors account for an estimated 3000 to 4000 clearly hereditary diseases, and heredity is a known risk factor in many birth defects, cancer, cardiovascular diseases, diabetes mellitus, neurological diseases, autoimmune disorders and susceptibility to infection (Collins, 1995; Guyer and Collins, 1995). Recent evidence also suggests a genetic role in certain instinctive and cognitive process such as the ability of mothers to nurture their young (Brown et al., 1996). The role of genes in complex or multigenetic disease will not be simple to identify. This class includes diseases with polygenic or quantitative inheritance, where several genes can contribute in incremental ways to the presence or absence of disease.

In the rapid advances in genetics in recent years too little attention has been paid to the complex relationship of genes and the environment. In many cases, diseases are the result of a combination of genetic and environmental factors and include some of the most common chronic diseases such as cancer, cardiovascular disease, diabetes and mental illness (Collins, 1995; Guyer and Collins, 1995).

Profound and troubling ethical, social and legal questions are raised by the rapid advances in genetics, particularly the development of genetic tests and gene therapy (Task Force on Genetic Testing, 1994). The predicted and potentially discriminatory uses of genetic tests, particularly those performed on healthy or apparently healthy people, have been a cause for concern. The promise of the early genetic research for the development of gene therapy is also of concern. The article by Hubbard and Lewontin (1996), included in chapter 4, illustrates the concerns now being expressed about genetic testing.

Space does not permit inclusion of articles on a number of other current public health issues including immunization, substance abuse and mental health or maternal and child health. Important papers in these areas include: "Present and Future Challenges of Immunizations on the Health of our Patients" (Gershon, 1995), "Nonfinancial Barriers to Care for Children and Youth" (Halfon, Inkelas, and Wood, 1995) and "Community-based Approaches for the Prevention of Alcohol, Tobacco, and Other Drug Use" (Aguirre-Molina and Gorman, 1996). These references are included in our list of Recommended Reading.

❖ The Food and Drug Administration's Regulation of Tobacco Products

David A. Kessler, Ann M. Witt,
Philip S. Barnett, Mitchell R. Zeller,
Sharon L. Natanblut, Judith P. Wilkenfeld,
Catherine C. Lorraine, Larry J. Thompson,
and William B. Schultz

On August 23, the Food and Drug Administration (FDA) issued a regulation restricting the sale and distribution of cigarettes and smokeless tobacco to children and adolescents.[1] This regulation, known as a rule, is the most far-reaching measure ever instituted to reduce the use of tobacco by young people. This article describes the investigation that led the FDA to assert its jurisdiction over cigarettes and smokeless tobacco and the policy considerations that shaped the final rule.

The FDA announced on February 25, 1994, that it was considering regulating tobacco products under the authority of the Federal Food, Drug, and Cosmetic Act.[2] Under the act, the decision to regulate tobacco products as drug-delivery devices for nicotine would depend on whether the products were "articles (except for food) intended to affect the structure or any function of the body." After its announcement, the agency extensively reviewed the effects of nicotine on the structure or function of the body and investigated whether cigarettes and smokeless tobacco are "intended" to deliver nicotine to consumers. The agency also investigated the effect of advertising and marketing by the tobacco industry on children and adolescents.

Eighteen months later, on August 10, 1995, President Bill Clinton announced that the agency's evidence and analysis supported a finding, subject to public comment, that the nicotine in cigarettes and smokeless-tobacco products is a drug and that these products are drug-delivery devices under the terms of the act.[3] Citing evidence that smoking begins in childhood as a "pediatric disease," the FDA proposed a regulatory program that would reduce the use of cigarettes and smokeless tobacco by young people by limiting their advertising and sale.[4]

The FDA received more than 700,000 comments on its finding of jurisdiction and on the proposed regulations—more comments than had been received about any other federal rule in history. These comments included 2500 pages of text and nearly 50,000 pages of exhibits from the cigarette and smokeless-tobacco industries alone. Among the hundreds of public health organizations, physicians, and other health professionals expressing views, virtually all agreed that cigarettes and smokeless tobacco should be regulated by the FDA. (The supporting documentation for this report can be found in the August 10, 1995, *Federal Register* and the administrative record supporting that publication; these documents, including both unpublished industry reports and scientific studies, are available for review at FDA headquarters.)

These tobacco regulations are historic for their importance to the public health, for the depth of the President's commitment, and for the extent of public support. They are aimed at protecting American children from a lifelong addiction that often leads to a premature death.

❖ The Investigation of Tobacco

In 1994, the FDA began an investigation to determine whether the pharmacologic effects of nicotine were "intended" by tobacco manufacturers. If they were, cigarettes and smokeless tobacco would fall within the agency's jurisdiction. At that early stage, agency officials understood very little of what the tobacco industry knew about its products or how it designed them. Piece by piece, a clearer picture emerged. Documents from the industry showed that it has known for decades that tobacco products have powerful pharmacologic effects, including addiction to nicotine. Moreover, the evidence revealed that tobacco manufacturers design their products to provide consumers with pharmacologically active doses of nicotine. The inevitable consequence has been to keep consumers addicted to these products.

Early Developments

Two developments prompted the FDA inquiry into whether the pharmacologic effects of cigarettes and smokeless tobacco were intended and should therefore be regulated under the authority of the Food, Drug, and Cosmetic Act. First, by the early 1990s, a scientific consensus had emerged that the nicotine in tobacco products is addictive and that the market for such products is based largely on this addiction.[5-11] The scientific definitions of addiction place their primary emphasis on the presence of highly controlled or compulsive use (despite a desire to quit or repeated attempts to do so); psychoactive effects produced by the action of the drug on the brain; and drug-seeking behavior caused by the "reinforcing" effects of the psychoactive substance.[12]

Second, the tobacco industry was introducing new products whose composition showed that the manufacturers could control the amount of nicotine delivered to the user or even remove the nicotine entirely. In 1988, for example, the R.J. Reynolds Tobacco Company introduced Premier, a novel product that heated, rather than burned, tobacco to deliver a carefully

controlled dose of nicotine.[13] One year later, Philip Morris test-marketed
Next, a cigarette that contained no nicotine.[14]

In the spring of 1994, the FDA observed a trend that strongly suggested
that the tobacco industry manipulated and controlled the levels of nicotine
in conventional cigarettes. Tobacco companies are required to report the
levels of nicotine and tar in their products to the Federal Trade Commission. When FDA investigators analyzed those reports, they found that the
amount of nicotine delivered has been increasing since 1982, with the
greatest increases in the lowest-tar cigarettes (Fig. 1).[15] These increases occurred without parallel increases in the delivery of tar, directly contradict-
ing the industry's claim that "nicotine follows the tar level" in "a near
perfect correlation."[16] It seemed unlikely that the delivery of nicotine could
increase independently of the delivery of tar unless the manufacturers had
made deliberate design decisions.

The agency's suspicions grew when FDA scientists learned that certain
cigarettes advertised as having the lowest tar content actually contained the
blends of tobacco richest in nicotine. For example, tests of three varieties of
Merit cigarettes—one delivering the regular amount of tar, one low in tar,
and one with ultra-low levels of tar—showed that the ultra-low-tar variety
had the highest concentration of nicotine in its tobacco blend.[17] This suggested that the manufacturers were compensating for the effects of filtration

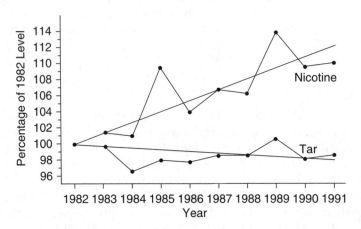

FIGURE 1   Changes in Mean Levels of Nicotine and Tar in Smoke from All Brands
of Cigarettes, 1982–1991, as a Percentage of 1982 Levels.

Data are based on calendar-year sales information for each brand, as reported to the Federal
Trade Commission. Nicotine and tar levels were measured by standard analytic techniques.
Because systematized data are available only beginning in 1982, that year was used as the
reference year. Each point represents the average of 35 to more than 300 samples collected
nationwide. Including brands sold as "high," "low," and "ultra-low" in tar. The measurements were averaged and weighted according to the volume of sales to give an estimate of
the average nicotine and tar content of all cigarettes sold that year. The straight lines indicate
the results of regression analyses showing trends in nicotine and tar content over the decade.

and ventilation, the principal variables in design used to reduce the delivery of tar, by using high-nicotine tobacco in the blends of their lowest-tar products.

A review of tobacco-industry patents also showed that since the early 1960s the industry has been conducting extensive research on methods of controlling the precise amount of nicotine a cigarette delivers.[18] As one patent stated, "maintaining the nicotine content at a sufficiently high level to provide the desired physiological activity, taste, and odor . . . can thus be seen to be a significant problem in the tobacco art."[19]

Inside the Tobacco Companies

The FDA's first important insights into the internal knowledge and actions of the tobacco companies came in the spring and summer of 1994. In April 1994, Victor DeNoble and Paul Mele, two former Philip Morris scientists, testified before Congress about that company's efforts in the early 1980s to find an analogue of nicotine that would "mimic nicotine's effect in the brain" but not have "cardiovascular liability."[20] The scientists explained that to identify the pharmacologic effects of nicotine on the brain, Philip Morris used "exactly the same tests" that the National Institute on Drug Abuse uses to determine whether a drug has a potential for abuse.[21] The company's experiments showed that rats would both self-administer nicotine and develop tolerance to it—two key properties of an addictive substance.[22] The experiments in rats also showed that nicotine served as a discriminative stimulus,[23] a finding predicting that a substance will have mood-altering effects in humans—another defining trait of addictive compounds.[24] Thus, it appeared that at least one tobacco company had knowledge of nicotine's potential for addiction.

In May 1994, further evidence of the industry's knowledge of nicotine's addictiveness emerged when *The New York Times* published an article describing confidential documents obtained from the Brown and Williamson Tobacco Corporation, the nation's third-largest tobacco company, and its British parent, BAT Industries, formerly the British-American Tobacco Company.[25] The documents showed that in the 1960s senior company officials had explicitly acknowledged that "smoking is a habit of addiction"[26] and stated that "we are, then, in the business of selling nicotine, an addictive drug."[27] The Brown and Williamson documents also showed that the companies had conducted dozens of studies of the drug-like properties of nicotine, leading company researchers to conclude that nicotine, is "pharmacologically active in the brain"[28] and "an extremely biologically active compound capable of eliciting a range of pharmacological, biochemical, and physiological responses."[29]

The FDA investigators also discovered that Brown and Williamson had created a new variety of tobacco grown in Brazil, code-named Y-1, with twice the normal level of nicotine.[30] Most important, company executives stated that Y-1 was intended as a "blending tool" to permit the design of cigarettes lower in tar but not in nicotine.[31] Company officials, however, said that they did not use it as such.

The next piece of evidence arrived anonymously in the mail—part of one company's handbook on leaf blending and product development. From it the agency learned that tobacco companies used chemical additives to affect the delivery of nicotine; for example, they added ammonia compounds to "liberate free nicotine from the blend, which is associated with increases in impact and 'satisfaction' reported by smokers."[32]

The Emerging Picture

The FDA investigation also revealed that for at least three decades manufacturers have conducted and funded extensive research into the pharmacokinetics of nicotine, its pharmacodynamics, and methods of delivery.[33] Through research, the industry learned that nicotine has potent pharmacologic effects on the brain, that that is the primary reason consumers use tobacco products, and that nicotine delivery can be manipulated and controlled through a wide array of methods, including the blending of tobacco, selective filtration and ventilation, and chemical manipulation.

In late July and early August 1995, shortly before the President announced the FDA's proposed tobacco regulations, important information became available about Philip Morris, the nation's largest tobacco company, when the contents of hundreds of pages of confidential company documents were disclosed to Congress.[34,35] These and other company documents showed that as early as 1969, Philip Morris researchers had told the company's board of directors that "the ultimate explanation for the perpetuated cigarette habit resides in the pharmacological effect of smoke upon the body of the smoker."[36] Throughout the 1970s, Philip Morris laboratories had conducted extensive research into both the pharmacology of nicotine and methods of nicotine manipulation.[37] Philip Morris researchers also "systematically manipulated tar and nicotine parameters of cigarettes . . . to predict nicotine/tar ratios for optimal cigarette acceptability."[38] In one 1972 document that emerged in a court case,[39] a senior Philip Morris researcher actually conceived of the cigarette as "a dispenser for a dose unit of nicotine."[40]

Numerous documents were submitted to the FDA during the period of public comment that followed the President's August 1995 announcement. According to one tobacco-company document, in the 1970s, R.J. Reynolds researchers stated that "the confirmed user of tobacco products is primarily seeking the physiological 'satisfaction' derived from nicotine"[41] and that "without any question, the desire to smoke is based on the effect of nicotine on the body."[42] In another document, William Farone, the former director of applied research at Philip Morris, informed the agency that "product developers and blend and leaf specialists at Philip Morris were responsible for manipulating and controlling the design and production of cigarettes in order to satisfy the consumer's need for nicotine."[43]

More Than Just Cigarettes

FDA laboratories and investigators also examined how manufacturers of smokeless tobacco manipulate the delivery of nicotine. The FDA learned that manufacturers of smokeless tobacco adjust the pH of their products to produce intentionally graduated nicotine deliveries.[44] The industry's "starter" products for new users have a low pH and consequently deliver a low level of "free" nicotine, limiting the absorption of the compound in the mouth. Smokeless-tobacco products intended for users who have already acquired a tolerance to nicotine have a high pH and consequently deliver a high level of free nicotine, increasing the amount of nicotine available for absorption. Indeed, internal documents from the United States Tobacco Company, the nation's largest smokeless-tobacco manufacturer, refer to an explicit "graduation process" designed to encourage users to progress from low-nicotine brands to high-nicotine ones.[45]

Asserting Jurisdiction

The agency's task in determining whether the FDA has jurisdiction over tobacco products has been part scientific inquiry and part detective work. Like investigators trying to solve a mystery, we examined the evidence from several perspectives. In the end, the evidence converged remarkably.

Under the Food, Drug, and Cosmetic Act, the agency can establish in several ways that a product is "intended to affect the structure or any function of the body" and hence that it meets the criteria for a drug or device subject to FDA jurisdiction. The agency may show that a reasonable manufacturer would foresee that the product will be used for pharmacologic purposes, that consumers actually use it for such purposes, or that the manufacturer expects or designs the product to be used in such a manner.

The agency's analyses of the intended use of cigarettes and smokeless tobacco according to these three independent legal standards all led to the same conclusion: that cigarettes and smokeless tobacco are delivery devices for the drug nicotine. Although evidence meeting any one of these standards would suffice to establish the FDA's jurisdiction over cigarettes and smokeless tobacco, the evidence met all three standards to support such a finding.

❖ The Regulation of Tobacco

The agency's investigation and its finding that the FDA has regulatory jurisdiction over cigarettes and smokeless tobacco raised a difficult question: What is the most appropriate way to regulate these products? To answer this question, we considered the public health consequences of tobacco consumption and the pattern of tobacco use in the United States.

Tobacco affects the public health profoundly. More than 50 million Americans smoke cigarettes,[46] and experts estimate that 77 to 92 percent of them are addicted to nicotine.[47-49] Tobacco use is the leading preventable cause of death in the United States.[50] Tobacco-related disease kills more than 400,000 Americans annually,[50] more people than die from AIDS, car accidents, alcohol, homicides, illegal drugs, suicides, and fires combined.[51]

The death and disease caused by tobacco use occur primarily in adulthood, but nicotine addiction usually begins in adolescence or before. Consequently, the addiction begins as a "pediatric" disease. Eighty-two percent of adults with any history of smoking had their first cigarette before the age of 18, and more than half of them had already become regular smokers by that age.[52]

New smokers and smokeless-tobacco users come primarily from the ranks of the young. Approximately 3 million American adolescents already smoke, and an additional 1 million adolescent boys use smokeless tobacco.[52] Nearly 3000 young people start smoking each day, or more than a million each year.[54] Despite a decline in adult smoking, adolescent smoking is on the rise, and studies show that children begin smoking at earlier and earlier ages.[55-57] Even more alarming, approximately one of every three such young smokers will die prematurely from a tobacco-caused disease.[58]

Given the level of addiction already present among adults, an outright ban would not be effective in preventing the use of tobacco. Instead, the FDA has decided to focus on breaking the cycle of addiction to nicotine. There is convincing evidence that the right policy is to stop children and adolescents from using tobacco in the first place.

Restricting Access to Tobacco

Each year young people purchase tobacco products worth an estimated $1.26 billion.[59] Despite laws in all 50 states that prohibit tobacco sales to minors, numerous studies show that adolescents have little difficulty purchasing these products. The 1994 report of the surgeon general examined 13 studies of over-the-counter sales and determined that approximately 67 percent of the time minors can buy cigarettes illegally.[60] Moreover, substantial numbers of young people successfully purchase smokeless tobacco as well, with 90 percent of such users in junior high and high school saying they buy their own smokeless tobacco.[61]

Studies show that minors who purchase cigarettes and smokeless-tobacco products in stores are infrequently asked for identification. In addition to over-the-counter sales, vending machines are a principal source of cigarettes for children. The 1994 surgeon general's report examined studies of vending-machine sales and found that children and adolescents were successful in purchasing cigarettes in that manner 88 percent of the time.[60] In addition, surveys show that vending machines are most popular with the youngest smokers. According to a study by the vending-machine industry itself, 22 percent of 13-year-olds who smoke purchase cigarettes from vending machines, as compared with 2 percent of 17-year-olds.[62]

Self-service displays also give young people easy access to cigarettes and smokeless-tobacco products, because they permit them to obtain these products quickly, easily, and independently. A study by the Institute of Medicine found that more than 40 percent of grade-school students who smoked daily had at some time shoplifted cigarettes from self-service displays.[63] Young people also obtain tobacco products by redeeming coupons for free or discounted cigarettes through the mail. As part of an investigation by his office, the attorney general of Massachusetts had 30 minors mail in coupons to manufacturers for free samples of smokeless tobacco. Virtually all of them received the samples.[64] Children and adolescents often obtain free samples of cigarettes that are distributed on street corners, at shopping malls, and at festivals, concerts, and other places frequented by youngsters. Despite the tobacco industry's voluntary code prohibiting the distribution of free samples to children, a number of surveys and reports demonstrate that young people can obtain them easily. Finally, "kiddie" packs, which typically contain 5, 10, or 15 cigarettes, are inexpensive and easy for young people to hide.

To limit young people's easy access to tobacco products, the FDA's rule prohibits the sale of tobacco products to anyone under 18 years old and requires retailers to check photographic identification, such as a driver's license, for everyone 26 or under. In addition, the access provisions of the rule prohibit tobacco vending machines and self-service displays, except in facilities, such as certain nightclubs, where the management ensures that no one under 18 will be present at any time. It also prohibits free samples, kiddie packs, and most sales of single cigarettes. And while permitting mail-order sales, it prohibits coupons for cigarettes or smokeless tobacco from being redeemed through the mail.

Reducing the Appeal of Advertising

Tobacco products are among the most heavily advertised and promoted commodities in this country. In 1993, tobacco companies' expenditures for advertising and promotion exceeded $6 billion.[65-67] Studies show that advertising substantially influences young people's smoking and use of smokeless tobacco.

Two reports on tobacco and young people, one by the surgeon general[68] and the other by the Institute of Medicine,[69] studied how advertising affects young people's use of tobacco and concluded that it was an important factor. Officials at the FDA reviewed scores of other reports examining the psychological and social factors affecting tobacco use. Collectively, the studies showed that young people are widely exposed to cigarette advertising, aware of it, and influenced by it. One study found that 30 percent of three-year-olds and 91 percent of six-year-olds could identify Joe Camel as a symbol of smoking.[70] Other studies have shown that young people's exposure to cigarette advertising is correlated with their smoking behavior and their intention to smoke. Still others suggest that cigarette advertising helps young people decide what behavior is normal or socially acceptable and that those who are led to overestimate the prevalence of smoking seem more likely to begin smoking and progress to regular smoking. Finally, such advertising appears to be particularly effective with children and adolescents. The three most heavily advertised brands are smoked by 86 percent of young smokers; by contrast, adults are far more likely to choose one of the "generic" brands, which are advertised less and are less expensive.[71]

Billboards are one of the most effective means of reaching young people with tobacco advertising. A survey conducted by BKG Youth for *Advertising Age* showed that 46 percent of children 8 to 13 years old said they most often saw cigarettes advertised on billboards, more than in magazines.[72] Furthermore, the billboard industry's own marketing materials emphasize the unavoidability of billboards, as in this statement: "Outdoor is right up there. Day and night. Lurking. Waiting for another ambush."[73]

Promotional items—such as T-shirts, caps, sporting goods, and other items displaying tobacco brand names or other types of product identification—have become particularly popular with young people. A Gallup survey found that about half of adolescents who smoke and one quarter of adolescents who do not smoke owned at least one such item.[74]

Lastly, studies show that sponsorship by cigarette and smokeless-tobacco companies associates the use of their products with events young people perceive as exciting, glamorous, or fun, such as car races and rodeos. Such sponsorship provides an opportunity for advertising to create a "friendly familiarity" between tobacco and sports enthusiasts, many of whom are children and adolescents. The leading source of data on television viewership estimates that motor vehicle sports are watched 64 million times a year by those under 18.[76] Whereas print advertisements are typically seen for only a few seconds, the brand name is viewed for hours at a time during sponsored events.

The many types of advertising and promotion of tobacco—billboards, printed advertisements, direct mail, promotional items, and sponsored events—give children and adolescents the misperception that the large majority of their peers and adults use tobacco. Children are constantly exposed to this message, which is funded by $6 billion in advertising and promotional expenditures. Teenagers look at *Rolling Stone* and see a cardboard Joe Camel pop out of the center of the magazine holding concert tickets in his hand.[76] Children walking home from school pass under billboards showing appealing images related to tobacco products. When they attend a car race or watch one on television, they see the bright-red Marlboro car and posters around the racetrack bear the brand name and its associated colors. On their friends' caps and T-shirts they see yet more ads for tobacco.

For these reasons, the regulation limits tobacco advertising in the media to a black-and-white, text-only format. This restriction preserves the textual information for adult smokers while at the same time eliminating the colorful imagery that makes advertising appealing and compelling to children and adolescents. There are a few exceptions. Advertising in publications read primarily by adults or that appears in places frequented only by adults is exempt from restrictions. In contrast, outdoor advertising within 1000 feet of schools or playgrounds is prohibited.

Tobacco companies will not be permitted to sell or distribute promotional items, such as T-shirts, caps, and sporting goods, that carry the brand name or logo of a tobacco product. Similarly, tobacco companies that sponsor sporting or other events, race cars, athletic teams, or the like will be restricted to using their corporate names only.

Educating Children about Tobacco

Young people are generally aware of the link between tobacco use and a variety of diseases. However, studies show that those who smoke do not usually see these long-term risks as applying to them personally and that, furthermore, they tend to discount the risks. For example, only half of highschool seniors who smoke, but three quarters of those who do not smoke, report that smoking a pack or more of cigarettes per day constitutes a serious health risk.[77]

In addition, although young people say that nicotine is addictive, there is evidence that those who begin to smoke do not believe that they themselves will become addicted. One study found that senior-high-school students' expectations about their own future smoking bore little relation to their actual smoking practices. Of students who smoked at least one pack a day and said they would probably or definitely not be smoking in five years, only 13 percent did in fact quit. More than 72 percent continued to smoke at least one pack a day.[78]

For these reasons, the FDA intends to require a national program of education, relying primarily on television messages, to help young people understand the health risks to which they are subjecting themselves if they use tobacco. Such messages proved effective in the late 1960s, when broadcasters were required to air them to counter the advertising for cigarettes that was then permitted on television. After the publication of this rule, the agency plans to notify the major cigarette and smokeless-tobacco companies that it will begin discussing a requirement that they fund an educational program in the mass media.

These regulations will be implemented over the next two years. The goal is to cut the use of tobacco among young people by half over a seven-year period. This reduction will improve the public health in general because as these children grow up, fewer and fewer adults will be addicted to nicotine.

In financial terms alone, the rule is expected to yield substantial health-related benefits ranging from $28 billion to $43 billion each year. The FDA estimates that implementing the rule will entail a one-time cost of $174 million to $187 million and annual operating costs of $149 million to $185 million. These economic benefits were calculated by estimating the number of adolescents who will not start smoking because of the rule and then, from existing risk data, predicting how much sickness and death caused by tobacco products will be prevented. These cost estimates were based on the public comments and on extensive economic analyses by the affected industries.

❖ Conclusions

This new FDA regulation presents a historic opportunity, giving the United States a chance to reduce the consumption of a product that kills more Americans each year than die from any other preventable cause. The approach is focused in the right place; sparing children and adolescents a lifetime of addiction to tobacco.

❖ About the Authors

David A. Kessler, M.D., Commissioner of the Food and Drug Administration (FDA) from 1990–1997, is Medical Director of the Albert Einstein University Hospital and faculty in the Department of Ambulatory and Community Medicine.

Ann M. Witt, Philip S. Barnett, Mitchell R. Zeller, Sharon L. Natanblut, Judith P. Wilkenfeld, Catherine C. Lorraine, Larry J. Thompson, and William B. Schulz are with the Food and Drug Administration, Rockville, Maryland.

REFERENCES

1. Department of Health and Human Services. Regulations restricting the sale and distribution of cigarettes and smokeless tobacco products to protect children and adolescents. Fed Regist 1996;61: 44396-618.

2. Kessler DA. Agency's response to Coalition on Smoking OR Health's outstanding petitions. Rockville, Md.: Food and Drug Administration, February 25, 1994.

3. Department of Health and Human Services, Food and Drug Administration. Analysis regarding the Food and Drug Administration. Analysis regarding the Food and Drug Administration's jurisdiction

over nicotine-containing cigarettes and smokeless tobacco products. Fed Regist 1995;60:41453.

4. *Idem.* Regulations restricting the sale and distribution of cigarettes and smokeless tobacco products to protect children and adolescents, Fed Regist 1995;60:41314-75.

5. Department of Health and Human Services, Office on Smoking and Health. The health consequences of smoking: nicotine addiction; a report of the Surgeon General, Washington, D.C.: Government Printing Office, 1988:13-4. (DHHS publication no. (CDC) 88-8406.)

6. Benowitz NL. Clinical pharmacology of inhaled drugs of abuse: Implications in understanding nicotine dependence. In: Chiang CN, Hawks RL, eds. Research findings on smoking of abused substances. NIDA research monograph 99. Washington, D.C.: Government Printing Office, 1990: 12-29.

7. Diagnostic and statistical manual of mental disorders. 3rd ed. rev. Washington, D.C.: American Psychiatric Association, 1987:159-60, 176-8.

8. Ethyl alcohol and nicotine as addictive drugs. In: 1993 AMA policy compendium. Chicago: American Medical Association, 1993:35.

9. World Health Organization. The ICD-10 classification of mental and behavioral disorders: clinical descriptions and diagnostic guidelines. Geneva: World Health Organization, 1992:76.

10. Health and Welfare of Canada, Health Protection Branch, Tobacco, nicotine, and addiction: a committee report. Ottawa: Royal Society of Canada, 1989:v-vi.

11. MRC field review of drug dependence. London: Medical Research Council, 1994:1L.

12. Department of Health and Human Services, Office on Smoking and Health, The health consequences of smoking: nicotine addiction: a

report of the Surgeon General, Washington, D.C.: Government Printing Office, 1988:7-8. (DHHS publication no. (CDC) 88-8406.)

13. Chemical and biological studies: new cigarette prototypes that heat instead of burn tobacco. Winston-Salem, N.C.: R.J. Reynolds Tobacco, 1988.

14. Dagnoli J. PM's denic may get more nicotine. Advertising Age. February 12, 1990:31.

15. Kessler DA. Statement. In: Regulation of tobacco products. Part 1. Hearings before the Subcommittee on Health and the Environment of the Committee on Energy and Commerce, House of Representatives. Washington, D.C.: Government Printing Office, 1994: Chart T. (Serial no. 103-149.)

16. Spears AW. Testimony. In: Regulation of tobacco products. Part 1. Hearings before the Subcommittee on Health and the Environment of the Committee on Energy and Commerce, House of Representatives. Washington, D.C.: Government Printing Office, 1994:143-4. (Serial no. 103-149.)

17. Department of Health and Human Services, Food and Drug Administration. Analysis regarding the Food and Drug Administration's jurisdiction over nicotine-containing cigarettes and smokeless tobacco products. Fed Regist 1995; 60:41723-4.

18. Regulation of tobacco products. Part 1. Hearings before the Subcommittee on Health and the Environment of the Committee on Energy and Commerce, House of Representatives. Washington, D.C.: Government Printing Office, 1995:Charts B–D. (Serial no. 103-149.)

19. Bavley A, Air D, Robb E II. Additive-releasing filter for releasing additives into tobacco smoke. 1966. (U.S. Patent No. 3,280,823.)

20. DeNoble VJ. Statement. In: Regulation of tobacco products. Part 2. Hearings before the Subcommittee

on Health and the Environment of the Committee on Energy and Commerce, House of Representatives. Washington, D.C.: Government Printing Office, 1994:33. (Serial no. 103-153.)

21. Regulation of tobacco products. Part 2. Hearings before the Subcommittee on Health and the Environment of the Committee on Energy and Commerce, House of Representatives. Washington, D.C.: Government Printing Office, 1994:17. (Serial no. 103-153.)

22. Regulation of tobacco products. Part 2. Hearings before the Subcommittee on Health and the Environment of the Committee on Energy and Commerce, House of Representatives. Washington, D.C.: Government Printing Office, 1994:17-8. (Serial no. 103-153.)

23. Regulation of tobacco products. Part 2. Hearings before the Subcommittee on Health and the Environment of the Committee on Energy and Commerce, House of Representatives, Washington, D.C.: Government Printing Office, 1994:6. (Serial no. 103-153.)

24. Department of Health and Human Services, Office on Smoking and Health. The health consequences of smoking: nicotine addiction: a report of the Surgeon General. Washington, D.C.: Government Printing Office. 1988:274-5. (DHHS publication no. (CDC) 88-8406.)

25. Hilts PJ. Tobacco company was silent on hazards. New York Times. May 7, 1994.

26. Ellis C. The smoking and health problem. In: Smoking and health—policy on research. Southampton, England: BATCO Research Conference, 1962:4.

27. Yeaman AY. Implications of Battelle Hippo I and II and the Griffith filter. Southampton, England: BATCO Research Conference, July 17, 1963:4.

28. Minutes of the BATCO Group R&D Conference on Smoking Behaviour, Southampton, England,

October 11 and 12, 1976. (BW-W2-02145.)

29. Minutes of the BATCO Group R&D Conference on Method of Nicotine and Cotinine in Blood and Urine, Southampton, England, May 21, 1980:2.

30. Federative Republic of Brazil, Ministry of Industry, Commerce and Tourism, National Institute for Industrial Property. Genetically stable tobacco variety and tobacco plant. Louisville, Ky.: Brown & Williamson Tobacco, 1993. (Publication no. PI 9203690A.)

31. Department of Health and Human Services, Food and Drug Administration. Analysis regarding the Food and Drug Administration's jurisdiction over nicotine-containing cigarettes and smokeless tobacco products. Fed Regist 1995; 60:41701.

32. Regulation of tobacco products. Part 3. Hearings before the Subcommittee on Health and the Environment of the Committee on Energy and Commerce, House of Representatives. Washington, D.C.: Government Printing Office, 1995:21. (Serial no. 103-171.)

33. Department of Health and Human Services, Food and Drug Administration. Analysis regarding the Food and Drug Administration's jurisdiction over nicotine-containing cigarettes and smokeless tobacco products. Fed Regist 1995; 60:416225-43.

34. Waxman HA. Remarks. Congressional Record (Daily ed.) 1995;141: H7470.

35. Idem. Congressional Record (Daily ed.) 1995;141:H8007.

36. Wakeham H. Smoker psychology research. In: Presentation to the Philip Morris board of directors. Richmond, Va.: Philip Morris, November 26, 1969;240.

37. Dunn WL. Plans and objectives—1979. Congressional Record (Daily ed.) 1995;141:h7668-70.

38. Idem. Smoker psychology/April 1–30, 1974. Memorandum, May 9,

1974. Congressional Record (Daily ed.) 1995;141:H8132.

39. Cipollone v. Liggett Group, Inc., et al. Civil Action No. 83-2864, U.S. District Court for the District of New Jersey.

40. Dunn WL. Motives and incentives in cigarette smoking. Richmond, Va.: Philip Morris, 1972:5.

41. Teague CE. Memorandum. Research planning memorandum on the nature of the tobacco business and the crucial role of nicotine therein. Winston-Salem, N.C.: RJ. Reynolds Tobacco, April 14, 1972.

42. Senkus M. Some effects of smoking. Winston-Salem, N.C.: R.J. Reynolds Tobacco, 1976/1977:4.

43. Department of Health and Human Services, Food and Drug Administration. Analysis regarding the Food and Drug Administration's jurisdiction over nicotine-containing cigarettes and smokeless tobacco products: reopening the comment period as to specific documents. Fed Regist 1996;61: 11419.

44. *Idem.* Analysis regarding the Food and Drug Administration's jurisdiction over nicotine-containing cigarettes and smokeless tobacco products. Fed Regist 1995;60: 41737.

45. Afriek J. Interview. Executive vice president of U.S. Tobacco Company and president of the international division. Up to Snuff. Winter 1986:2.

46. Department of Health and Human Services. National household survey on drug abuse: population estimates 1993. Rockville, Md.: Substance and Mental Health Services Administration, 1994:89, 95. (DHHS publication no. SMA 94-3017.)

47. Cottler LB. Comparing DSM-Ill-R and ICD-10 substance use disorders. Addiction 1993;88:689-96.

48. Hughes JR, Gust SW, Pechacek TF. Prevalence of tobacco dependence and withdrawal. Am J Psychiatry 1987;144:205-8.

49. Woody GE, Cottler LB, Cacciola J. Severity of dependence: data from the DSM-IV field trials. Addiction 1993;88:1573-9.

50. Department of Health and Human Services, Centers for Disease Control. Cigarette smoking—attributable mortality and years of potential life lost—United States, 1990. MMWR Morb Mortal Wkly Rep 1993;42:645-9.

51. Institute of Medicine. Growing up tobacco free—preventing nicotine addiction in children and youths. Washington, D.C.: National Academy Press, 1994:3.

52. Department of Health and Human Services. Preventing tobacco use among young people: a report of the Surgeon General. Washington, D.C.: Government Printing Office, 1994:65. (S/N 017-001-00491-0.)

53. *Idem.* Preventing tobacco use among young people: a report of the Surgeon General. Washington, D.C.: Government Printing Office, 1994: 5. (S/N 017-001-00491-0.)

54. Pierce JP, Fiore MC, Novotny TE, Hatziandreu EJ, Davis RM. Trends in cigarette smoking in the United States: projections to the year 2000. JAMA 1989;261:61-5.

55. Cigarette smoking among adults—United States, 1993. MMWR Morb Mortal Wkly Rep 1994;43:925-9.

56. Johnston LD, O'Malley PM, Bachman JG. National survey results on drug use from the Monitoring the Future Study 1975–1993. Vol 1. Secondary school students. Rockville, Md.: National Institutes of Health, 1994:9, 19, 79, 80, 101. (NIH publication no. 94-3809.)

57. Smoking rates climb among American teen-agers, who find smoking increasingly acceptable and seriously underestimate the risks. Ann Arbor: University of Michigan News and Information Service, July 17, 1995.

58. Ericksen MP. Tobacco mortality estimates from the Centers for Disease Control and Prevention. CDC Fact Sheet. August 7, 1995.

59. DiFranza JR, Tye JB. Who profits from tobacco sales to children? JAMA 1990;263:2784-7.

60. Department of Health and Human Services. Preventing tobacco use among young people: a report of the Surgeon General, Washington, D.C.: Government Printing Office. 1994:249, (S/N 017-001-00491-0.)

61. Department of Health and Human Services, Office of Inspector General. Youth use of smokeless tobacco: more than a pinch of trouble. Washington, D.C.: Government Printing Office. 1986:4. (Publication no. P-06-86-0058.)

62. Response Research. Findings for the study of teenage cigarette smoking and purchasing behavior. Chicago: National Automatic Merchandising Association, June/July 1989. (Exhibit 22.)

63. Institute of Medicine. Growing up tobacco free—preventing nicotine addiction in children and youths. Washington, D.C.: National Academy Press, 1994:215.

64. Harshbarger S. Comment. In: Proposed regulations restricting the sale and distribution of cigarettes and smokeless tobacco products, Rockville, Md.: Food and Drug Administration, 1996. (Docket 95N-0253. No. C29885.)

65. Federal Trade Commission. Report to Congress for 1993; pursuant to the Federal Cigarette and Advertising Act, Washington, D.C.: Government Printing Office, 1995:Table 3D.

66. *Idem.* Report to Congress; pursuant to the Comprehensive Smokeless Tobacco Health Education Act of 1986. Washington, D.C.: Government Printing Office, 1995: 25-35.

67. Teinowitz I. Add RJR to list of cigarette price cuts. Advertising Age. April 26, 1993:3, 46.

68. Department of Health and Human Services. Preventing tobacco use among young people: a report of the Surgeon General. Washington, D.C.: Government Printing Office, 1994. (S/N 017-001-00491-0.)

69. Institute of Medicine. Growing up tobacco free—preventing nicotine addiction in children and youths. Washington, D.C.: National Academy Press, 1994.

70. Fischer PM, Schwartz MP, Richards JW Jr, Goldstein AO, Rojas TH. Brand logo recognition by children aged 3 to 6 years: Mickey Mouse and Old Joe the Camel. JAMA 1991;266:3145-8.

71. Changes in the cigarette brand preferences of adolescent smokers—United States, 1989–1993. MMWR Morb Mortal Wkly Rep 1994;43:577-81.

72. Levin G. Poll shows Camel ads are effective with kids; preteens best recognize brand. Advertising Age. April 27, 1992:12.

73. Outdoor: it's not a medium, it's a large. Washington, D.C.: Outdoor Advertising Association of America.

74. Teen-age attitudes and behavior concerning tobacco—report of the findings. Princeton, N.J.: George H. Gallup International Institute, 1992:17, 59.

75. Slade J. Tobacco product advertising during motor sports broadcasts: the quantative assessment. Paris: 9th World Conference on Tobacco and Health, 1994.

76. Advertising supplement between pages 12 and 13. Rolling Stone. March 7, 1996:12, 13.

77. Department of Health and Human Services. Preventing tobacco use among young people: a report of the Surgeon General. Washington, D.C.: Government Printing Office, 1994:80. (S/N 017-001-00491-0.)

78. *Idem.* Preventing tobacco use among young people: a report of the Surgeon General. Washington, D.C.: Government Printing Office, 1994:86. (S/N 017-001-00491-0.)

❖ Dietary Guidance for the 21st Century: New Approaches

MARION NESTLE

❖ Introduction

Nutrition educators face formidable challenges. Despite more than 15 years of federal advice, diet-related chronic diseases remain leading causes of death and disability among Americans,[1] and the risk factors for these conditions continue to rise, especially among individuals of low income, social status, and education.[2]

Today, federal policies to help the public reduce chronic disease risk factors are expressed in the Dietary Guidelines for Americans,[3] and its implementation guide, the Food Guide Pyramid.[4] These guides call for diets with more fruit, vegetables, and grains; lean meats and low-fat dairy foods; and limited fats and sweets.

Although Americans have adopted some of this advice, overall dietary patterns still do not meet recommendations. In an environment in which taste is the most important factor affecting food selection, consumers say they are making dietary changes to improve their health, but they are not always doing so; for example, surveys variously report that 94% of respondents claim that they are making dietary changes for health reasons,[5] but also state that they are eating about the same amount of fruit, vegetables, and grains as they did 10 years ago.[6] When their diets are compared to the pyramid pattern, survey respondents are found to be consuming the recommended number of meat and dairy servings but are eating more daily servings of fats and sweets than of fruit and vegetables.[7]

Reporters describe early signs of a "nutritional backlash"—widespread public hostility to dietary advice. They observe that Americans are becoming less concerned about diet and health, are dismissing the "health craze" as "history,"[8] and are returning to the coronary-inducing dietary patterns of the 1950s.[9] If such trends continue, it seems quite unlikely that national nutrition objectives for reduced fat and increased fruit, vegetable, and grain intake will be achieved by the year 2000.[10]

Many reasons of taste, culture, and socioeconomics might explain why Americans do not follow dietary advice. This viewpoint focuses on just one of them: ambiguities in federal dietary guidance messages. These ambiguities also have many causes. If nutrition education is to succeed in helping the public reduce chronic disease risk factors, dietary messages will need to be based on an understanding of these causes and should be stated more explicitly than is now the case.

91

❖ Ambiguous Recommendations

Current dietary trends should stimulate nutrition educators to critically examine nutrition messages. To do so, it is necessary to review existing information on consumer perceptions of dietary advice. Unfortunately, information on this subject is scant. Available research and anecdotal evidence reveal widespread public confusion about dietary advice,[11] and profound misunderstanding of dietary guidelines,[12] advice about fat and cholesterol,[13] words such as "moderation,"[14] and the size of servings recommended in the pyramid.[15] As the following indicates, the wording of dietary guidelines may well contribute to such confusion.

Variety. Consumers correctly understand the variety guideline to imply that foods should be selected from all food groups, but are uncertain about the nature of those groups.[13] Research has demonstrated that variety in food intake improves dietary adequacy[16] as well as overall health.[17] Individuals who consume a greater variety of foods, however, eat more foods in greater quantities;[18] they consume more fruit and vegetables, but they also consume more fats and sweets.[11,19] Therefore, to encourage a dietary pattern that meets recommendations, the variety guideline should specify: "eat a variety of foods low in fat, saturated fat, cholesterol, sugar, and salt," or, more generally, "eat a variety of healthful foods."

Fruit, Vegetables, and Grains. Despite strong evidence for the protective effects of fruit and vegetable consumption against chronic diseases,[20] consumption levels fall far short of recommendations.[7] Ambiguities in dietary advice about these foods have been reviewed previously.[21] The word "plenty" in the guideline correctly suggests "more," as does the triangular design of the pyramid, but if energy intake is to remain constant, eating more from this group necessarily requires eating less from the others—meat, dairy, and fats and sweets. Furthermore, eating more fruit and vegetables does not necessarily lead to a reduction in fat intake; it is also necessary to eat less of meat, dairy, and processed foods or to choose those that are low in fat.[20] If meat and dairy foods become less prominent contributors to food intake, diets begin to approach the near-vegetarian. Research has shown that people who consume vegetarian or near-vegetarian diets are healthier as a group than those who consume high-fat meat and dairy products. Vegetarians, for example, exhibit lower rates of heart disease and diet-related cancers than the average population[22] and do not demonstrate higher rates of osteoporosis, whether or not they eat dairy products.[23] Thus, this recommendation might say: "obtain most of your daily energy from plant foods."

Fat, Saturated Fat, and Cholesterol. Meat and dairy foods (including eggs) contribute about 40% of the total fat, 60% of the saturated fat, and 100% of the cholesterol in the American diet.[24] Therefore, a reduction in intake of these substances necessarily demands a reduction in meat and dairy products. Nevertheless, federal dietary guidance materials continue to suggest 2 to 3 daily servings each from the meat and dairy groups, without any indication that this amount should be considered as an upper limit. A less ambiguous guideline might say: "eat less meat and fewer high-fat dairy products." At the very least, the guideline should more strongly emphasize the choice of lower-fat options from these groups.

❖ Reasons For Ambiguous Messages

Shift in Disease Patterns. The earliest Department of Agriculture (USDA) food group recommendations may not appear very different from those in current use, but the reasons for them have changed. Until the late 1970s, USDA guides were designed to help the public prevent nutritional deficiencies through daily intake of foods selected from various groups; the number and composition of food groups varied over the years, but all guides promoted consumption of the full range of American agricultural products. When diet-related chronic diseases became recognized as leading causes of death shortly after World War II, dietary advice began to include restrictions on intake of fat and other factors associated with those diseases. As guidelines shifted from "eat more" to "eat less," the producers of foods affected by such advice and their supporters in Congress began to protest.[25] In part, protesters used science to justify their complaints; they questioned the validity of the evidence relating diet to chronic diseases. Indeed, scientific consensus only was achieved in the late 1980s, with publication of the surgeon general's report on nutrition and health and the National Research Council's diet and health study.[26]

Political Pressures. Politics, however, was a more pressing basis for protests against dietary guidelines. As I have described elsewhere,[27,28] political pressures on dietary advice have been unrelenting, and are best illustrated by experience with the meat recommendation. From the beginning, advice to "eat less meat" elicited such strong protests from meat producers and their congressional supporters that the statement was soon replaced with its euphemism "choose lean," but even these words were considered controversial. Protests stopped only in 1990 when the third edition of the Dietary Guidelines stated the recommendation in positive terms: "have two or three servings, with a daily total of about six ounces."[3] When the USDA attempted to release its pyramid in 1991, however, meat producers protested the location of their products in the design, and were at least in part responsible for a year-long delay in publication.[29] This level of protest must be considered a tribute to the clarity with which the design of the pyramid conveys the message that fruit, vegetables, and grains constitute the basis of recommended diets, and that meat, dairy products, and processed foods should be consumed in much smaller amounts.

Food Marketing Issues.   The reasons for food producer opposition to dietary guidelines are not difficult to understand. This country vastly overproduces food, and the food marketing system is fiercely competitive.[30] In 1990, the U.S. food supply provided an average of 3700 kcal per day for every man, woman, and child in the country.[31] Most adults need one half to two thirds of that amount, and most children even less. Overproduction means that any choice of one food product necessarily implies rejection of another. Food marketers encourage consumers to choose their particular products through $36 billion of advertising, and through the development of 15,000 new food products each year.[32] Any suggestion to reduce intake of a food component for reasons of health threatens the competitive advantage of any product containing that component.

Weak Lobbying For Plant Foods.   Although it might seem reasonable to expect that the producers of fruit, vegetables, and grains would also attempt to lobby for their products, they have not yet done so effectively. The principal food-industry supporters of plant-based diets have conflicts of interest, as most of the grain produced in this country is used to feed animals. Furthermore, producers of fruit and vegetables tend to view each other as competitors, and focus on the differences among the various kinds of fruit and vegetables rather than on their similarities. Such views help to explain the rather low level of support given to the Produce for Better Health Foundation, the industry arm of the 5 A Day program.[33]

❖ Constancy Of Dietary Advice

The public commonly perceives that dietary advice changes constantly. This perception is particularly unfortunate because today's guidelines for prevention of diet-related chronic diseases have hardly changed at all since they were first proposed. On the basis of diet-disease

---

TABLE 1   Dietary Recommendations for Healthy Diets.*

Do not get fat; if you are fat, reduce.
Restrict saturated fats—the fats in beef, pork, lamb sausages, margarine, solid
    shortenings, fats in dairy products.
Prefer vegetable oils to solid fats, but keep total fats under 30% of your diet
    calories.
Favor fresh vegetables, fruits, and nonfat milk products.
Avoid heavy use of salt and refined sugar.
Get plenty of exercise and outdoor recreation.
Be sensible about cigarettes, alcohol, excitement, business strain.
See your doctor regularly, and do not worry.

---

*Adapted from Ancel and Margaret Keys, 1959.[34]

patterns observed in the Mediterranean region, Dr. and Mrs. Ancel Keys described the benefits—and pleasures—of largely vegetarian diets in a 1959 cookbook for heart disease prevention. Their "best advice" for healthy diets is summarized in Table 1.[34] Although written 18 years before the Dietary Goals, and 31 years before the most recent Dietary Guidelines, the Keys' precepts are consistent with both. Public—and professional—ignorance of the constancy of such recommendations may be due to the fact that nutrition research so often focuses on single nutrients such as fat, cholesterol, fiber, or one or another antioxidant vitamin. Advice about intake of foods to reduce chronic diseases has not changed at all since diet-related chronic conditions were first recognized as a public health problem.

❖ 1995 Dietary Guidelines

This review should make it clear that ambiguities in dietary messages are due at least in part to political pressures. The more straightforward the message, the more it is likely to threaten food marketers and, therefore, to cause trouble. The 1995 Dietary Guidelines have been under strong political pressure from the outset. By far, the vast majority of comment and testimony has come from food industry representatives openly requesting elimination or weakening of any statement that suggests that the public eat less fat, saturated fat, cholesterol, salt, sugar, or alcohol, or avoid any products containing such substances. Advocates for strengthening the guidelines and making them more explicit have been few in number and not nearly so assertive.

This situation closely follows the tradition of previous editions. In 1990, committee members changed the wording of the guidelines to make them more positive. They used the word "choose" rather than "avoid" so that advice to "avoid too much fat" became "choose a diet low in fat," and "choose lean meat" became "have two or three servings." The committee made these changes to help overcome public misperceptions that there are good and bad foods, and to emphasize the benefits of following the guidelines as opposed to the risks of not following them.[35]

From the standpoint of health, however, some foods *are* better than others. As noted earlier, there is ample scientific justification for recommendations to eat less meat, dairy, and processed foods that contain so much of the fat, sugar, and salt in the American diet.

Whether even the most unambiguous messages will overcome the impact of food advertising and lobbying efforts is uncertain. Because researchers have not addressed such questions, the impact of changes made in the 1990 Guidelines remains uncertain. In the absence of such research, the 1995 Guidelines committee also will be making its decisions on the basis of members' personal responses to the information they receive—much of it from food industry representatives with vested interests.

If, indeed, the public perceives healthful diets as a lost cause and blames nutritionists for constantly changing dietary messages, our profession has even more work to do than any of us might have anticipated. The development and funding of research on consumer understanding of dietary guidelines, and on the impact of dietary advice on consumer behavior, must become a major priority for nutrition educators. Without such research, we will not be able to overcome political pressures to eliminate or dilute dietary messages. The 5 A Day research initiatives on the impact of information about fruit and vegetable consumption are a welcome step,[36] but broader issues of message communication also require careful—and immediate—investigation.

It is now too late to influence the statements in the 1995 Dietary Guidelines, but it is not too early to begin establishing a research basis for dietary guidelines for the year 2000. Such research should be easy to justify; health promotion is at the forefront of national policy debates, and the role of nutrition in health is well established. As always, the health of the American people should be our first priority.

❖ About the Authors

Marion Nestle, Ph.D., M.P.H., is Professor, Department of Nutrition and Food Studies, New York University.

REFERENCES

1. McGinnis JM, Foege WH. Actual causes of death in the United States. JAMA 1993;270:2207–12.
2. Kuczmarski RJ, Flegal KM, Campbell SM, Johnson CL. Increasing prevalence of overweight among US adults: the national health and nutrition examination surveys, 1960–1991. JAMA 1994;272:205–11.
3. US Department of Agriculture and US Department of Health and Human Services. Nutrition and your health: dietary guidelines for Americans, 3rd Ed. HG 232. Washington, DC:USDA, 1990.
4. US Department of Agriculture. The food guide pyramid. HG 252. Hyattsville, MD:USDA, 1992.
5. Trends in the United States: consumer attitudes & the supermarket 1994. Washington, DC: Food Marketing Institute, 1994.
6. The prevention index: a report card on the nation's health. Emmaus, PA: Rodale Press, 1994.
7. Eating in America today: a dietary pattern and intake report, 2nd Ed. II. National Life Stock and Meat Board, 1994.
8. Woodbury R. The great fast-food pig-out. Time 1993;28 June:51.
9. Hamlin S. Eating in 1994: the year beef came back. New York Times 1994; Dec 28:C6.
10. US Department of Health and Human Services. Healthy people 2000: national health promotion and disease prevention objectives. Washington, DC, 1991.
11. Gallup Organization. How are Americans making food choices?—1994 update. Chicago, IL and Washington, DC: American Dietetic Association and International Food Information Council, 1994.

12. Achterberg C. Consumer interpretation of the US dietary guidelines. Proc Nutr Soc NZ 1991;16:15–30.

13. Auld GW, Achterberg CL, Getty VM, et al. Misconceptions about fats and cholesterol: implications for dietary guidelines. Ecol Food Nutr 1994;33:15–25.

14. Havala S. How do you define moderation? Vegetarian J 1992; Jul/Aug:8–13.

15. Sugarman C. A hard pyramid to swallow? Washington Post 1993; Apr 28:E1, E8–9.

16. Krebs-Smith SM, Smiciklas-Wright H, Guthrie HA, Krebs-Smith J. The effects of variety in food choices on dietary quality. J Am Diet Assoc 1987;87:897–903.

17. Kant AK, Schatzkin A, Harris TB, et al. Dietary diversity and subsequent mortality in the First National Health and Nutrition Examination Survey Epidemiologic Follow-up Study. Am J Clin Nutr 1993;57:434–40.

18. Rolls BJ. Experimental analyses of the effects of variety in a meal on human feeding. Am J Clin Nutr 1985;45:932–39.

19. Kant AK, Block G, Schatzkin A, Nestle M. Association of fruit and vegetable intake with dietary fat intake. Nutr Res 1992:12:1441–54.

20. Willett WC. Diet and health: what should we eat? Science 1994;264: 532–7.

21. Domel SB, Leonard SB, Baranowski T, Baranowski J. "To be or not to be . . ." fruits and vegetables. J Nutr Educ 1993;25:352–8.

22. Johnston PK, ed. Second international congress on vegetarian nutrition: proceedings of a symposium held in Arlington, VA, June 28–July 1, 1992. Am J Clin Nutr 1994; 59 (Suppl 5):1099s–1262s.

23. Kushi LH, Lenart EB, Willett WC. Health implications of Mediterranean diets in the light of contemporary knowledge. I. Plant foods and dairy products. Am J Clin Nutr 1995;61(Suppl):14075–155.

24. Raper NR, Zizza C, Rourke J. Nutrient content of the US food supply, 1909–1988. Home Econ Res Rep 50. Washington, DC: USDA, 1992.

25. Nestle M, Porter DV. Evolution of federal dietary guidance policy: from food adequacy to chronic disease prevention. Caduceus 1990;6:43–67.

26. McGinnis JM, Nestle M. The surgeon general's report on nutrition and health: policy implications and implementation strategies. Am J Clin Nutr 1989;49:23–8.

27. Nestle M. Food lobbies, the food pyramid, and US nutrition policy. Int J Health Serv 1993;23:483–96.

28. Nestle M. Editorial: the politics of dietary guidance—a new opportunity. Am J Public Health 1994;84: 713–4.

29. Nestle M. Dietary advice for the 1990s: the political history of the food guide pyramid. Caduceus 1993;9:136–53.

30. Stillings BR. Trends in foods. Nutr Today 1994;29:6–13.

31. Putnam JJ, Allshouse JE. Food consumption, prices and expenditures, 1970–92. Statistics Bulletin 867. Washington, DC: USDA, 1993.

32. Gallo AE. The food marketing system in 1991–92. Agricultural Information Bulletin 659. Washington, DC: USDA, 1992.

33. Gov't & industry launch fruit and vegetable push; but NCI takes back seat. Nutr Week 1992;22:1–2.

34. Keys A, Keys M. Eat well & stay well. Garden City, NY: Doubleday, 1959.

35. US Department of Agriculture. Report of the dietary guidelines advisory committee on the dietary guidelines for Americans. No. 261–463/20444. Washington, DC: USDA, 1990.

36. Havas S, Heimendinger J, Reynolds K, et al. 5 A Day for better health: a new research initiative. J Am Diet Assoc 1994;94:32–6.

❖ Surgeon General's Report on Physical Activity and Health
Chapter 1 Introduction, Summary, and Chapter Conclusions
US DEPARTMENT OF HEALTH
AND HUMAN SERVICES

❖ Introduction

This is the first Surgeon General's report to address physical activity and health. The main message of this report is that Americans can substantially improve their health and quality of life by including moderate amounts of physical activity in their daily lives. Health benefits from physical activity are thus achievable for most Americans, including those who may dislike vigorous exercise and those who may have been previously discouraged by the difficulty of adhering to a program of vigorous exercise. For those who are already achieving regular moderate amounts of activity, additional benefits can be gained by further increases in activity level.

This report grew out of an emerging consensus among epidemiologists, experts in exercise science, and health professionals that physical activity need not be of vigorous intensity for it to improve health. Moreover, health benefits appear to be proportional to amount of activity; thus, every increase in activity adds some benefit. Emphasizing the amount rather than the intensity of physical activity offers more options for people to select from in incorporating physical activity into their daily lives. Thus, a moderate amount of activity can be obtained in a 30-minute brisk walk, 30 minutes of lawn mowing or raking leaves, a 15-minute run, or 45 minutes of playing volleyball, and these activities can be varied from day to day. It is hoped that this different emphasis on moderate amounts of activity, and the flexibility to vary activities according to personal preference and life circumstances, will encourage more people to make physical activity a regular and sustainable part of their lives.

The information in this report summarizes a diverse literature from the fields of epidemiology, exercise physiology, medicine, and the behavioral sciences. The report highlights what is known about physical activity and health, as well as what is being learned about promoting physical activity among adults and young people.

❖ Development of the Report

In July 1994, the Office of the Surgeon General authorized the Centers for Disease Control and Prevention (CDC) to serve as lead agency for preparing the first Surgeon General's report on physical activity and health. The CDC was joined in this effort by the President's Council on Physical Fitness and Sports (PCPFS) as a collaborative partner representing the Office of the Surgeon General. Because of the wide interest in the health effects of physical activity, the report was planned collaboratively with representatives from the Office of the Surgeon General, the Office of Public Health and Science (Office of the Secretary), the Office of Disease Prevention (National Institutes of Health [NIH]), and the following institutes from the NIH: the National Heart, Lung, and Blood Institute; the National Institute of Child Health and Human Development; the National Institute of Diabetes and Digestive and Kidney Diseases; and the National Institute of Arthritis and Musculoskeletal and Skin Diseases. CDC's non-federal partners—including the American Alliance for Health, Physical Education, Recreation, and Dance; the American College of Sports Medicine; and the American Heart Association—provided consultation throughout the development process.

The major purpose of this report is to summarize the existing literature on the role of physical activity in preventing disease and on the status of interventions to increase physical activity. Any report on a topic this broad must restrict its scope to keep its message clear. This report focuses on disease prevention and therefore does not include the considerable body of evidence on the benefits of physical activity for treatment or rehabilitation after disease has developed. This report concentrates on endurance-type physical activity (activity involving repeated use of large muscles, such as in walking or bicycling) because the health benefits of this type of activity have been extensively studied. The importance of resistance exercise (to increase muscle strength, such as by lifting weights) is increasingly being recognized as a means to preserve and enhance muscular strength and endurance and to prevent falls and improve mobility in the elderly. Some promising findings on resistance exercise are presented here, but a comprehensive review of resistance training is beyond the scope of this report. In addition, a review of the special concerns regarding physical activity for pregnant women and for people with disabilities is not undertaken here, although these important topics deserve more research and attention.

Finally, physical activity is only one of many everyday behaviors that affect health. In particular, nutritional habits are linked to some of the same aspects of health as physical activity, and the two may be related lifestyle characteristics. This report deals solely with physical activity; a Surgeon General's Report on Nutrition and Health was published in 1988.

Chapters 2 through 6 of this report address distinct areas of the current understanding of physical activity and health. Chapter 2 offers a historical perspective: after outlining the history of belief and knowledge about physical activity and health, the chapter reviews the evolution and content of physical activity recommendations. Chapter 3 describes the physiologic responses to physical activity—both the immediate effects of a single episode of activity and the long-term adaptations to a regular pattern of activity. The evidence that physical activity reduces the risk of cardiovascular and other diseases is presented in Chapter 4. Data on patterns and trends of physical activity in the U.S. population are the focus of Chapter 5. Lastly, Chapter 6 examines efforts to increase physical activity and reviews ideas currently being proposed for policy and environmental initiatives.

❖ Major Conclusions

1. People of all ages, both male and female, benefit from regular physical activity.
2. Significant health benefits can be obtained by including a moderate amount of physical activity (e.g., 30 minutes of brisk walking or raking leaves, 15 minutes of running, or 45 minutes of playing volleyball) on most, if not all, days of the week. Through a modest increase in daily activity, most Americans can improve their health and quality of life.
3. Additional health benefits can be gained through greater amounts of physical activity. People who can maintain a regular regimen of activity that is of longer duration or of more vigorous intensity are likely to derive greater benefit.
4. Physical activity reduces the risk of premature mortality in general, and of coronary heart disease, hypertension, colon cancer, and diabetes mellitus in particular. Physical activity also improves mental health and is important for the health of muscles, bones, and joints.
5. More than 60 percent of American adults are not regularly physically active. In fact, 25 percent of all adults are not active at all.
6. Nearly half of American youths 12–21 years of age are not vigorously active on a regular basis. Moreover, physical activity declines dramatically during adolescence.
7. Daily enrollment in physical education classes has declined among high school students from 42 percent in 1991 to 25 percent in 1995.
8. Research on understanding and promoting physical activity is at an early stage, but some interventions to promote physical activity through schools, worksites, and health care settings have been evaluated and found to be successful.

❖ Summary

The benefits of physical activity have been extolled throughout western history, but it was not until the second half of this century that scientific evidence supporting these beliefs began to accumulate. By the 1970s, enough information was available about the beneficial effects of vigorous exercise on cardiorespiratory fitness that the American College of Sports Medicine (ACSM), the American Heart Association

(AHA), and other national organizations began issuing physical activity recommendations to the public. These recommendations generally focused on cardiorespiratory endurance and specified sustained periods of vigorous physical activity involving large muscle groups and lasting at least 20 minutes on 3 or more days per week. As understanding of the benefits of less vigorous activity grew, recommendations followed suit. During the past few years, the ACSM, the CDC, the AHA, the PCPFS, and the NIH have all recommended regular, moderate-intensity physical activity as an option for those who get little or no exercise. The *Healthy People 2000* goals for the nation's health have recognized the importance of physical activity and have included physical activity goals. The 1995 *Dietary Guidelines for Americans,* the basis of the federal government's nutrition-related programs, included physical activity guidance to maintain and improve weight—30 minutes or more of moderate-intensity physical activity on all, or most, days of the week.

Underpinning such recommendations is a growing understanding of how physical activity affects physiologic function. The body responds to physical activity in ways that have important positive effects on musculoskeletal, cardiovascular, respiratory, and endocrine systems. These changes are consistent with a number of health benefits, including a reduced risk of premature mortality and reduced risks of coronary heart disease, hypertension, colon cancer, and diabetes mellitus. Regular participation in physical activity also appears to reduce depression and anxiety, improve mood, and enhance ability to perform daily tasks throughout the life span.

The risks associated with physical activity must also be considered. The most common health problems that have been associated with physical activity are musculoskeletal injuries, which can occur with excessive amounts of activity or with suddenly beginning an activity for which the body is not conditioned. Much more serious associated health problems (i.e., myocardial infarction, sudden death) are also much rarer, occurring primarily among sedentary people with advanced atherosclerotic disease who engage in strenuous activity to which they are unaccustomed. Sedentary people, especially those with preexisting health conditions, who wish to increase their physical activity should therefore gradually build up to the desired level of activity. Even among people who are regularly active, the risk of myocardial infarction or sudden death is somewhat increased during physical exertion, but their overall risk of these outcomes is lower than that among people who are sedentary.

Research on physical activity continues to evolve. This report includes both well-established findings and newer research results that await replication and amplification. Interest has been developing in ways to differentiate between the various characteristics of physical activity that improve health. It remains to be determined how the interrelated characteristics of amount, intensity, duration, frequency, type, and pattern of physical activity are related to specific health or disease outcomes.

Attention has been drawn recently to findings from three studies showing that cardiorespiratory fitness gains are similar when physical activity occurs in several short sessions (e.g., 10 minutes) as when the same total amount and intensity of activity occurs in one longer session (e.g., 30 minutes). Although, strictly speaking, the health benefits of such intermittent activity have not yet been demonstrated, it is reasonable to expect them to be similar to those of continuous activity. Moreover, for people who are unable to set aside 30 minutes for physical activity, shorter episodes are clearly better than none. Indeed, one study has shown greater adherence to a walking program among those walking several times per day than among those walking once per day, when the total amount of walking time was kept the same. Accumulating physical activity over the course of the day has been included in recent recommendations from the CDC and ACSM, as well as from the NIH Consensus Development Conference on Physical Activity and Cardiovascular Health.

Despite common knowledge that exercise is healthful, more than 60 percent of American adults are not regularly active, and 25 percent of the adult population are not active at all. Moreover, although many people have enthusiastically embarked on vigorous exercise programs at one time or another, most do not sustain their participation. Clearly, the processes of developing and maintaining healthier habits are as important to study as the health effects of these habits.

The effort to understand how to promote more active lifestyles is of great importance to the health of this nation. Although the study of physical activity determinants and interventions is at an early stage, effective programs to increase physical activity have been carried out in a variety of settings, such as schools, physicians' offices, and worksites. Determining the most effective and cost-effective intervention approaches is a challenge for the future. Fortunately, the United States has skilled leadership and institutions to support efforts to encourage and assist Americans to become more physically active. Schools, community agencies, parks, recreational facilities, and health clubs are available in most communities and can be more effectively used in these efforts.

School-based interventions for youth are particularly promising, not only for their potential scope—almost all young people between the ages of 6 and 16 years attend school—but also for their potential impact. Nearly half of young people 12–21 years of age are not vigorously active; moreover, physical activity sharply declines during adolescence. Childhood and adolescence may thus be pivotal times for preventing sedentary behavior among adults by maintaining the habit of physical activity throughout the school years. School-based interventions have been shown to be successful in increasing physical activity levels. With evidence that success in this arena is possible, every effort should be made to encourage schools to require daily physical education in each grade and to promote physical activities that can be enjoyed throughout life.

Outside the school, physical activity programs and initiatives face the challenge of a highly technological society that makes it increasingly convenient to remain sedentary and that discourages physical activity in both obvious and subtle ways. To increase physical activity in the general population, it may be necessary to go beyond traditional efforts. This report highlights some concepts from community initiatives that are being implemented around the country. It is hoped that these examples will spark new public policies and programs in other places as well. Special efforts will also be required to meet the needs of special populations, such as people with disabilities, racial and ethnic minorities, people with low income, and the elderly. Much more information about these important groups will be necessary to develop a truly comprehensive national initiative for better health through physical activity. Challenges for the future include identifying key determinants of physically active lifestyles among the diverse populations that characterize the United States (including special populations, women, and young people) and using this information to design and disseminate effective programs.

❖ Chapter Conclusions

Chapter 2: Historical Background and Evolution of Physical Activity Recommendations

1. Physical activity for better health and well-being has been an important theme throughout much of western history.
2. Public health recommendations have evolved from emphasizing vigorous activity for cardiorespiratory fitness to including the option of moderate levels of activity for numerous health benefits.
3. Recommendations from experts agree that for better health, physical activity should be performed regularly. The most recent recommendations advise people of all ages to include a minimum of 30 minutes of physical activity of moderate intensity (such as brisk walking) on most, if not all, days of the week. It is also acknowledged that for most people, greater health benefits can be obtained by engaging in physical activity of more vigorous intensity or of longer duration.
4. Experts advise previously sedentary people embarking on a physical activity program to start with short durations of moderate-intensity activity and gradually increase the duration or intensity until the goal is reached.
5. Experts advise consulting with a physician before beginning a new physical activity program for people with chronic diseases, such as cardiovascular disease and diabetes mellitus, or for those who are at high risk for these diseases. Experts also advise men over age 40 and women over age 50 to consult a physician before they begin a vigorous activity program.

6. Recent recommendations from experts also suggest that cardiorespiratory endurance activity should be supplemented with strength-developing exercises at least twice per week for adults, in order to improve musculoskeletal health, maintain independence in performing the activities of daily life, and reduce the risk of falling.

Chapter 3: Physiologic Responses and Long-Term Adaptations to Exercise

1. Physical activity has numerous beneficial physiologic effects. Most widely appreciated are its effects on the cardiovascular and musculoskeletal systems, but benefits on the functioning of metabolic, endocrine, and immune systems are also considerable.
2. Many of the beneficial effects of exercise training—from both endurance and resistance activities—diminish within 2 weeks if physical activity is substantially reduced, and effects disappear within 2 to 8 months if physical activity is not resumed.
3. People of all ages, both male and female, undergo beneficial physiologic adaptations to physical activity.

Chapter 4: The Effects of Physical Activity on Health and Disease

Overall Mortality

1. Higher levels of regular physical activity are associated with lower mortality rates for both older and younger adults.
2. Even those who are moderately active on a regular basis have lower mortality rates than those who are least active.

Cardiovascular Diseases

1. Regular physical activity or cardiorespiratory fitness decreases the risk of cardiovascular disease mortality in general and of coronary heart disease mortality in particular. Existing data are not conclusive regarding a relationship between physical activity and stroke.
2. The level of decreased risk of coronary heart disease attributable to regular physical activity is similar to that of other lifestyle factors, such as keeping free from cigarette smoking.
3. Regular physical activity prevents or delays the development of high blood pressure, and exercise reduces blood pressure in people with hypertension.

Cancer

1. Regular physical activity is associated with a decreased risk of colon cancer.

2. There is no association between physical activity and rectal cancer. Data are too sparse to draw conclusions regarding a relationship between physical activity and endometrial, ovarian, or testicular cancers.
3. Despite numerous studies on the subject, existing data are inconsistent regarding an association between physical activity and breast or prostate cancers.

Non–Insulin-Dependent Diabetes Mellitus

1. Regular physical activity lowers the risk of developing non–insulin-dependent diabetes mellitus.

Osteoarthritis

1. Regular physical activity is necessary for maintaining normal muscle strength, joint structure, and joint function. In the range recommended for health, physical activity is not associated with joint damage or development of osteoarthritis and may be beneficial for many people with arthritis.
2. Competitive athletics may be associated with the development of osteoarthritis later in life, but sports-related injuries are the likely cause.

Osteoporosis

1. Weight-bearing physical activity is essential for normal skeletal development during childhood and adolescence and for achieving and maintaining peak bone mass in young adults.
2. It is unclear whether resistance- or endurance-type physical activity can reduce the accelerated rate of bone loss in postmenopausal women in the absence of estrogen replacement therapy.

Falling

1. There is promising evidence that strength training and other forms of exercise in older adults preserve the ability to maintain independent living status and reduce the risk of falling.

Obesity

1. Low levels of activity, resulting in fewer kilocalories used than consumed, contribute to the high prevalence of obesity in the United States.
2. Physical activity may favorably affect body fat distribution.

Mental Health

1. Physical activity appears to relieve symptoms of depression and anxiety and improve mood.
2. Regular physical activity may reduce the risk of developing depression, although further research is needed on this topic.

Health-Related Quality of Life

1. Physical activity appears to improve health-related quality of life by enhancing psychological well-being and by improving physical functioning in persons compromised by poor health.

Adverse Effects

1. Most musculoskeletal injuries related to physical activity are believed to be preventable by gradually working up to a desired level of activity and by avoiding excessive amounts of activity.
2. Serious cardiovascular events can occur with physical exertion, but the net effect of regular physical activity is a lower risk of mortality from cardiovascular disease.

Chapter 5: Patterns and Trends in Physical Activity

Adults

1. Approximately 15 percent of U.S. adults engage regularly (3 times a week for at least 20 minutes) in vigorous physical activity during leisure time.
2. Approximately 22 percent of adults engage regularly (5 times a week for at least 30 minutes) in sustained physical activity of any intensity during leisure time.
3. About 25 percent of adults report no physical activity at all in their leisure time.
4. Physical inactivity is more prevalent among women than men, among blacks and Hispanics than whites, among older than younger adults, and among the less affluent than the more affluent.
5. The most popular leisure-time physical activities among adults are walking and gardening or yard work.

Adolescents and Young Adults

1. Only about one-half of U.S. young people (ages 12–21 years) regularly participate in vigorous physical activity. One-fourth report no vigorous physical activity.

2. Approximately one-fourth of young people walk or bicycle (i.e., engage in light to moderate activity) nearly every day.
3. About 14 percent of young people report no recent vigorous or light-to-moderate physical activity. This indicator of inactivity is higher among females than males and among black females than white females.
4. Males are more likely than females to participate in vigorous physical activity, strengthening activities, and walking or bicycling.
5. Participation in all types of physical activity declines strikingly as age or grade in school increases.
6. Among high school students, enrollment in physical education remained unchanged during the first half of the 1990s. However, daily attendance in physical education declined from approximately 42 percent to 25 percent.
7. The percentage of high school students who were enrolled in physical education and who reported being physically active for at least 20 minutes in physical education classes declined from approximately 81 percent to 70 percent during the first half of this decade.
8. Only 19 percent of all high school students report being physically active for 20 minutes or more in daily physical education classes.

Chapter 6: Understanding and Promoting Physical Activity

1. Consistent influences on physical activity patterns among adults and young people include confidence in one's ability to engage in regular physical activity (e.g., self-efficacy), enjoyment of physical activity, support from others, positive beliefs concerning the benefits of physical activity, and lack of perceived barriers to being physically active.
2. For adults, some interventions have been successful in increasing physical activity in communities, worksites, and health care settings, and at home.
3. Interventions targeting physical education in elementary school can substantially increase the amount of time students spend being physically active in physical education class.

❖ How Fast Do We Age?
Exercise Performance Over Time as a Biomarker

WALTER M. BORTZ IV AND WALTER M. BORTZ II

The heterogeneity of older people is well acknowledged. The dichotomization of aging into "usual" or "successful" recognizes that the population of old people contains a segment that does not exhibit the same rate of deteriorative change found in the majority (1). This recognition prompts the question as to whether the findings derived from usual and average older people include agencies above and beyond those from successful and unusual older people (2).

The frequently referenced figure first presented by Shock and colleagues in 1960 recorded declines of 15 to 90% in nine functional capacities (renal, respiratory (two), cardiac (two), metabolic (two); nerve conduction velocity, and cell water) from age 35 to age 90 (3). Later analyses, however, have shown that much of the data from which the above figure was derived were contaminated by changes that were due to disease or disuse and not aging. Lindeman et al. (4), for example, reported that one-third of older people exhibited no diminution in renal function with age. Similarly, Lakatta (5) has shown that much of the previously believed decrease in cardiovascular function with age is due instead to the disuse of physical inactivity. Fiatarone et al. (6) have reversed the supposed age-dependent loss in muscle size and strength in a group of nonagenarians by a weight-lifting protocol. The density of brain dendritic branching is dependent also on the principle of active use (7).

It is with the advantage of hindsight that the supposed time-dependent declines in function with age are shown not to be so steep as originally thought. In order to tease out true biomarkers for aging, a study cohort free of the artifacts of disease and disuse is desired. The Masters athlete emerges as the person who best represents this ideal. Older athletes until recently were considered to be oddities, but the increased participation of persons over 50 years of age (nearly 5000 ran the 1994 New York Marathon), even into their nineties, provides a data source of rich opportunity.

Athletic endeavor involves most of the major body systems. By observing the rate of change of records with age, it is proposed that no subtending cellular organ or system function can deteriorate at a rate faster than the exercise performance, or that function would become rate-limiting. Athletic records thereby constitute a possible biomarker of aging.

❖ Methods

Running data were provided by the Masters Track and Field Organization for the 100-yard dash and the marathon (8). Swimming data for the 1500-meter swim were obtained from the U.S. Masters Swimming Congress (9). Inasmuch as open-water rowing events do not lend themselves to composite records, the rowing data for the 2500-meter row were derived from records established on a rowing machine, Concept II. This effort draws tens of thousands of participants of all ages (10).

Because participation and records in these events depend on large numbers, only data derived from males are presented. The age of 35 is selected as the reference age because the Masters Track and Field records commence at this age. The performance at age 35 is taken to represent 100% for all events, and the subsequent age performances are conformed to this age. These athletic data are cross-sectional in character. Although longitudinal records are preferred, few are available and those which are, are distorted by differences in training intensity, possible cohort differences, and other factors over the life span. Data for $\dot{V}O_2$ max are longitudinal, however, as are those of Kasch et al. (11). Their measurements were obtained using both treadmill and bicycle ergometer loads, and were conducted at roughly 5-year intervals over the testing period.

Age and athletic performance records may be criticized as having been derived from an elite subset of people, as indeed they are. But it is argued that whereas the records represent specific performance levels, it is not the absolute levels that are of interest to this report, but instead the rate of their change. It seems likely that the background rate of age change would be similar in athletes, and that the calculation is thereby appropriate to non-athletes as well, albeit at a lower level.

❖ Results

Figure 1 displays the age records for three endurance athletic events, the 100-meter dash, and the declines in $\dot{V}O_2$ max over time. At age 60 the average decline in performance of the four activities was 12.9%, or roughly one half percent per year over the 25 years. The strikingly similar slopes of these events and physiologic functions from ages 35 to 65 are apparent. After the age of 65 it is evident that the linearity of decline of approximately 0.5% per year accelerates. It is uncertain how much of this more rapid decline is the result of true physiologic decay, and how much is due to lessened participation (12). The predominance of the latter function is suggested by the generalized observation of regular lowering of the records at the upper ages, and the stability of the records at lower ages.

Whitten (13) calculated an 11% fall in swimming dash times from ages 35 to 65 (0.3% per year). Notable too is the fact that for both the running and swimming events, the dashes show slower declines than the longer distances at upper ages (8). The field event performances (e.g., shotput, high jump) decline at faster rates than the running events (8), indicating the possibility that power-requiring activities have a faster decay than aerobic activities.

Whereas a number of studies purport to represent the relationship between age and $\dot{V}O_2$ max, nearly all are cross-sectional in nature (14,15). Early reports such as that of Dil et al. (16) recorded data from individuals who were athletes and subsequently were retested years later. However, it is clear that the intensity of training was not sustained. In only one case was there a fall of only 0.5% per year, similar to the observation of Kasch et al. (11), whose work represents fit and unfit individuals followed longitudinally over several decades. This report followed 15 trained individuals from age 44 to 68 and 15 untrained from 51 to 69. Rogers et al. (17) reported an annual .54% fall in $\dot{V}O_2$ max from ages 62 to 70 in their group of Masters athletes, which is similar to the .56% figure of Kasch et al. (11). Health et al. (18) have also concluded that 0.5% per year is the rate of decline in $\dot{V}O_2$ max in fit individuals.

❖ Discussion

Study of the biology of life span has until recently lacked rigor. The infinite complexities found in older persons rendered analysis difficult and conclusions imprecise. Usual and successful aging were inadvertently admixed so that any attempt to perceive orderly process was impossible.

From the cellular to the whole body level of organization, biomarkers for aging have been difficult to establish. $\dot{V}O_2$ max has been nominated as being one of the most useful parameters to assess biologic age (19). This function is critical insofar as it represents an expression of how the organism extracts oxygen from the environment at work. It represents a global measure, not only of basal circulatory, respiratory, thermoregulatory, metabolic, musculoskeletal, and neurologic functions, but those under an exercise load. Numerous workers have reported that $\dot{V}O_2$ max is highly dependent on physical conditioning. The data of Kasch et al., presented in Figure 1, are consistent with many others (14–18). Kasch et al. (11) concluded that two-thirds of the decline in $\dot{V}O_2$ max with age noted in untrained persons is due to disuse, and only one-third (0.5% per year) is due to age per se.

The close coincidence of the $\dot{V}O_2$ max data to the decline in several diverse athletic events from ages 35 to 70 gives support to the proposition that 0.5% per year represents a key biomarker for the aging process. This assertion derives more support from analysis of a broad range of age changes reported from the cellular to the whole body hierarchical levels and includes structural and functional age findings. At the cellular level, division of human skin fibroblasts decreases at the rate of 0.5% per year (20), as does the length of their telomeres (21). DNA repair is reported as decreasing at the rate of 0.6% per year (22). Cerebral metabolism (23) has likewise been calculated to decrease at 0.6% per year. Maximum pulse rate (24) and rate of nail growth (25) decrease 0.5% per year. Numbers of muscle

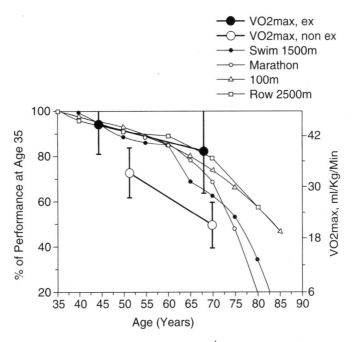

Figure 1 Change in exercise performance and $\dot{V}O_2$ max over time.

cells in the thigh (26) and appendicular bone calcium decrease at 0.5% per year (27). Notable, however, is the rate of loss of calcium from the axial skeleton, which can be several times this rate, similar to the observation of $\dot{V}O_2$ max, again sensitive to the effects of physical conditioning. The rate of loss of irregularity of the pulse rate decreases at 0.5% per year (28). Flow medicated dilation of arteries has been shown to decrease at .49% per year in women, and .21% per year in men (29).

The 0.5% per year figure closely approximates declines in cognitive competence reported by Schaie (30).

The coherence of the rates of change with age of a wide variety of physical and functional parameters suggests that 0.5% per year may represent a common biomarker for age. This value is lower than many earlier proposed, and if true has important implications to the delineation of usual from successful aging. It is assumed that maximal biologic function exists at the end of the maturation growth phase (± age 30) and that age exerts its deteriorative effects from that moment on at the rate of 0.5% per year. At this rate, after 60 years (age 90) only 30% of maximal function will have been lost. On the other hand, if function is lost at the rate of 2% per year after 35 years (age 65), 70% of maximal vitality will have been lost and the frailty barrier of 30% of maximal function reached (31). It is unknown whether changes due to age alone would remain linear at higher ages.

Gavrilov and Gavrilova (32) suggest the likelihood of a cascade effect in which the rate of catabolic change would increase, possibly reflected in the decreased athletic performance seen at the higher ages in this study.

It is significant to note that the differences between the proposed rate of age changes of successful (0.5% per year) and usual (2% per year) are so small over a short time that the observance of the effect of intervention efforts may be small as well. Yet, when the 1.5% per year difference is multiplied by several decades, the difference becomes profound.

Acknowledgments

We acknowledge the review of the manuscript by Drs. Leonard Hayflick and F. Eugene Yates, and the statistical assistance of Dr. Byron Brown.

❖ About the Author

Walter M. Bortz, IV, M.D., is in the Department of Medicine, University of North Carolina Medical Center, Chapel, Hill, North Carolina

Walter M. Bortz, II, M.D., is at the Palo Alto Medical Foundation, Internal Medicine Department, Palo Alto, California.

REFERENCES

1. Rowe JW, Kahn RL. Human aging: usual and successful. Science 1987; 243:143–9.
2. Bortz W. Redefining human aging. J Am Geriatr Soc 1989;37:1092–6.
3. Shock NW. Mortality and measurement of aging. In: Strehler B, Ebert J, Glass H, Shock NW, eds. The biology of aging. Washington, DC: American Institute of Biological Sciences, 1960.
4. Lindemann R, Tobin J, Shock N. Longitudinal studies and the rate of decline in renal function with age. J Am Geriatr Soc 1985;33:278–85.
5. Lakatta E. Alterations in the cardiovascular system that occur in advanced age. Fed Proc 1979;38: 163–7.
6. Fiatarone M, Marx E, Ryan N, et al. High intensity strength training in nonagenarians: effects on skeletal muscle. JAMA 1990;263:3029–39.
7. Jacobs B, Schall M, Scheibel AB. A quantitative dendritic analysis of Wernicke's area in humans. II. Gender, hemispheric and environmental factors. J Comp Neurol 1993;327:97–111.
8. Masters Age Records 1991. Compiled by Peter Mundle, Venice, CA, 1992.
9. Masters Swimming Records 1992. Compiled by Walter Reed, Tacoma, WA.
10. Ergo Update Publication of Concept II, Rowing Records. Morrisville, VT, 1992.
11. Kasch FW, Boyer JL, van Camp SP, Verity LS, Wallace SP. The effect of physical activity and inactivity on aerobic power in older

men (a longitudinal study). J Physician Sports Med 1990;18:73–83.

12. Fair RC. How fast do old men slow down? Working paper 3757. Cambridge, MA: National Bureau of Economic Research, 1991.

13. Whitten P. Just how much do we decline with age? Swim 1992;July–Aug: 17–20.

14. Dehn MM, Bruce RA. Longitudinal variation in max oxygen intake with age and activity. J Appl Physiol 1972;33:805–7.

15. Pollock ML, Foster C, Knapp D, Rod JL, Schmidt DH. Effect of age and training on aerobic capacity and body composition of masters athletes. J Appl Physiol 1987;62:725–31.

16. Dil DB, Robinson S, Ross JC. A longitudinal study of 16 champion runners. J Sports Med Phys Fitness 1967;7:4–27.

17. Rogers MA, Hagberg J, Martin SH, Eksani AA, Holloszy JO. Decline in VO$_2$ max with aging in masters athletes and sedentary men. J Appl Physiol 1990;68:2195–9.

18. Heath G, Hagberg J, Ehsani AA, Holloszy JO. Physical comparison of young and old endurance athletes. J Appl Physiol 1981;51:634–40.

19. Dean W. Biologic aging measurement: its rationale, history, and current status. In: Balin AK, ed. Human biologic age determination. Boca Raton, FL: CRC Press, 1994:9.

20. Martin G, Sprague C, Epstein J. Replication of life span of cultivated human cells: effect of donor's age, tissue and genotype. Lab Invest 1970;23:86–92.

21. Hardy C, Futcher A, Greider C. Telomeres shorten during aging of human fibroblasts. Nature 1990;345:458–60.

22. Wei Q, Matanoski GM, Farmer ER, Hedayato MA, Grossman L. DNA repair and aging in basal cell carcinoma: a molecular epidemiologic study. Proc Natl Acad Sci USA 1993;90:1614–18.

23. Marchal G, Rioux P, Petit-Tabove M, et al. Regional cerebral oxygen consumption. Blood flow, blood volume. Health, Human Aging Arch Neurol 1992;49:1013–20.

24. Fox S. Haskell W. The detection of coronary heart disease as a challenge to the work physiologist. In: Proceedings of Research Conference in Applied Physiology. Buffalo, NY. 1968:283–306.

25. Orentreich N, Markovskyi J, Vogelmer J. The effect of aging on the rate of linear nail growth. J Invest Derm 1979;73:126–30.

26. Lexell J, Henriksson-Larsen K, Wimblad B, Sjostron M. Distribution of different fiber types in human skeletal muscle. Effect of aging studied in whole muscle cross sections. Muscle Nerve 1983;6:588–95.

27. Riggs BL, Wahner W, Dumas FM, et al. Differential changes in bone mineral density of the appendicular and axial skeleton with aging. J Clin Endocrinol 1981;67:328–35.

28. Ryan S, Goldberger A, Pincus S, Mietus J, Lipsitz L. Gender and age related differences in heart rate dynamics: are women more complex than men? J Am Coll Cardiol 1994;24:1700–7.

29. Celerunger D. Aging is associated with endothelial dysfunction in healthy men years before the age-related decline in women. J Am Coll Cardiol 1994;24:471–6.

30. Schaie KW. The course of adult intellectual development. Am Psychol 1994;49:304–19.

31. Kerlan R. Health and fitness through physical activity. In: Pollock M, Wilmore J, Fox S, eds. Health and fitness through physical activity. New York: John Wiley, 1978:22.

32. Gavrilov L, Gavrilova N. The biology of life span. Chur, Switzerland: Harwood, 1991.

❖ International Aspects of the AIDS/HIV Epidemic

ANN MARIE KIMBALL, SETH BERKLEY,
ELIZABETH NGUGI, AND HELENE GAYLE

❖ The Importance of AIDS

The importance of AIDS is, in part, due to the societal effect of the prolonged course of the illness affecting young adults, and the eventual complete fatal outcome of the disease. Only now is the international development community becoming cognizant of the social, political, and economic impacts of AIDS worldwide. The World Health Organization has projected that over 13 million people are now infected and that 18 million people will succumb to clinical AIDS by the year 2000 (83). More than two million people have died thus far. Other authors characterize these estimates as too conservative (45). Moreover, the world population (estimated at 5.3 billion at the time of this writing) is not uniformly infected. Thus, as discussed below, some regions and certain population groups will be much more adversely affected by morbidity and mortality from AIDS. Nonetheless, the economic costs, estimated to reach $350 billion by the year 2000 (4), will be felt worldwide. This figure approximates the current gross national product of Australia.

The international policy dialogue has begun to reflect an understanding of the profundity of the challenge still before us, particularly as issues of equity are highlighted in vaccine development efforts (32). The coordination of multiple UN agency programs into a single effort is aimed at broadening and strengthening the international response (72) through a new joint cosponsored program. Nonetheless, intractable global economic and political questions remain: Are international strategies beyond promotion and advocacy needed to insure timely protective action by individual governments? What is the most appropriate form of international relief for those countries hardest hit by the pandemic? How will this relief be financed? How should counterproductive and ethically unacceptable strategies (e.g. quarantine of the HIV positive and restrictions on the travel and employment of infected persons) be met by the international public health community? We aim to provide a framework for this broad, ongoing dialogue.

❖ The Transmission of HIV

It is now thought that the late 1970s were the apparent starting point of intense HIV spread (1). The initiation of HIV spread appears to have occurred simultaneously in at least two distinct geographic areas—Central Africa and the United States/Caribbean, but was not heralded until 1982 when the first cluster of clinical illness was reported in the medical literature (11a). In retrospect, endemic African disease patterns had clearly been shifting for some time during the 1980s, possibly in response to the incursion of HIV and resultant immunocompromise. For example, cryptococcal meningitis in tropical areas increased, with changing ecology of the agent (ref. 6a). The advent of more sophisticated diagnostic techniques revealed that sporadic cases of clinical AIDS occurred in North America and Africa prior to the reported cluster (27).

In the mid-1980s, WHO scientists classified regions into three patterns of epidemic spread of HIV in an attempt to clarify the distinct regional modes of HIV transmissions. However, it has subsequently become apparent that such classification represents a "snapshot" of an epidemiologic global phenomenon that is characterized more by continual change than by its ability to be classified.

The mechanisms of HIV transmission are limited: sexual intercourse; exposure to contaminated blood products or body fluids, including the use of unclean needles for injection; vertical transmission from an infected mother to her child prior to or at delivery; and transmission from an infected mother to her child through breast-feeding. Estimates of the efficiency for each route vary from about 0.1% per sexual contact to over 90% for blood-borne transmission via transfusion. However, wide regional variations occur—for reasons that remain unclear. For example, recent research in Thailand suggests there is a much higher risk of 3–6% per homosexual contact compared with the estimate of 0.1% for North America (47). However, these findings have been recently questioned (20a). To calm fears of contagion, it has been as important to define the routes of nontransmission as to define the routes of transmission. Casual transmission is very rare even in settings of substandard hygiene and of direct nursing of the sick. Nor has transmission by mosquitoes been demonstrated (43). Malaria itself, rather than its vector, has contributed to HIV transmission through the anemia it causes. Transfusion of children with malaria promotes HIV transmission if blood screening for HIV is not available (34) and HIV is prevalent.

Insight gained through behavioral research and the application of microbiological tools indicates that the transmission dynamics of this global academic are more complex than initially suspected. Our understanding of the nature of different strains of HIV and their apparent segregation by certain transmission routes continues to evolve.

Heterosexual transmission accounts for an estimated 70–80% of global transmission of HIV. Nonetheless, other routes also figure prominently in the global picture because of their social repercussions. Infected mother-to-infant transmission of the virus is increasing worldwide. However, not all children born from infected mothers are infected. This rate of vertical transmission is estimated to be 25–50% in lesser developed countries (Table 2) compared with 20–30% in developed countries. Maternal-to-infant

TABLE 2   Rates of Maternal/Infant Transmission

Collected African Studies		
Location	% Transmission	Reference
Klasbasa, Zaire	39	63a
Lusaka, Zambia	39	30a
Brazzaville, Congo	32	41a
Kigall, Rwanda	25.7	42a

transmission can occur preparation, and HIV has been found in fetuses aborted in the first trimester of pregnancy (59). Transmission definitely occurs during delivery; contrary to previous findings, a recent study of mode of delivery suggested caesarean section may decrease transmission by up to 50% (22a, 76), but these studies await confirmation.

The risk of transmission from mother to infant through breast-feeding is a difficult issue internationally. During the late 1970s, it was demonstrated that bottle-feeding clearly placed infants at increased risk of diarrheal disease mortality, especially during periods of epidemic diarrheal disease (28). In response, the World Health Organization, UNICEF, and other agencies recommended and actively promoted breast-feeding in the developing world as a means of improving child survival. The first definitive report of transmission of HIV through breast-feeding was published in 1985 (92). Subsequent studies have shown high rates of infant HIV infections through breast-milk transmission when the mother seroconverts during the breast-feeding period. A prospective study in Kigali of 212 mothers seronegative at delivery identified nine maternal seroconversions, of which five (56%) resulted in infant seroconversion via breast-milk transmission (75). In a recent review, Dunn et al estimated that additional risk of maternal-to-infant transmission from breast-feeding (above and beyond that measured in delivery) to be 14% (21). Based on such data, the policy recommendation in favor of breast-feeding has been repeatedly re-examined (35). Latin American countries are adopting guidance similar to that of the United States and the United Kingdom, which do not promote breast-feeding when the mother is infected with HIV. Universal recommendation of breast-feeding remains in countries where access to clean water and hygiene are problematic.

The role that infected blood plays in the spread of HIV worldwide varies by region. In Latin America, blood screening is virtually complete, whereas in Africa estimates of screened transfusions do not exceed 50%. In Africa the attributable risk of unscreened blood is thought to be small (less than 10% overall); nonetheless, this is a preventable route of transmission that contributes to transmission (10). Before the implementation of blood screening in 1985, large numbers of infections were transmitted by transfusions, particularly to infants where one donor could infect multiple patients. (Other methods besides screening have been employed to reduce the risk of transmission through blood transfusion. These include decreasing the use of transfusions through early treatment of predisposing conditions, thereby eliminating unnecessary use of transfusion, and obtaining blood from low-risk donors.

Shared use of needles for recreational drug use is a major route of transmission. The use of injections for treatment worldwide is routine both in traditional and modern practice, and the reuse of needles is common in resource-poor settings because of limited supply and the absence of sterile technique. Concern that contaminated needles used in health care settings may play a major role in HIV transmission has not been borne out by research. A careful review of the limited data on parenteral transmission of HIV from epidemiologic studies and age-specific HIV infection rates suggests that, even if occasional transmission of HIV does occur, such injections are not a major route of transmission (5), with the possible exception of the Romanian epidemic among institionalized children (90a). Certainly the link has been demonstrated between vaccination programs in Africa or Latin America and HIV transmission, probably due to the strong emphasis during training of medical personnel regarding the supply and use of sterile needles.

❖ The AIDS Pandemic: A Series of Regional Epidemics

AIDS in Africa

At the same time that the first cases of AIDS were being identified in homosexual populations in the United States and Europe, cases of a wasting illness with a high mortality and an unknown etiology were occurring in villages in Central Africa (58, 66, 74). Physical examination, including routine examination of the oral cavity, plays a major role in diagnosing diseases in these communities. The occurrence of oro-pharyngeal candidiasis together with the occurrence of wasting disease in adults portended the appearance of a new disease for the region and was noted by clinicians in the early 1980s. The advent of HIV testing in 1985 enabled Eastern and Central African countries such as Rwanda, Tanzania, Uganda, and Zaire to confirm HIV and relate this illness to the newly described disease of AIDS in the United States and Europe.

Coincidentally, virology researchers in Senegal identified a similar virus, which was not initially associated with disease. This agent, now known as HIV2, was originally thought by some in the West African scientific community to be protective against HIV1, since HIV2 was present and HIV1 was not apparent in the mid-1980s in West Africa. Subsequent studies have demonstrated that HIV2 is pathogenic, and causes AIDS. Some studies suggest that the severity of HIV2 disease may be somewhat less than HIV1 disease (18).

These discoveries focused international attention on AIDS in Africa. Serologic testing using the early generation of tests led to excessive and inaccurate estimates of infection as a result of cross-reactivity with serum that had high concentrations of nonspecific antibodies from exposure to other infectious agents (65). As a result, Africa was unfairly identified as the origin of HIV infection worldwide. The results from these serologic surveys, later retracted, damaged international confidence in predictions of the epidemic. This mistrust may have facilitated denial once the true magnitude of infection became clear. Behaviors associated with transmission in the West, such as homosexuality, use of intravenous drugs, and anal intercourse, were absent in the vast majority of AIDS cases in Africa. Studies demonstrated a male-to-female ratio of close to 1:1—very different from the overwhelmingly male presentation seen at that time in North America and Europe. Subsequent studies in areas where the epidemic is long-standing, like Uganda and Tanzania, have shown infection rates to be higher in women than in men (2, 6). In addition, females are infected at a younger age than males—on average 5 years—in virtually all African populations studied, a finding also seen among populations in the Caribbean and South America.

The epidemic has clearly spread much more widely in the heterosexual population in Africa than in North America or Europe. Careful studies have suggested that the transmission cannot be explained solely by more sexual exposure but rather that the actual efficiency of transmission appears to be higher. This hypothesis has led to a search for risk factors that could explain a higher risk of transmission. Studies in Africa have shown other sexually transmitted infectious diseases (STDs) (both ulcerative and nonulcerative), male noncircumcision, and young age among females to increase the risk of transmission. Some studies have also shown sex during menses, use of intravaginal preparations, and oral contraceptives to be risk factors. These effects are not consistent across studies. Female circumcision, although biologically plausible as a risk factor, is not common in the areas with the highest rate of transmission and probably contributes little to attributable risk.

The initial report of an almost exclusively urban location of HIV has been misleading.

The spread of AIDS is devastating to individuals, families, communities, and countries. AIDS has a powerful effect beyond the actual numbers of infected and dying. It affects people during their economically most productive adult years when they are typically responsible for the support and care of others. The chronic nature of the illness and its high cost of treatment magnify its societal impact. In addition, because of its sexual spread there is clustering among certain households, with both the husband and wife—or wives, in a polygamous family—commonly infected. Simulations by the World Bank indicate an annual slowing of growth of income per capita by an average of 0.6 percentage point per country in the 10 worst affected countries in sub-Saharan Africa (87).

AIDS in the Western Hemisphere

In the Caribbean, the first reports of clinical AIDS in 1983 indicated that the initiation of infection in the United States and the Caribbean was temporally closely related. The earliest group at risk in the Caribbean, as in the United States, consisted of gay and bisexual men. In fact, reports of illness were confined to this group until 1985, when a transition to more heterosexual transmission began. As in the United States, the advent of HIV seroprevalence testing in the mid-1980s confirmed a high seroprevalence among gay and bisexual males, but also demonstrated a rapid rise among other high-risk groups such as commercial sex workers and intravenous drug users.

For reasons that are not completely understood, the transition to a heterosexual pattern of disease was extremely rapid in the Caribbean in the mid-1980s. This shift has been discussed in relation to a variety of factors: Bisexuality is more common than an exclusively homosexual orientation; populations are more proximate and urbanized in port city settings; there are high levels of endemic sexually transmitted disease; the characteristics of the HIV strains that were introduced; and the background of other retroviruses that predated HIV in this population (3).

Synergistic linkage with sexually transmitted diseases (78) is one plausible mechanism behind the shift in risk to heterosexual populations, given the high rates of sexually transmitted diseases in the Caribbean. Biases for these data include the increased ascertainment that occurs in these island settings with relatively small, accessible populations. The rates of gonorrhea are threefold, for syphilis twofold, and for chancroid 15-fold higher in the Caribbean than in Latin America. In addition, an epidemic of crack cocaine in the Bahamas was shown to be closely related temporally to an epidemic of genital ulcer disease and a marked increase in HIV seroprevalence (26). These kinds of interactions among STDs are well-known contributors to infectivity and severity of HIV/AIDS (77).

The other countries in Central and South America have remained less affected by the pandemic than either the U.S. or the Caribbean. In general, rates of disease in Central America and in urban centers on the eastern coast of South America are two- to fourfold higher than those found elsewhere on the continent. In all areas, the annual incidence rates for clinical AIDS have been climbing year to year since reporting started in 1988. Within countries active commercial urban centers generally are foci of AIDS.

The transition to heterosexual transmission with increasing cases among women is seen in surveillance data from South America as well as the Caribbean. Two groups—bisexual males and intravenous drug users—are thought to serve as "bridge" groups in the generalization of transmission. The community of gay and bisexual men most affected in Latin America is difficult both to research and to reach with public health interventions because of social stigmatization. Recent studies in Mexico suggest that the risk of infection in partner pools is a stronger predictor of individual risk in that group than individual behavior (33), but research in gay populations is too limited to confirm this observation.

Seroprevalence rates among intravenous drug users in urban centers in Brazil and Argentina are similar to those of the eastern seaboard in the United States (38). As early as 1989, seroprevalences between 20% and 62% were reported in a series of surveys of intravenous drug injectors carried out in Buenos Aires, as well as 29% in Mexico City and 73% in Santos City, Brazil. Selection biases make international comparisons difficult. Because intravenous drug users in Latin America are socially stigmatized, with limited treatment available for their addiction, they are only identified late in their course. Thus studies of seroprevalence may reflect a heavier exposure to HIV through nonsterile needle use over a longer period of time than for North American users, who are often tested in the setting of drug-treatment centers. Nonetheless, the high infection rates seen in intravenous drug injectors in Latin America represent an important target group for prevention strategies. No recent studies have been published on this high-risk group.

The dramatic increase in HIV transmission to women in Central America is facilitated by their subservient social role. Perhaps the major risk factor for women is conduct by her sexual partner—conduct that she is not in a position to question, given the prevailing social norms. For example, a study in Costa Rica found the typical woman with AIDS was a housewife who reported no knowledge of any risk factors that may have caused her infection (30). This suggests that these women may have been unaware because the risky conduct was actually that of the husband.

The relationship between cervical pathology and HIV transmission merits study in this setting. Women in Latin America and the Caribbean have high rates of cervical disease including cervical cancer. The mortality rates from cervical cancer are between 1.6 and 6.1 times higher than in Canada, Cuba, and the United States. These data reflect a stagnation of services to women.

HIV transmission to women in Latin America was intensified by the earlier lack of blood screening. Mexico, as of 1991, attributed 63% of cumulative cases of AIDS in women to blood transfusion, whereas this route was cited for only 6% of men. The risk to women is higher because of the higher incidence of transfusion at childbirth. Blood screening has been shown to be an effective strategy for reducing risk of HIV in women in Latin America (41). Systematic blood screening has been a cornerstone of most national programs in the region. Private blood banks, such as those operating in some Andean countries, have been more difficult to regulate than those in the public sector.

An alarming result of the shift of the epidemic to women is the consequent increase in perinatal transmission around the region. Increasing numbers of such cases are being reported, although the absolute numbers remain small. Studies from Brazil suggest that a high proportion of transmission is related to intravenous drug use by the mother or her partner (30, 44).

Prevention strategies for women in Latin America will be enhanced when barrier or virucidal methods under the control of women themselves are available (40). Social norms make disclosure of previous risk behavior by men to their female partners unlikely, and the ability of women to negotiate regular condom use even less likely. In this setting, the need for new research on HIV prevention that works for women is compelling.

❖ Newer Epidemics

Asia and the Pacific

The history of the HIV / AIDS epidemic in the world cannot yet be written. The epidemic is continuing to advance, with the most dramatic recent growth occurring in Asia. Two major routes of transmission, intravenous drug use and sexual intercourse, have combined to create rapid increases in transmission in that region. Two countries, Burma and Thailand, are instructive as examples of this new epidemic; the US Census bureau has recently published a detailed discussion (80). Data from Burma suggest that the rate of infection in some groups of intravenous drug users increased from 17% in 1989 to 76% in 1991. Data for women at high risk (commercial sex workers) indicate recent seroprevalence has reached 11%.

Thailand put into place an extensive surveillance system for seroprevalence studies that has facilitated meticulous tracking of the epidemic. Incursion of the virus was seen first among intravenous drug users, gay males, and commercial sex workers in the Northern and Central regions of the country. Coincident surveillance documented a near doubling of infection in urban STD clinic attendees throughout the country between 1990 and 1993, with the highest level seen in the North, and 8% seroprevalence in 1992 among military recruits in the North. The prevalence among low-charge female commercial sex workers has increased steadily from 3% in 1989 to 29% in 1993 (5a).

There is continued paucity of surveillance information about high-risk groups from the rest of Asia. Serosurveillance among intravenous drug injectors reveals a high incidence of infection in China (15%) (91) and Malaysia (30%) (67), but not among injectors tested in Hong Kong (86). Other countries apparently are not reporting on seroprevalence in this high-risk group. Commercial sex workers in Bombay, India, are heavily infected, but information about other countries is lacking. Given the explosive rise in infection seen in these groups in Africa, the Caribbean, and Latin America, additional studies in the newer epidemic areas of Asia and Oceania are needed.

If seroprevalence is as low as the limited available information suggests, there is still opportunity for timely prevention campaigns. Singapore has mounted a particularly active educational campaign (67), conducted under the close collaboration of government and nongovernmental sectors. Thailand has documented success with its "100% condom" campaign among prostitutes. Operations research in South China has demonstrated the potential efficacy of harm-reduction strategies using bleach for needles (89). Such efforts represent a hopeful start.

The World Health Organization estimates that the implementation of effective prevention in Asia could dampen the rate of transmission, with more than 2 million infections prevented by the year 2000.

In Asia, the early development of a broad response to the epidemic, not limited to the health sector, is encouraging. Increasingly, the HIV/AIDS issue is being successfully incorporated into the policy agenda of development, trade, and commerce. The US/Japan Agreement for Cooperation for Economic Development includes AIDS cooperation in the Asia Pacific region as a point for the agenda (73). Both of these major economies have pledged several billion dollars in support of AIDS prevention. Business councils have been formed in the Asian capitals of Kuala Lumpur, Hong Kong, Taipei, Bangkok, and Djakarta to address the threat of AIDS. The 10th International Conference on AIDS in Yokohama, Japan, included satellite sessions on business and AIDS in the Asia Pacific region, including the founding of an intersectoral network of corporations and public health organizations (Asia Pacific Alliance Against AIDS). The costs of HIV/AIDS to business have been detailed (23). Business interests are central to the economic development of the Asia Pacific region, so the costs of an uncontrolled epidemic in this region may further spur prevention activity.

❖ Information Systems/Case Reporting

Reporting completeness varies widely around the globe. Routine disease-reporting systems in most African countries are extremely limited. Estimates suggest that only 10–30% of actual AIDS cases are being reported. In Latin America and the Caribbean, it is estimated that between 30% and 50% of cases are reported. To monitor the spread of infection, WHO has piloted a number of sentinel reporting systems to follow infection rates over time in selected populations.

Differences in the presentation of the disease in Africa and the lack of sophisticated diagnostic facilities have made the use of the standard CDC/WHO case definition for AIDS problematic. In 1985 the World Health Organization convened a meeting in Bangui, Central African Republic, to develop a simple case definition for use in Africa (82). The Pan American Health Organization (PAHO) convened a similar meeting in Caracas, Venezuela, to tailor the definition of AIDS to regional diagnostic capabilities. The Bangui definition requires no laboratory or pathologic testing to establish the diagnosis, whereas that developed in Venezuela includes HIV testing. The Bangui definition is moderately specific (92%), but is not sensitive (52%) (85). The clinical diagnosis of pediatric cases of AIDS in international settings presents even more of a problem. A companion to the Bangui definition for children has a sensitivity of 35% and a specificity of 87%, modifications have not led to substantial improvements (16). It is hoped that a new generation of tests will improve the ability at least to diagnose infection in infants.

❖ Theories of Emergence: A Continuing Search

The emergence of HIV as a major human pathogen is an area of ongoing investigation. The close timing of the apparent initiation of transmission in Africa and the New World—two geographically remote sites—continues to provoke theories of origin, which are published both in the lay press and the scientific literature. Improving genetic techniques indicate that the HIV2 virus is close genetically to simian retroviruses. However, HIV1 is "centuries away" from SIV in genetic terms. The disparate sites of its first occurrence and additional genetic detailing through microepidemiologic techniques still leave questions about how this major pandemic started. Some level of man-made facilitation through the imperfect incubation of unrelated vaccines in monkey cells has been posited by some authors, but convincingly refuted by others (22). Recent modeling of genetic variation suggests that the rate of "escape mutant" production of HIV strains is higher than previously believed. This high degree of genetic variability may have figured in its emergence as a major pathogen.

HIV has been present in Africa for decades. The earliest documented infection with HIV in Africa was from a serum sample from Equateur Province in Northern Zaire from 1976. HIV was isolated from serum collected and frozen during a serosurvey investigation of the epidemic of Ebola fever in 1976. Another study of stored serum from Africa detected antibodies reactive to HIV by ELISA and Western blot from a frozen serum from Kinshasa from 1959 (51). However, virus isolation was never attempted.

The HIV pandemic can be seen as a sentinel event in the history of global disease. Given the increasing international linkages between communities through travel, trade, and migration, the emergence of new infectious diseases such as AIDS will become more frequent (42). Thus, gaining as much insight into the factors that brought the HIV pandemic to its current level of devastation will be central to our ability to cope with future pandemics.

❖ The International Response

Prevention Challenges

Prevention remains the only effective way to protect individuals, families, and communities from HIV transmission, and the eventual sequelae of AIDS. Despite a decade of research, cures and preventive vaccines remain elusive, and will remain so for resource-poor settings for the foreseeable future. Initial efforts at prevention in Africa were hampered by (a) unavoidably tardy initiation relative to the timing of transmission, (b) the "vertical" nature of the effort and its heavy reliance on external expertise, (c) the difficulty in defining culturally acceptable and appropriate interventions, and (d) the lack of cheap diagnostic testing or infrastructure for testing. As a result, current levels of infection are highest in Africa, and still rising, and the ongoing challenges to prevention continue to be very serious.

Despite its relative inefficiency, transmission of HIV through sexual intercourse is by far the most prevalent transmission worldwide. Most communities maintain a culture of silence about sexuality, and sexual practices that may increase the risk of HIV have been difficult to identify and are often culturally based (57). There is a general suspicion of the introduction of sexual education in schools, despite studies demonstrating the efficacy of this approach in delaying the initiation of sexual activity (90) and in promoting sexual responsibility, as evidenced by the use of contraceptives (64).

Accurate information is often particularly deficient for teenagers. For example, one schoolgirl in Kenya reported a classmate attempting to persuade her that her womb would burst in later pregnancy if she were not "cleansed" through sexual intercourse in girlhood (EN Ngugi, personal observation). Thus the provision of accurate and comprehensible information is, appropriately, a centerpiece of educational efforts to prevent AIDS around the world.

In the Americas, frank educational campaigns directed at young adults have been equally difficult to mount. School-based information campaigns have been successfully put in place in some countries, such as Bahamas.

Gender inequality is an obstacle to AIDS prevention internationally, as is generally true in political, economic, and social development. In Africa, the Caribbean, and Latin America (39), cases of AIDS occur earlier in life in women than in men. This difference, labeled the "demographic imperative" for enhancing prevention in women, has been ascribed to (a) male preference for younger partners less likely to already be infected, (b) the relative disfranchisement of young women in poor societies that makes them economically dependent on older men for survival, (c) traditional marriage practices which foster child marriage and emphasize fertility, and (d) physiologic increased risk of receptive sex especially with the presence of juvenile cervical ectopy. It has been documented that women have a relatively higher risk than men per sexual encounter with an infected partner.

International prevention efforts are grappling with the need to address issues specific to women. Abstinence, reduction of sexual partners, and condom use are the three behavioral changes that have been associated with reduced HIV transmission. As seen in the discussion of the Latin American epidemic, participation in these strategies by women is not straightforward because of their position in their society. Some educational strategies can help some women, for example the increasing emphasis on client education in prevention programs for commercial sex workers. Female-based barrier or virucidal methods will be necessary additions if prevention is to be effective (68).

For the near future, the continuing social disparity of the sexes will continue to hamper effective prevention. Studies in Kenya show that economic and social barriers compel women to wait twice as long as men to address symptoms of sexually transmitted disease infection (48a). This delay prolongs the increased vulnerability to HIV transmission that such coinfection represents. Health service schemes to treat these diseases continue to be inaccessible financially and logistically, as well as culturally unacceptable in most international settings.

As we review the regional epidemics, the increasing infection of women has led in all settings to an increasing number of vertically transmitted infections in their infants. The successful use of AZT in chemical trials in the U.S. to interrupt such transmission could presage help in preventing such transmission. Given an early efficacy of over 60% (17), this intervention merits discussion and study in settings where vertical transmission is highest.

The concept of targeting "core group" members is gaining acceptance in international efforts. This concept, first put forward based on experience gained in New York City (63), has been refined in international modeling and research. A recent analysis by the World Bank contrasting "core" with "non-core" approach to prevention projected tenfold greater impact in averting cases of sexually transmitted diseases (56). Developing country researchers have confirmed the cost-effectiveness of focused interventions for core group transmitters (60). However, after a certain population prevalence is reached the effectiveness of such an approach is more difficult to demonstrate. In addition, in some settings the stigmatization of high-risk individuals as potential "core group" members has resulted in repeated and frequent testing without real programmatic benefit.

In Europe and the United States, counseling, testing, and partner notification are central and effective strategies in HIV-transmission control. These strategies have not been employed to any great extent in developing countries. Access to individual HIV testing is problematic because of cost and difficulties in defining appropriate counseling strategies. Thus prevention strategies in resource-poor settings are not focused as specifically on individuals at risk. Often caregivers are reluctant to reveal the results of HIV testing if such testing is positive, an overwhelming obstacle to public health workers who are attempting follow-up counseling (53). Even in some research studies in Africa, commercial sex workers have not been advised of their seropositivity, with the rationale that resources did not permit adequate counseling or support if the information was shared. Thus the targeting of core groups in many developing countries has relied on anonymous serosurveillance information and generalization of research results rather than on individual testing.

In Asia and Latin America, individual testing and counseling are available, although concerns over confidentiality render governmental involvement in such activities less acceptable. Most counseling and testing activity is being carried out by the nongovernmental sector. New testing technologies may make testing more accessible and less costly, for instance by using two different rapid tests and foregoing the more costly Western blot confirmation, as outlined by WHO (84).

Harm-reduction strategies are increasingly gaining acceptance and recognition for their effectiveness in developed countries (20). These strategies have also been successful when applied in resource-poor settings. Unfortunately, intravenous drug use prior to AIDS had been stereotyped internationally as a western, or US, problem. As HIV serosurveillance has unmasked the true extent of this public health problem worldwide, most countries face the AIDS pandemic without the diagnostic, prevention, or treatment capabilities to combat injection drug use. Politically, services for this group are not seen as a priority, with the result that the implementation of needle exchange or bleach programs has lagged far behind the imperative presented by the level of transmission. Many Latin American and Asian urban centers, particularly those located on illicit international drug-trafficking routes, are at tremendous risk of HIV transmission related to intravenous drug use in the next decade.

Condom promotion is one of the few effective strategies available to combat HIV transmission in developing countries. Because there is no knowledge of infection status, there is only general promotion of condoms, with more intense promotion for risk groups such as commercial sex workers and their clients. Work in population and family planning programs in the previous decade had resulted in a very low international acceptance of the condom as a method of birth control. More modern approaches of "social marketing" of condoms have had some additional success. Labor intensive condom promotion to certain groups has been successful among commercial sex workers in Zaire and Thailand. In the latter case, a "100% condom" program coupled with the authority and enforcement of law demonstrated a dramatic drop in sexually transmitted diseases as condom use increased (29).

In summary, the range of prevention strategies available to public health workers in the developing countries is limited. In fact, technical and financial resources available to prevent HIV transmission in most settings now witnessing the pandemic are inadequate to the challenge. An analysis of governmental expenditures on HIV/AIDS in the United States and the rest of the hemisphere revealed that at least $90 was spent in 1990 on HIV prevention and control in the U.S. for every one dollar spent in Latin America (69). This difference may well reflect the debt crisis that has severely limited public health expenditures in Latin American countries over the past decade. This international disparity of the ability to invest in the power of prevention will be further discussed below.

New Technologies

Although the origin of the HIV/AIDS pandemic continues to elude definition, new diagnostic tools have increased the understanding of transmission and pathophysiology of the disease. Increasingly scientists are able to map the genome of the HIV virus and define the variants that are affecting different geographical regions of the world. In addition, technology for detecting virus and identifying the number of virus particles ("viral load") affecting an individual has improved greatly (24, 70, 71). These technologic advances are allowing microepidemiologic studies of HIV as well as studies of the host response to infection. This technology is increasingly being applied to the areas where HIV transmission has proved most intractable to prevention, such as Africa, through collaborative research efforts.

The developing countries of the world serve as source of genetic variants of HIV under study. Increasingly, researchers in these countries are participating in the application of these sophisticated techniques to the epidemiologic puzzles of transmission among their populations. Recent studies in Thailand, for example, have teamed Thai and US researchers in an effort to understand the significance of two separate strains of HIV isolated in Thailand. It appears that each strain has a preferred route of transmission, a finding which may, if confirmed, have implications for prevention.

Techniques being developed hold promise for improving the application of HIV diagnostic tests globally, as well as for defining the epidemiology of transmission. Current barriers to use such as cost, the need for centrifugation and refrigeration, and laboratory training may be mitigated as development moves forward. This could enhance the specificity of prevention targeting in resource-poor settings as discussed above.

HIV Vaccines

An affordable AIDS vaccine could significantly increase the capacity for prevention in resource-poor settings. Since the discovery of the responsible viral agent of AIDS in 1984, there has been a concerted effort to develop an AIDS vaccine. The limited success of behavioral and social prevention efforts makes it crucial to assure a continuing full-fledged effort to develop a vaccine for worldwide use. A vaccine is potentially most cost-effective in halting the spread of the epidemic. The initiative can be broadly divided into the development of a preventive vaccine (i.e. given before infection either to prevent infection or to prevent the development of disease in those infected), or a therapeutic vaccine (i.e. given to an infected person to slow or stop progression of disease).

There has been an unprecedented gain in knowledge about the virus, its biology, and its mechanisms of action over the past decade. Numerous vaccine strategies are being explored in the laboratory and in animal models. However, certain critical scientific obstacles have retarded the development of a vaccine.

Given these major problems, vaccine development should use traditional empirical approaches with early movement from the laboratory to testing in humans. Unfortunately, the long latency period from infection to illness, the fact that the virus integrates into host DNA, and the risk related to the oncogenic potential of retroviruses have made vaccine developers wary in their approach to vaccine development and testing in humans. As a result, such classical approaches of vaccine development as live attenuated or whole killed virus were given low priority for development. The long time required to develop, test, and register any vaccines has led many manufactures to accord low priority to HIV vaccine development in general. Most vaccines under development are protein or peptide subunit vaccines made from US or European strains, with the logic that companies need a proof of efficacy before increasing investment to deal with other strains. If these approaches are successful, the resultant vaccines will probably be expensive to produce, will have limited immunologic protection, and may not be useful for those with infections with non-US, non-European strains. Such vaccines will, therefore, have limited, if any, usefulness for those living in developing countries where 90% of the new HIV infections are occurring.

At this juncture, current product development activity should be supplemented with approaches and strains that are more likely to be useful for those living in developing countries, and with policy determinations to finance and distribute newly developed vaccines to those who need them most. A new international venture is underway that hopefully will provide some solutions to these difficult problems (62).

In summary, considerable progress has been achieved in understanding the biology of the Human Immunodeficiency Virus (HIV). Although the possibility of a vaccine remains elusive, there are encouraging signs. Various vaccine development strategies are under way in the laboratory, although their movement into testing is limited by scientific and economic forces. The current initiative on vaccine development is insufficient in scope given the magnitude of the problem. Furthermore, the gap between the spread of the disease and the amount of effort on vaccine development is widening. New strategies are imperative to speed this effort and to assure that any vaccines that are developed will be made available to those who need it most—those living in developing countries.

❖ Care: The Challenge Broadens
Current Therapies

Outside of affluent countries, the response of caring for persons with HIV in developing countries has been limited. Use of antiretroviral therapies has been limited to the wealthy who are able to travel or import medicines for use in their treatment. Experience with these medications is minimal in most developing countries. One exception is the Brazilian program, which began purchasing zidovidine at public expense for HIV/AIDS patients in 1992, just as evidence for longterm benefit from AZT has become disappointing.

Increasingly, the limitation of the international support to prevention has become unacceptable to health workers in developing countries. Strategies are needed to assist in coping with the care of persons with HIV/AIDS (19). This argument is reinforced with the finding that AZT may prove an effective tool to prevent vertical transmission. Pressure on valuable hospital resources, now monopolized by AIDS patients, could be eased by community nursing programs. This call for help has been met with concern that resources will be diverted from prevention to care, and the discussion continues (8).

Despite the reluctance to invest in care, there is eagerness to study the high-prevalence populations of the developing world. The resulting ethical crisis is being addressed through the leadership of WHO and other international organizations. Issues of research are being discussed at the international level. Minimum ethical standards have been defined, including the expectation that drugs or vaccines tested in poor populations will be made available on a continuous basis to such populations. These requirements may be playing some role in the slow pace of research for cure, and new incentives are being considered to promote research.

Tuberculosis

HIV is reversing the gains made in tuberculosis control throughout the world. The pervasive nature of tuberculosis as a coinfection with HIV is only now being documented. A recent study of wasting ("Slim's Disease") in Ivory Coast suggests that up to one half of such clinical cases are coinfection of TB and HIV (13). Based on notification and annual risk estimates, CDC and WHO estimate that 7.5 million incident cases of clinical tuberculosis occurred in 1990, and that this number will increase to 11.9 million by the year 2005.

❖ Predicting the Future of the HIV/AIDS Pandemic

Various sophisticated modeling techniques have been brought into play to help define the future of this ongoing international calamity. Asia is predicted to show rapidly increasing incidence, with Africa continuing to see high incidence. Transmission is continuing in the earliest areas of the HIV/AIDS epidemic such as Uganda. The potential efficacy of prevention and control efforts will probably be greatest in new areas of epidemic activity. The World Bank has included scenarios based on differing investment assumptions in the 1993 Development Report. Increased resource availability could halve the annual infections projected for Asia in the year 2000. A great deal of work clearly remains if global efforts are to succeed. At present there is a mismatch with 90% of resources being spent where only 10% of global HIV infections occur.

As the epidemic has widened in geographic reach and deepened in the number of persons and groups affected in each country, the economic and social toll has become more pronounced. Although global estimates vary, a recent estimate of $350 billion by the year 2000 has been put forward (4), based on a well-accepted proprietary trade-linked model of economic systems. The model allows the examination of shared impact among trading economies, reflecting the increasing interdependence of world economies. The weakness of this work is its reliance on a proprietary tool which prevents independent validation of the methodology used. Nonetheless, there is general acceptance that the economic cost of AIDS is high. These costs include the following:

1. *Direct costs of treatment and care* These costs include the opportunity cost in poor countries of using scarce hospital beds for an illness with no cure. In some areas in Central Africa 70–80% of beds are occupied by persons with AIDS (37). In Thailand, similar occupancy rates are seen in the Northern region according to recent unpublished reports.
2. *Indirect costs of the epidemic* These costs are as much as ten times larger than the direct costs. They include the loss in productivity, loss in purchasing power through diversion of personal resources into care expense, and an increase in the dependency of societies through the loss of adults and increases in orphaned children and elderly with no identified support.

Indirect costs vary by economic setting. Experience in the United States has demonstrated the impact of AIDS on a developed, market economy, a harbinger for the effect on the market economies of Asia over the next two decades. Initial studies are underway (9).

Despite progressive recommendations by the United Nations organizations such as WHO, ILO, and others, the societal response to the deepening world crisis of HIV has created concerns about human rights and has not been cost-effective. Travel restrictions that mandate HIV testing for visitors or immigrants are widespread. Although such screening of immigrants may limit care expenditure (93), this consideration can be effectively limited through other means. Travel restrictions serve no public health function in limiting the introduction or spread of HIV, and have a general "chilling" effect on international travel that is difficult to quantify. More restrictive measures have been put into place in Cuba: A system of sanatoria has been established and widespread mandatory testing has been carried out with over 10 million tests performed under governmental auspices since the initiation of the program. This system has proved to be unsustainable in its social and economic costs, and the recent efforts to reintroduce internees into society have met with difficulty. In addition, although rates of infection have remained relatively low in Cuba, similar rates are found in Nicaragua, which did not implement isolation programs. The similarity suggests that being off the route of trade and travel may be more responsible for the slow unfolding of the HIV epidemic in these settings. Thus, beyond the human rights concerns that sanitoria efforts provoke, there is increasing evidence that quarantine cannot serve as an efficient control of HIV transmission.

In summary, the international pandemic of HIV is continuing to progress in all regions of the globe. The epidemiological trends show that women and children are increasingly affected. Asia has become the newest major area of epidemic activity. The epidemic has taught us that AIDS prevention strategies and the technologies they rely on need to be made accessible on a global basis for successful disease control. Early investment in effective strategies for prevention is cost-effective (7). Broadening the societal response to AIDS beyond the health sector may improve the world's ability to stem the inexorable transmission of HIV into new areas and new population groups.

❖ About the Authors

Ann Marie Kimball, Department of Health Services and Epidemiology, University of Washington, Seattle, Washington.

Seth Berkly, Health Sciences Division, Rockefeller Foundation, New York

Elizabeth Ngugi, Department of Community Health, Strengthening STD/HIV Control Project, Nairobi, Kenya.

Helene Gayle, M.D., is Director of the Centers for Disease Control and Prevention, Atlanta.

LITERATURE CITED

1. Anderson, RM, May RM. 1992. Understanding the AIDS pandemic. *Sci. Am.* 266:58–66.
2. Barongo LR, Borgdorff MW, Mosha FF, Nicholl A, Grosskurth H, et al. 1992. The epidemiology of HIV-1 infection in urban areas, roadside settlements and rural villages in Mwanza Region, Tanzania. *AIDS* 6:1521–28
3. Bartholemew C, Cleghorn G. 1989. Retroviruses in the Caribbean. In *AIDS: Profile of an Epidemic*, ed. F Zacarias. Washington, DC: PAHO
4. Behravesh N. 1993. *Measuring the global economic impact of the AIDS epidemic.* DRI/McGraw-Hill Insight Rep.
5. Berkley SF. 1991. Parenteral transmission of HIV in Africa. *AIDS* 5:S87–S92
6. Berkley S, Naamara W, Okware S, Downing R, Kondelue J, et al. 1990. AIDS and HIV infection in women in Uganda—are women more infected than males? *AIDS* 4:1237–42
7. Berkley S, Piot P, Schopper D. 1994. AIDS: Invest now or pay more later. *Fin. Dev.* 31:40
8. Biggar RJ. 1993. When ideals meet reality—the global challenge of HIV/AIDS. *Am. J. Public Health* 83:1383–84
9. Bloom DE, Lyons JV. 1993. *Economic Implications of AIDS in Asia.* UN Dev. Program. Rep.
10. Butler D. 1994. Concern over the "invisible problem" of HIV blood in developing countries. *Nature* 369:429
11. Cantwell MF, Binkin N. 1994. *Tuberculosis in Subsaharan Africa: can a good tuberculosis control program make a difference?* Presented at 43rd Annu. EIS Conf., Cent. Dis. Control, Atlanta, April
11a. Cent. Dis. Control. 1982. Persistent, generalized lymphadenopathy among homosexual males. *Morbid Mortal. Wkly. Rep.* 31: 249–51
12. Cent. Dis. Control. 1993. Estimates of future global tuberculosis morbidity and mortality. 1993. *Morbid Mortal. Wkly. Rep.* 42:961–64
13. Cent. Dis. Control. AIDS Clearinghouse. 1994. TB underestimated in HIV Wasting, Daily rep. June 11
14. Central Africa 1959. *Lancet* 1: 1279–80
15. Chin J, Mann J. 1990. HIV infections and AIDS in the 1990s. *Annu. Rev. Public Health* 11:127–42
16. Colebunders RI, Greenberg A, Nguyen-Dinh P, Francis H, Kabote N, et al. 1987. Rapid communication: evaluation of a clinical case definition of AIDS in African children. *AIDS* 1:151–53
17. Connor EM, Sperling RS, Gelber R, Kiselev P, Scott G, et al. 1994. Reduction of maternal-infant transmission of human immunodeficiency virus type 1 with zidovudine treatment. *N. Engl. J. Med.* 331:1173–80
18. DeCock KM, Adjorlolo G, Ekpine E, Sibailly T, Kouadio J, et al. 1993. Epidemiology and transmission of HIV-2. Why there is no HIV-2 pandemic. *J. Am. Med. Assoc.* 270:2083–86
19. DeCock KM, Luca SB, Lucas S, Agness J, Kadio A, Gayle HD. 1993. Clinical research, prophylaxis, therapy and care for HIV disease in Africa. *Am. J. Public Health* 83:1385–89
20. Des Jarlais DC, Friedman SR, Ward TP. 1993. Harm reduction: a public health response to the AIDS epidemic among injecting drug users. *Annu. Rev. Public Health* 14:413–50
20a. Duerr A, Xia Z, Nagachinta T, Tovanabutra S, Tansuhaj A, et al. 1994. *Probability of male-to-female HIV transmission among married couples in Chiang Mai, Thailand.*

Presented at Int. Conf. AIDS, 10th, Yokohama, Japan

21. Dunn DT, Newell ML, Ades AE, Peckham CS. 1992. Risk of human immunodeficiency virus type 1 transmission through breastfeeding. *Lancet* 340:585–88

22. Editor. 1992. Poliovaccine and AIDS origin link very unlikely. *Lancet* 340:1090–91

22a. European Collaborative Study. 1994. Caesarian section and risk of vertical transmission of HIV-1 infection. *Lancet* 343:1464–67

23. Farnham P. 1994. Defining and measuring the costs of the HIV epidemic to business firms. *Public Health Rep.* 109:311.

24. Ferre F, Marchese AL, Griffin SL, Daigle AE, Richieri SP, et al. 1993. Development and validation of a polymerase chain reaction method for the precise quantiation of HIV-1 DNA in blood cells from subjects undergoing a 1-year immunotherapeutic treatment. *AIDS* 7:S21–27 (Suppl. 2)

25. Getchell JP, Hicks DR, Svinivasan A, Heath JL, York DA, et al. 1987. Human immunodeficiency virus isolated from a serum sample collected in 1976 in Central Africa. *J. Infect. Dis.* 156:833–37

26. Gomez P, Kimball A, Orlander H, Bain RM, Fisher L, Hoemes K. 1995. Epidemic crack cocaine use, linked with genital ulcer disease and heterosexual HIV infection in the Bahamas. Submitted

27. Grmek M. 1990. *History of AIDS: The Emergence of a Modern Pandemic*, p. 124. Princeton, NJ: Princeton Univ. Press

28. Gunn RA, Kimball AM, Pollard RA, Feeley JC, Feldman RA, et al. 1979. Bottle feeding as a risk factor for cholera in infants. *Lancet* 2:730–32

29. Hanenberg RS, Rojanapithayakorn W, Kunasol P, Sokal DC. 1994. Impact of Thailand's HIV-control programme as indicated by the decline of sexually transmitted diseases. *Lancet* 344:243–45

30. Herrera G. 1990. *Characteristics of women with AIDS in Costa Rica.* Costa Rica Natl. AIDS Program. San Juan, Costa Rica

30a. Hira SK, Kamanga J, Bhat GJ, Mwale C, Tembo G, et al. 1989. Perinatal transmission of HIV1 in Zambia. *Br. Med. J.* 299:1250–52

31. Hughes A, Corrah T. 1990. Human immunodeficiency virus type 2 (HIV-2). *Blood Rev.* 4:158–64

32. Int. Forum AIDS Research. 1990. *Toward an AIDS Vaccine: The Policy Supporting the Research.* Washington, DC: Inst. Med. Proc., Sept.

33. Iszazola JA, Valdespino-Gomez SL, Gortmaker SL, Townsend J, Becker J, et al. 1991. HIV-1 seropositivity and behavioral and sociological risks among homosexual and bisexual men in six Mexican cities. *J. Acquired Immune Defic. Syndr.* 4:614–22

34. Jager H, Ngaly B, Perriens J, Nseka K, Davaci F, et al. 1990. Prevention of transfusion-associated HIV transmission in Kinshasa, Zaire: HIV screening is not enough. *AIDS* 4:571–74

35. Kennedy KI, Fortney JA, Bonhomme MG, Potts M, Lamptey P, Carswell W. 1990. Do the benefits of breastfeeding outweigh the risk of postnatal transmission of HIV via breastmilk? *Trop. Doctor* 20:25–29

36. Killewo J, Nyamuryekunge K, Sandstrom A, Bredbergraden U, Wall S. et al. 1990. Prevalence of HIV-1 infection in the Kagera Region of Tanzania: a population-based study. *AIDS* 4:1081–85

37. Kimball AM. 1991. *Impact of HIV/AIDS on social and economic development in Africa.* Testimony before the US House of Representatives, Comm. For. Aff., Subcommittee on Africa, Nov. 6. US. GPO

38. Kimball AM, González RS, Betts CM, eds. 1990. *Annu. HIV/AIDS Surveillance Rep., 1991.* Washington, DC: PAHO

39. Kimball AM, González RS, Zacarías F. 1991. AIDS among women in Latin America and the Caribbean. *Bull. PAHO* 25:367

40. Kimball AM, González RS, Zacarías F. 1993. Women and the AIDS epidemic: an impending crisis for the Americas. In *Gender, Women and Health in the Americas*. PAHO Sci. Publ. 541

41. Koifman R, Monteiro G, Rodriques R. 1990. *Epidemiologic characteristics of AIDS in women in Rio de Janeiro, Brazil.* Presented at 6th Int. Conf. AIDS, San Francisco

41a. Lallemant M, Cheynier D, Nzingoul S, Jourdain G, Sinet M, et al. 1992. Characteristics associated with HIV1 infection in pregnant women in Brazzaville, Congo. *J. Acquired Immune Defic. Syndr.* 5: 270–85

42. Lederberg J, Shope RE, Oaks SC Jr, eds. 1992. *Emerging Infections: Microbial Threats to Health in the United States.* Washington, DC: Natl. Acad. Press

42a. Lepage P, Vandeper P, Msellati O, Hittimand DG, Simonon A, et al. 1993. Mother-to-child transmission of human immunodeficiency virus type 1 (HIV1) and its determinants: a cohort study in Kigali, Rwanda. *Am. J. Epidemiol.* 137:589–99

43. Lifson AR. 1988. Do alternate modes for transmission of human immunodeficiency virus exist? *J. Am. Med. Assoc.* 259:1353–56

44. Lima ES, Bastos FI, Teller PR, Friedman SR. 1993. HIV infection and AIDS among drug injectors at Rio de Janeiro: perspectives and unanswered questions. *Bull. Narc.* 45:107–15

45. Mann J, Tarantola DJ, Netter TW, eds. 1992. *AIDS in the World: The Global AIDS Policy Coalition*, pp. 25–32. Cambridge, MA: Harvard Univ. Press

46. Mascola JR, Louwagie J, McCutchan FE, Fischer CL, Hegerich PA, et al. 1994. Two antigenically distinct subtypes of human immunodeficiency virus type 1: viral genotype predicts neutralization serotype. *J. Infect. Dis.* 169:48–54

47. Mastro TD, Satten GA, Nopkesorn T, Sangkharomya S, Logini IM. 1994. Probability of female-to-male transmission of HIV-1 in Thailand. *Lancet* 343:204–7

48. Ministry of Health, Thailand 1992. *100% condom program*. Rep. to GPA/WHO

48a. Moses S, Ngugi EN, Bradley J, Njeru E, Eldridge G, et al. 1994. Health care-seeking behavior related to the transmission of sexually transmitted diseases. *Am. J. Public Health* 84:1947–51

49. Moss RB, Ferre F, Trauger R, Jensen FC, Daigle A, et al. 1994. Inactivated HIV-1 immunogen: impact on markers of disease progression. *J. AIDS* 7:S21–27 (Suppl. 1)

50. Mulder D, Kamali A, Nakyinge J, et al. 1993. HIV-1 associated mortality in a rural Ugandan Cohort: results at two year follow-up. *Proc. 9th Int. Conf. AIDS, Berlin* (Abstr. WS-CO3-6)

51. Nahmias AJ, Weiss J, Yao X, Lee F, Kodsi R, et al. 1986. Evidence for human infection with an HTLV III/LAV-like virus in Central Africa. *Lancet* 1:1279–80

52. Narain JP, Raviglione MC, Kochi A. 1992. HIV associated tuberculosis in developing countries: epidemiology and strategies for prevention. *Tubercle Lung Dis.* 73: 311–21

53. Ngugi EN, Njenga E, Anderson S, et al. 1994. Preliminary results of a feasibility study to integrate community based care of people with HIV/AIDS into existing urban health services in Nairobi.

54. Nowak MA, McLean AR. 1991. A mathematical model of vaccination against HIV to prevent the development of AIDS. *Proc. R. Soc. London Ser. B* 246:141–46

55. Nzilambi N, DeCock KM, Forthal DN, Francis D, Ryder RW, et al. 1988. The prevalence of infection

with human immunodeficiency virus over a 10 year period in rural Zaire. *New Engl. J. Med.* 318: 276–79

56. Over M, Piot P. 1993. HIV infection and sexually transmitted diseases. In *Disease Control Priorities in Developing Countries.* New York: World Bank/Oxford Univ. Press

57. PANOS. 1994. *The Practice of Dry Sex.* World AIDS

58. Piot P, Taelman H, Minlangu KB, Mbendi N, Ndangi K, et al. 1984. Acquired immunodeficiency syndrome in a heterosexual population in Zaire. *Lancet* 2:65–69

59. Plebani A, Biolchini A, Bucceri A, Buscaglia M, Pardi G, Semprini AE. 1990. Prenatal immune status of fetuses of HIV-seropositive mothers. *Gynecol. Obstet. Invest.* 29:108–11

60. Plummer FA, Nagelkerke NJD, Moses A, Ndinya-Achola JO, Bwayo J, Ngugi E. 1991. The importance of core groups in the epidemiology and control of HIV-1 infection. *AIDS* 5:S169–76 (Suppl. 1)

61. Raggi R, Blanco GA. 1992. Epidemic model of HIV infection and AIDS in Argentina. Status in 1990 and predictive estimates. *Medicina* 52:225–35

62. Rockefeller Found. 1994. *HIV vaccines—accelerating the development of preventive HIV vaccines for the world,* Bellagio, Italy, March 7–11

63. Rothenberg RA. 1983. The geography of gonorrhae: empirical demonstration of core group transmission. *Am. J. Epidemiol.* 117:688–94

63a. Ryder RW, Nsa RW, Hassig SE, Behets F, Rayfield M, et al. 1989. Perinatal transmission of the human immunodeficiency virus type 1 to infants of seropositive women in Zaire. *New Engl. J. Med.* 320:1637–42

64. Sakondhavat C, Kanato M, Leungtongkum P, Kuchaisit C. 1988. KAP study on sex, reproduction and contraception in Thai teenagers. *J. Med. Assoc. Thailand* 71:649–53

65. Saxinger WC, Levine PH, Dean AG, Dethe G, Langewantzin G, et al. 1985. Evidence for exposure to HTLV-III in Uganda before 1973. *Science* 227:1036–38

66. Serwaada D, Sewankambo NK, Caswell JW, Bayley AC, Tedders RS, et al. 1985. Slim disease: a new disease in Uganda and its association with HTLV-III infection. *Lancet* 2:849–52

67. Singh S, Crofts D, Gertig D. 1993. HIV infections among IDUs in North East Malaysia. *9th Int. Conf. AIDS, Berlin,* Poster Present.

68. Stein ZA. 1990. HIV prevention: the need for methods women can use. *Am. J. Public Health* 80:460–62

69. Suarez R, Kimball A. 1992. *What would be the cost of AZT for Latin America and the Caribbean.* Presented at 2nd Pan Am. Conf. AIDS, Santo Domingo

70. Trauger RJ, Ferre F, Daigle AE, Jensen FC, Moss RB, et al. 1994. Effect of immunization with inactivated gp120-depleted Human Immunodeficiency Virus Type 1 (HIV-1) immunogen on HIV-1 immunity, viral DNA, and percentage of CD4 cells. *J. Infect. Dis.* 169:1256–64

71. Trauger RJ, Giermakowska WK, Ferre F, Duffy PC, Wallace MR, et al. 1993. Cell-mediated immunity to HIV-1 in Walter Reed stages 1–6 individuals: correlation with virus burden. *Immunology* 78:611–15

72. UN Resolution. 1994. *(ECOSOC) E/1994/18/Rev 1,* July 20

73. US Japan Cooperative Framework for Economic Development 1993. Point 5

74. Van de Perre P, Lepage P, Kestelyn P, Hekker AC, Pouvroy D, et al. 1984. Acquired immunodeficiency syndrome in Rwanda. *Lancet* 2:62–65

75. Van de Perre P, Simonson A, Msellati P, Hitimana DG, Vaira

D, et al. 1991. Postnatal transmission of human immunodeficiency virus type one from mother to infant. *New Engl. J. Med.* 325:593–98

76. Villari P, Spino C, Chalmers TC, Lau J, Sacks HS. 1993. Cesarean section to reduce perinatal transmission of human immunodeficiency virus. A metaanalysis. *J. Curr. Clin. Trials* July 8

77. Wald A, Corey L, Handsfield HH, Holmes HK. 1993. Influence of HIV infection on manifestations and natural history of other sexually transmitted diseases. *Annu. Rev. Public Health* 14:19–42

77a. Wasserheti JN. 1989. The significance and scope of reproductive tract infections among third world women. *Int. J. Gynecol. Obstet.* 3:145–68 (Suppl.)

78. Wasserheit JN. 1992. Epidemiologic synergy: interrelationships between human immunodeficiency virus infection and other sexually transmitted diseases. *Sex. Transm. Dis.* 19:61–77

79. Wawer MJ, Serwadda D, Musgrave SD, Kondelule JK, Musagara M, et al. 1991. Dynamics of spread of HIV-1 infection in a rural district of Uganda. *Br. Med. J.* 303:1303–6

80. Way P, Stanecki K. 1993. *Trends and Patterns of HIV/AIDS Infection in Selected Developing Countries.* Res. Note No. 12. US Census Bur.

81. Weninger BG, Quinhoes EP, Sereno AB, Deperez MA, Krebs JW. 1992. A simplified case definition of AIDS derived from empirical data. *J. Acquired Immune Defic. Syndr.* 12:1212–13

82. WHO. 1985. *Workshop on AIDS in Central Africa.* Bangui, Central African Republic, Oct. 22-24

83. WHO. 1994. Current global situation of the HIV/AIDS pandemic. *Wkly. Epidmiol. Rec.* 69:7–8

84. WHO Evaluation Unit. 1994. Strategies for laboratory HIV testing strategies that do not require use of the Western blot approach. *Bull. WHO* 72:129–34

85. Widy-Wirski R, Berkley S, Downing R, Okware S, Recine U, et al. 1988. Evaluation of the WHO clinical case definition for AIDS in Uganda. *J. Am. Med. Assoc.* 260:3286–89

86. Wong K, Lee SS, Lim WL. 1993. HIV surveillance among drug users in Hong Kong. *9th Int. Conf. AIDS, Berlin,* Poster Present.

87. World Bank. 1993. *Investing in Health, The 1993 World Development Rep.* New York: Oxford Univ. Press

88. *World Development Report.* 1993. New York: Oxford Univ. Press

89. Xia M, Kreiss J, Holmes K. 1993. *Risk factors for HIV infection among drug users in Yunan Province, China: association with intravenous drug use and protective effect of boiling reusable needles and syringes.* Presented at ISSTDR, Finland

90. Zabin LS, Hirsch MB, Smith EA, Street R, Hardy JB. 1986. Evaluation of a pregnancy prevention program for urban teenagers. *Fam. Plan. Perspect.* 18:119–26

90a. Zaknum D, Oswald HP, Zaknun J, Mayersbach P, Sperl W, et al. 1991. Effects of health and medical undertreatment on the clinical status and social behavior of infants and small children in a Romanian orphanage. *Padiatr. Padol.* 26:65–67

91. Zheng XW, Zhang JP, Tian CQ, Cheng HH, Yang XZ, et al. 1993. Cohort study of HIV infection among drug users in Ruili, Longchuan and Luxi of Yunnan Province, China. *Biomed. Environ. Sci.* 6:348–51

92. Ziegler JB, Johnson RO, Cooper DA, Gold J. 1985. Postnatal transmission of AIDS associated retrovirus from mother to infant. *Lancet* 1:896–98

93. Zowall H, Coupal L, Fraser RD, Gilmore N, Deutsch A, Grover SA. 1992. Economic impact of HIV infection and coronary heart disease in immigrants to Canada. *Can. Med. Assoc. J.* 147:1163–72

❖ Surveillance in Environmental Public Health: Issues, Systems, and Sources

Stephen B. Thacker, Donna F. Stroup, R. Gibson Parrish, and Henry A. Anderson

❖ Introduction

For federal, state, and local health departments, environmental health—the prevention and control of health problems related to the environment—is an essential function. The process by which an agent—biological, chemical, or physical—in the environment produces an adverse outcome in a host can be depicted in a "hazard-exposure-outcome" axis (Figure 1). While all steps in this axis are necessary for an agent to produce an adverse outcome, both the relative importance of each step and the time necessary to move from one step to the next may vary among agents.

Public health surveillance has been defined as the ongoing systematic collection, analysis, and interpretation of data on specific health events affecting a population, closely integrated with the timely dissemination of these data to those responsible for prevention and control.[1] While this definition focuses on health outcomes (e.g., diseases, disabilities, or injuries), surveillance of hazards (or risk factors) and exposures is also critical to environmental public health practice (Figure 1). Hazard surveillance is the "assessment of the occurrence of, distribution of, and the secular trends in levels of hazards (toxic chemical agents, physical agents, biomechanical stressors, as well as biological agents) responsible for disease and injury."[2] Exposure surveillance is the monitoring of individual members of the population for the presence of an environmental agent or its clinically inapparent (e.g., subclinical or preclinical) effects.

Three of the functions of a surveillance system are critical to its usefulness for environmental public health.[1] First, the system must enable measurement of specific hazards (e.g., air pollutants), exposures (e.g., blood lead), or health outcomes (e.g., asthma). Second, it must produce an ongoing data record; although one-time surveys or sporadic epidemiologic studies are valuable to public health, they are distinct from surveillance activities. Third, it must produce timely and representative data that can be used in planning, implementing, and evaluating public health activities.

The uses of surveillance data can be categorized according to timeliness. For detecting epidemics, unusual clusters of specific birth defects (by use of automated triggers defined by sentinel health events) signal instances in

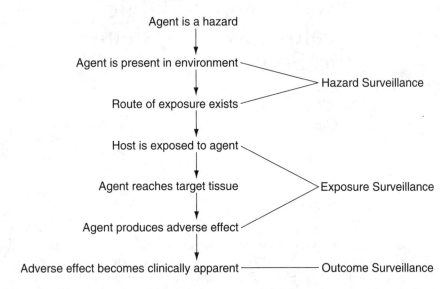

Figure 1   The process by which an environmental agent produces an adverse effect and the corresponding types of public health surveillance.

which public health officials should respond immediately.[3] In addition, such a system may enable detection of newly emerging conditions[4] (e.g., toxic shock syndrome). Detection of changes in health practice could be signaled by an increase in the use of over-the-counter medications for asthma. Changes in antibiotic-resistance patterns may lead physicians to change their prescription practices or researchers to alter their priorities. Data from the Environmental Protection Agency, the US Bureau of the Census, and the National Health Interview Survey can be used to relate risk of illness among defined populations (e.g., asthma in children) to air quality.[5]

In the United States, decisions affecting public health policy and allocation of resources usually are made yearly in conjunction with government budgets. Timely annual data summaries would provide immediate estimates of the magnitude of a health problem, thus assisting policymakers to modify priorities and plan intervention programs.[6] These same data would be useful to those assessing control activities and would help researchers establish priorities in applied epidemiology and laboratory research. In addition, reviewing surveillance data annually can facilitate the testing of hypotheses related to prevention and intervention efforts (e.g., ocular injuries associated with fireworks).[7] As intervention programs are evaluated and priorities are set, policymakers must evaluate the effects of the programs on populations (e.g., protective measures to reduce the threat of lead toxicity in workplaces[8]).

Surveillance data should be retained in readily accessible archival form, not only to document the evolving health status of a population but also to help us understand the predictors of disease and injury. These data should be of the best possible quality and should be made available for research, including that conducted by individuals not affiliated with the government. Carefully maintained archival data can provide the most accurate portrayal of the natural history of a disease in a population. For example, mortality attributed to smoking in women in the United States has now surpassed mortality attributed to breast cancer. To measure effectively the long-term effects of public policies or social changes, researchers must have access to archival surveillance and health information systems. For example, the effect of programs encouraging women to stop smoking could be apparent from archival data on lung cancer mortality.[9] In addition, archival surveillance information can be used to validate interim data.

The surveillance of infectious diseases, chronic disease, injuries, and occupational health has been treated elsewhere.[10–12] In this paper, we focus on those aspects of environmental public health surveillance that have not been considered adequately (e.g., exposure to environmental toxicants). First, we address special issues related to environmental public health surveillance. Second, we present a framework for categorizing systems for environmental public health surveillance and illustrate the framework with examples. We also list selected data sources for those conducting environmental public health surveillance (see Table 1).

❖ Special Issues in Environmental Public Health Surveillance

While not unique to environmental public health, four issues are of particular concern to those who practice in this arena. First, our ability to identify the specific environmental causes of many adverse outcomes is limited. This is especially true for adverse outcomes that occur long after exposure and are caused by an agent that does not persist in the body; does not produce an easily detected, unique effect or marker; or does not occur in a setting (e.g., occupational) where there is a readily identifiable, significant hazard. Although adverse outcomes have been linked to many biological and physical agents, very few of the millions of known chemical agents have been studied adequately.[13] Although the causes of some adverse outcomes may be unique (e.g., mercury poisoning, which causes acrodynia among children), many adverse outcomes have multiple causes, some of which may not be environmental.[14]

Second, data collected for other purposes may not be sufficient for environmental public health surveillance.[15] For example, data from vital records or disability claims rarely contain sufficient information to meet a case definition for a condition caused by an environmental exposure. Other limitations of such data sources may include lack of timeliness of data collection or data availability, incomplete data on outcomes, nonrepresentativeness of the population, and problems with data quality.[16]

Third, although all public health decisions are made in a social context, in environmental public health, public alarm is quite common and may often be out of proportion to the hazard itself.[17] Thus, sentiment rather than science may influence environmental public health policy disproportionately.

Fourth, biological markers are likely to become critical elements of environmental exposure surveillance, just as they are critical to surveillance of infectious diseases.[18] Like most infectious biological agents, some chemical agents and noninfectious biological agents can be measured directly or produce a specific immune response in their host that usually persists after the adverse outcome (e.g., chronic renal problems linked to cadmium exposure or various allergenic dusts).[19,20]

❖ A Framework for Environmental Public Health Surveillance

To address these issues, we propose three types of surveillance for use in environmental public health: hazard surveillance, exposure surveillance, and outcome surveillance. If a clear link has been documented between a hazard and an adverse health outcome, there is a route of exposure to the hazard, and the hazard can be readily monitored in the environment, then hazard surveillance offers the best potential for early intervention and prevention. If the hazard cannot be monitored readily but there is a marker for exposure to the hazard, then exposure surveillance would provide information to inform the earliest opportunity for intervention. Finally, if an important public health outcome has a suspected (but undocumented) relationship to an environmental hazard, then outcome surveillance, in combination with etiologic studies, is warranted.

It is important to emphasize that these types of surveillance are complementary, and the optimal strategy for preventing or reducing the impact of a specific public health problem often dictates the use of all three types of surveillance. For example, outcome surveillance may be used to document the disease burden on the population.[10] Hazard surveillance may be used to identify new relationships between hazards and outcomes. Exposure and outcome surveillance may also provide valuable information for evaluating the effectiveness of hazard reduction programs.[21] We illustrate this framework with examples of each type of surveillance from environmental public health practice.

Hazard Surveillance: Air Pollutants

Environmental air monitoring data from more than 4200 state and local monitoring sites in the United States are collected and published routinely for six air pollutants covered by national air quality standards (carbon monoxide, lead, nitrogen dioxide, ozone, particulate matter, and sulfur dioxide).[22] These data are used to monitor compliance with standards for these six pollutants under the Clean Air Act.[23] The data are also used to enforce emission control laws for cars,[24] and, in some cities, they provide the basis for hazard alerts or press releases to encourage restricted work and other outdoor activity on days when pollutants are forecast to exceed federal standards. Better collaboration between state air pollution agencies and state and local health departments could lead to even more effective use of these environmental public health surveillance data.

Exposure Surveillance: Childhood Lead Poisoning

The results of blood lead testing among children are used to monitor exposure to lead and to assess the effectiveness of programs designed to reduce environmental lead hazards.[25] The use of these data for program management is illustrated by the system implemented by the New Mexico Department of Health.[26] The New Mexico prevention program developed legislation, documented lead poisoning outside high-risk metropolitan areas, and provided hypotheses to investigators seeking to identify sources of lead other than paint (e.g., traditional medicines and ceramic ware). Complementary data from repeated administrations of the National Health and Nutrition Examination Survey have documented the national impact of reduction of lead in gasoline on the incidence of lead poisoning.[27]

Outcome Surveillance: Birth Defects

The Metropolitan Atlanta Congenital Defects Monitoring Program, together with data from 28 state birth defect monitoring programs, are used to monitor trends in specific birth defects or combinations of defects.[28] Because there is population-based ascertainment of both case and control subjects, these data facilitate epidemiologic research and have been used to study the teratogenicity for several exposures of potential public health concern, including exposure to spray adhesive,[29] airport noise,[30] and military service in Vietnam.[31]

Combination of Data Sources

Environmental public health surveillance often requires more information than is available from a single source and is complicated by the limited availability of incidence data, incomplete case ascertainment, and changes in record keeping. The combination of monitoring data for environmental hazards and data from vital records, recurrent exposure surveys, registries, and office records may be necessary to assess the occurrence of and trends in environmental hazards and their related outcomes.

The national surveillance system for asthma illustrates the use of multiple data sources for outcomes to monitor a particular health problem. This system uses data from vital records, the National Hospital Discharge Survey, the National Ambulatory Medical Care Survey, and the National Health Interview Survey to show an increase during the 1980s in the burden of asthma in the United States as measured by morbidity, mortality, and disability, especially among urban and minority populations.[32]

An example of a surveillance program combining hazard, exposure, and outcome data is that for environmental lead and its effects. Lead is one of the six priority air pollutants monitored all over the country.[33]; surveys of selected housing stock are done regularly in some cities to identify housing with a lead hazard,[34] and lead is monitored in the air in some workplaces.[35,36] Exposure to lead is monitored in blood screening programs for children[37] and in workers at risk.[38] Vital statistics systems can be used to identify deaths due to lead poisoning.[39]

❖ Discussion

In the United States, all states monitor food, air, and water, as mandated by law. The exposure levels set by this legislative mandate, however, may still permit environmentally related illness.[40,41] According to a recent survey, only eight state health departments have responsibility for environmental public health; in other states, departments of the environment or of natural resources are separate from the health department.[42] Furthermore, lead poisoning and pesticide poisoning are the only two environmental health conditions for which states routinely conduct surveillance in the general population.[43] Unless the interaction between practicing public health professionals and their counterparts in environmental public health is fostered, the use of surveillance data for disease prevention and health promotion may be constrained.[44]

For example, environmental public health surveillance should take advantage of what has been learned by those conducting surveillance in occupational health. First, there is a need to establish outcomes on the basis of their public health importance and amenability to prevention or control measures. Thus, the National Institute for Occupational Safety and Health has focused its surveillance efforts on 10 leading work-related diseases and injuries.[45] Second, the most successful use of surveillance in prevention and control of occupational diseases and injuries has been in those situations in which there is a clearly recognized relationship, usually demonstrated through epidemiologic or laboratory studies, between a hazard and an adverse outcome (e.g., lead-based paint and blood lead levels).[46] Third, a combination of hazard, exposure, and outcome surveillance is optimal once a relationship has been established between a specific hazard and a specific outcome. Hazard surveillance should form the foundation of prevention and control efforts,[2,47] and exposure and outcome surveillance can serve to identify failures of—and the need to institute, modify, or enforce—prevention and control programs.[36] Finally, data from outcome surveillance can be used to identify increases in diseases or injuries of unknown or previously unrecognized causes and, when used in conjunction with data from hazard or exposure surveillance, may suggest relationships to specific hazards that warrant further study (e.g., house dust and childhood asthma).[48]

National, state, and local health and environmental agencies should move rapidly to establish effective systems of environmental public health surveillance. As an initial step, local, state, and national environmental health practitioners should identify health conditions associated with exposure to environmental hazards and determine, through a consensus, which conditions and hazards should have priority in surveillance efforts. While priority setting is always challenging and sometimes contentious, the national experience with the development of health status indicators suggests that such endeavors can be undertaken effectively.[49] That experience also illustrates the need to retain the flexibility to modify priorities over time.

Next, health officials need to identify useful existing data systems, as well as gaps in these data systems that need to be filled by new sources. In addition to the effort to establish health status indicators, the process used by the Occupational and Environmental Health Committee of the Council of State and Territorial Epidemiologists may serve as a model, both for setting priorities and for identifying gaps on existing data systems.[50] Finally, analytic methods to aid in the identification of associations between environmental hazards and adverse health events need to be explored aggressively.[51] Development of this "public health surveillance infrastructure" could produce a coordinated system for preventing and controlling disease, injury, and disability related to the interaction between people and their environment.

❖ About the Authors

Stephen B. Thacker and Donna F. Stroup are with the Epidemiology Program Office, Centers for Disease Control and Prevention, Atlanta, Ga. R. Gibson Parrish is with the National Center for Environmental Health. Centers for Disease Control and Prevention. Henry A. Anderson is with the Wisconsin Department of Health and Social Services, Madison.

REFERENCES

1. Thacker SB, Stroup DF. Future directions of comprehensive public health surveillance and health information systems in the United States. *Am J Epidemiol.* 1994;140: 1–15.

2. Wegman DH. Hazard surveillance. In: Halperin W, Baker EL Jr, eds. *Public Health Surveillance.* New York, NY: Van Nostrand Reinhold Co; 1992:62–75.

3. Centers for Disease Control.

Guidelines for the investigation of clusters. *MMWR.* 1990;39(RR-11): 1–16.

4. Kilbourne EM. Informatics in public health surveillance: current issues and future perspectives. *MMWR.* 1992;41(suppl):91–99.

5. White R. Rappaport S, Lieber K, et al. Children at risk from ozone air pollution—United States, 1991–1993. *MMWR Morb Mortal Wkly Rep.* 1995;44:309–311.

6. Centers for Disease Control and Prevention. Smoking-attributable mortality—Mexico, 1992. *MMWR Morb Mortal Wkly Rep.* 1995;44: 372–381.

7. Centers for Disease Control and Prevention. Serious ocular injuries associated with fireworks—United States, 1990–1994. *MMWR Morb Mortal Wkly Rep.* 1995;44:449–451.

8. Centers for Disease Control and Prevention. Controlling lead toxicity in bridge workers—Connecticut, 1991–1994. *MMWR Morb Mortal Wkly Rep.* 1995;44:76–89.

9. Centers for Disease Control. Cigarette smoking among adults—United States, 1990. *MMWR* 1992; 41:354–355, 361–362.

10. Thacker SB, Stroup DF, Rothenberg RB, Brownson RC. Public health surveillance for chronic conditions: a scientific basis for decisions. *Stat Med.* 1995;14:629–642.

11. Graitcer PL. The development of state and local injury surveillance systems. *J Safety Res.* 1988;18:191–198.

12. Baker EL. Surveillance in occupational health and safety. *Am J Public Health.* 1989;79(suppl):1–63.

13. National Research Council. *Toxicity Testing. Strategies to Determine Needs and Priorities.* Washington, DC: National Academy Press; 1984.

14. Rothman KJ. *Modern Epidemiology.* Boston, Mass: Little Brown & Co Inc; 1986:10–16.

15. Goldman LR, Gomez M, Greenfield S, et al. Use of exposure databases for status and trends analysis. *Arch Environ Health.* 1992;47: 430–438.

16. Holzner CL, Hirsh RB, Perper JB. Managing workplace exposure information. *Am Ind Hyg Assoc J.* 1993;54:15–21.

17. Omenn GS. The role of environmental epidemiology in public policy. *Ann Epidemiol.* 1993;3:319–322.

18. Hulka BS, Wilcosky TC, Griffith JD. *Biological Markers in Epidemiology.* New York, NY: Oxford University Press Inc; 1990.

19. Mueller PW, Paschal DC, Hammel RR, et al. Chronic renal effects in three studies of men and women occupationally exposed to cadmium. *Arch Environ Contam Toxicol.* 1992;23:125–136.

20. Groopman JD, Skipper PL. *Molecular Dosimetry and Human Cancer.* Boca Raton, Fla: CRC Press; 1991.

21. Mage D. A comparison of the direct and indirect methods of human exposure. In: *New Horizons in Biological Dosimetry.* New York, NY: Wiley-Liss; 1991:443–454.

22. *National Air Quality and Emissions Trends Report, 1991.* Research Triangle Park, NC: US Environmental Protection Agency, Office of Air Quality Planning and Standards; 1992. EPA publication 450-R-92-001.

23. Schwartz J. Air pollution and daily mortality in Birmingham, Alabama. *Am J Epidemiol.* 1993;137: 1136–1147.

24. Centers for Disease Control. Air pollution information activities at state and local agencies—United States, 1992. *MMWR Morb Mortal Wkly Rep.* 1993;41:967–969.

25. Centers for Disease Control. Surveillance of children's blood lead levels—United States, 1991. *MMWR.* 1992;41:620–622.

26. Merians D. *Prevalence of Blood Lead Levels for Children, New Mexico 1992.* Santa Fe, NM: New Mexico Department of Health; 1993.

27. Brody DJ, Pirkle JL, Kramer RA, et al. Blood lead levels in the U.S.

population from phase 1 of the Third National Health and Nutrition Examination Survey. *JAMA.* 1994;272:277–283.

28. Edmonds LD, Layde PM, James LM, et al. Congenital malformations surveillance: two American systems. *Int J Epidemiol.* 1981;10: 247–252.

29. Hanson JW, Oakley GP Jr. Spray adhesives and birth defects. *JAMA.* 1976;236:1010.

30. Edmonds LD, Layde PM, Erickson JD. Airport noise and teratogenesis: a negative study. *Arch Environ Health.* 1979;34:243–247.

31. Erickson JD, Mulinare, J, McClain PW, et al. Vietnam veterans' risks for fathering babies with birth defects. *JAMA.* 1984;252:903–912.

32. Centers for Disease Control and Prevention. Asthma—United States, 1982–1992. *MMWR.* 1995; 43:952–955.

33. DeRosa CT, Choudhury H, Peirano WB. An integrated exposure/pharmacokinetic based approach to the assessment of complex exposures. Lead: a case study. *Toxicol Ind Health.* 1991;7:231–248.

34. Daniel K, Sedlis MH, Polk L, et al. Childhood lead poisoning, New York City, 1988. *MMWR.* 1990; 39(SS-4):1–7.

35. Seta JA, Sundin DS, Pederson DH. *National Occupational Exposure Survey: Field Guidelines.* Cincinnati, Ohio: US Dept of Health and Human Services, Public Health Service; 1988. DHHS publication NIOSH 88–106.

36. Schwartz BS, Ford DP, Yodaiken R. Analysis of OSHA inspection data with exposure monitoring and medical surveillance violations. *J Occup Med.* 1992;34:272–278.

37. Briss P, Rosenblum LS. Screening strategies for lead poisoning. *JAMA.* 1993;270:2556–2557. Comment.

38. Lofgren JP, Fowler MS, Payne S, et al. Adult blood lead epidemiology and surveillance—United States, fourth quarter 1994. *MMWR Morb Mortal Wkly Rep.* 1995;44: 286–287.

39. Staes C, Matte T, Staehling N, Rosenblum L, Binder S. Lead poisoning deaths in the United States, 1979 through 1988. *JAMA.* 1995; 273:847–848. Letter.

40. Reilly MJ, Rosenman KD, Watt FC, et al. Surveillance for occupational asthma—Michigan and New Jersey, 1988–1992. *MMWR CDC Surveill Summ.* 1994;43:9–17.

41. Addiss DG, Arrowood MJ, Bartlett ME, et al. Assessing the public health threat associated with waterborne cryptosporidiosis: report of a workshop. *MMWR Morb Mortal Wkly Rep.* 1995;44(RR-6): 1–19.

42. Burke T. Innovative environmental health strategies: meeting tomorrow's challenges. Presented at the 121st Annual Meeting of the American Public Health Association, October 1993, San Francisco, Calif.

43. Public Health Foundation. States report minimal efforts to track environmental diseases. *Public Health Macroview,* 1995;7:4–5.

44. Forbes GI. National recording of environmental incidents in Scotland. *J R Soc Health.* 1993;113:295–297.

45. Ordin DL. Surveillance, monitoring, and screening in occupational health. In: Last JM, Wallace RB, eds. *Public Health & Preventive Medicine.* Norwalk, Conn: Appleton & Lange; 1992.

46. Staes C, Matte T, Copley CG, Flanders D, Binder S. Retrospective study of the impact of lead-based paint hazard remediation on children's blood lead levels in St. Louis, Missouri. *Am J Epidemiol.* 1994;139:1016–1026.

47. Markowitz S. The role of surveillance in occupational health. In: Rom WN, ed. *Environmental and Occupational Medicine.* 2nd ed. Boston, Mass: Little Brown & Co Inc; 1992;19–28.

48. Sporik R, Holgate ST, Platts-Mills TAE, Cogswell JJ. Exposure to house-dust mite allergen and the development of asthma in childhood. *N Engl J Med.* 1990;323:502–507.

49. Centers for Disease Control. Health objectives for the nation. Consensus set of health status indicators for the general assessment of community health status—United States. *MMWR.* 1991;40:449–451.

50. Council of State and Territorial Epidemiologists. *Guidelines: Minimum and Comprehensive State-Based Activities in Occupational Safety and Health.* Washington, DC: Association of State and Territorial Health Officials; 1993.

51. Prentice RL, Thomas D. Methodologic research needs in environmental epidemiology: data analysis. *Environ Health Perspect.* 1993;101:39–48.

❖ Pitfalls of Genetic Testing

RUTH HUBBARD AND R.C. LEWONTIN

Genes have become the preferred way to explain all types of ill health and unwanted behavior. Some of the attributions seem fairly clear-cut, but many are being embraced uncritically and oversold. This situation can be troubling for clinicians, as well as for the general public. It is often hard to be sure that genes do account for someone's complex condition, such as circulatory problems or cancer. But even when such an association seems fairly clear, it is hard to know what practical conclusions to draw. Unfortunately, many of these uncertainties arise from the way genes function, not just from shortcomings of technique.

At present, our increased knowledge about the DNA sequences that constitute genes is transforming the concepts of wild-type, or "normal," genes and their mutations. The relations between such sequences of nucleotides and their clinical manifestations can be complex and unpredictable, even in conditions with mendelian patterns of inheritance. A sequence of bases is designated as the gene "for" a particular trait when it can be correlated with that phenotype, but it turns out that sequences in the same gene can vary considerably from one person to another. The only differences that are acknowledged as mutations, however, are those associated with noticeable consequences. What this means is that a gene (together with its regulatory regions) is simply the locus of the various DNA sequences that are manifested in a trait and its variant forms. This definition does not imply that the appearance of the same trait in different people corresponds to the presence of an identical sequence of DNA bases. Conversely, although the sequence of bases may offer predictive information—in Tay-Sachs disease, for example—in most cases it does not predict the way a trait will be manifested phenotypically, for two reasons.

First, even for the relatively predictable familial conditions that we designate as mendelian traits, the actual nucleotide sequences—the DNA patterns—are much more variable than the phenotypic manifestations. More than 200 different nucleotide variations appear to produce the symptoms of hemophilia B, for example.[1] And of the many variants that constitute what is called the cystic fibrosis gene, some are associated with phenotypically different symptoms, but the symptoms associated with others are indistinguishable.[2]

Conversely, people with the same DNA pattern can have a range of clinical manifestations, or none at all. An example is autosomal dominant retinitis pigmentosa, a condition in which retinal rod cells typically degenerate over time. One form of this condition has been associated with a gene

147

on chromosome 3 that is involved in coding for rhodopsin, the light-sensitive visual pigment of the retinal rods. Currently, changes in about one fifth of the amino acids in this protein have been linked to autosomal dominant retinitis pigmentosa. In one family containing two sisters with the same mutation, however, one is blind, whereas the other (the older one) drives a truck even at night. Furthermore, in both the autosomal dominant and the recessive forms of retinitis pigmentosa, the rod cells do not degenerate at a uniform rate across the entire retina, and some base changes are typically associated with the destruction of only the lower half of the retina.[3,4]

Fortunately for the development of molecular genetics, interest in the field was sparked by what we now realize to be the highly unusual case of sickle cell anemia. The transformation of ordinary hemoglobin into sickle cell hemoglobin (hemoglobin S) depends on a change of only one base in what we call the hemoglobin gene. But the simplicity of this one case may have misled researchers and clinicians so that they expect similarly simple correlations between other DNA sequences and the diseases we associate with them. Even for this mutation, however, there is a considerable range in the expression of sickle cell disease among different people, as well as in the same person at different times. The phenotypes depend on a variety of circumstances, including the concentration of hemoglobin in the blood corpuscles, the degree of hydration, the state of constriction of capillaries, and so on. Another point to bear in mind is that the simplicity of the alterations in the base sequence and hemoglobin associated with sickle cell anemia has not yielded therapeutic benefits. And many DNA variants are involved in another hemoglobinopathy, β-thalassemia.

By current estimates, human beings appear to be heterozygous for about $\frac{1}{10}$ of 1 percent of the nucleotides in their DNA. Assuming that there are about 3 billion nucleotides in human chromosomes, each of us is heterozygous for about 3 million of them, and none of us are homozygous for the sequence of bases in any one gene. Only a small fraction of this nucleotide variation is translated into differences in amino acid sequences, although we cannot be sure that it does not have some other effect. Nor do all differences in amino acid sequences have phenotypic importance.

The conclusion we are forced to accept is that even in the case of so-called simple mendelian variations, the relation between the DNA sequence of a gene and the corresponding phenotype is far from simple. When we move from the relatively rare conditions whose patterns of inheritance follow Mendel's laws (such as cystic fibrosis, phenylketonuria, and Huntington's disease) to the more prevalent and usually late-onset conditions that sometimes have familial components (such as diabetes, coronary heart disease, Alzheimer's disease, and certain cancers), the situation becomes even more complicated. In these diseases, the patterns of transmission are unpredictable and seem to depend on various other factors, be they social, economic, psychological, or biologic. The notion that health or illness can be predicted on the basis of DNA patterns because highly questionable. For each condition, extensive, population-based research would be needed in order to establish the existence and extent of correlations between specific DNA patterns and overt manifestations over time. Furthermore, the correlations are likely to have only a degree of statistical validity, not absolute validity. Therefore, DNA tests cannot usually help clinicians or benefit patients—and not only because the techniques are still inadequate, but also because biologic phenomena result from multiple and complex interactions.

Serious difficulties arise from the relative ease with which information on DNA sequences can be acquired, when adequate knowledge of its correct interpretation is lacking. This can be seen in relation to the so-called breast-cancer genes BRCA1 and BRCA2. These two DNA sequences have both been linked to increased susceptibility to breast or ovarian cancer. To date, more than 100 variants of BRCA1 and several variants of BRCA2 have been identified. Only a few of them, however, have been shown to be associated with tumor growth. They have been found predominantly among the small percentage of women who belong to families in which there is an unusually high incidence of one or both types of cancer or in whom breast cancer develops at an unusually young age. Yet about 90 percent of women with breast or ovarian cancer do not fall into these categories.

We must therefore ask how the predictive tests now being developed on the basis of variants of BRCA1 are relevant to most women. The fact that a woman from a "cancer-prone" family tests positive for one of the cancer-linked DNA variants does not mean that she will definitely have a tumor, even though her lifetime risk of breast cancer may be as high as 85 percent, and that of ovarian cancer as high as 45 percent. Clearly, other factors are also involved. If the woman tests negative for cancer-linked DNA variants, her risk of having a tumor is similar to that of any woman in the general population. Furthermore, it is not clear what a woman should do if she tests positive, whatever her family history, since there are no effective measures of prevention. "Early detection" is problematic because it is uncertain what is actually being detected, and even such extreme measures as "prophylactic" bilateral mastectomy and oophorectomy provide no assurance that a tumor will not develop in the residual tissue. Given the uncertainty of what being "susceptible" signifies, it is hard to know how to counsel women who are trying to decide whether to be tested for a cancer-associated variant of BRCA1. It is also hard to know how to help women integrate the information they may receive from such a test into the context of their lives.[5,6]

Despite the biologic uncertainties and the potential for discrimination and other social and personal problems, biotechnology companies have begun to develop tests for DNA variants thought to be linked to "cancer susceptibilities." OncorMed, a company in Maryland, is marketing tests for BRCA1 and colon cancer directly to physicians. Myriad Genetics in Utah plans to offer a BRCA1 test, at first only for clinical trials conducted by cancer centers, but for commercial purposes later in 1996. Indeed, Dr. Joseph D. Schulman has just announced that his commercial laboratory, the Genetics and I.V.F. Institute of Fairfax, Virginia, will sell women a test for a *BRCA1* variant that appears to occur with unusual frequency among Jews of Eastern European extraction. Although there is no evidence linking this variant to nonfamilial breast or ovarian cancer, Schulman says he is offering the test because women have a right to know whether they carry the variant. At present, the only thing certain is that each test will bring in $295 to Dr. Schulman's company.[7]

These companies are not required to involve the Food and Drug Administration, because they are using their own reagents and performing the tests in their own laboratories. This means, however, that there has been no external certification of the quality of the procedures or the proper way to interpret the results. (Both the American Society for Human Genetics and the National Breast Cancer Coalition, an advocacy organization, are opposed to susceptibility testing outside controlled clinical trials.)

Physicians are soon likely to confront extremely awkward situations. Worried patients, encouraged by overly optimistic claims by researchers, biotechnology companies, and the media, may want to have genetic tests performed whose validity has not been established. At the same time, physicians may legitimately feel at sea about the meaning, reliability, and predictiveness of the tests. For the foreseeable future, perhaps the best they can do is to alert patients about the underlying uncertainty associated with the tests themselves and their actual prognostic value, and to point out that usually no practical consequences can be drawn from the information gained, however the test comes out. In the meantime, the test results can have disastrous implications for the psychological well-being, family relationships, and employability and insurability of those tested. All the same, some people will want to be tested because they want to know whether they carry a particular variant. Recent studies and testimony, however, show that people's decisions about whether to undergo DNA tests often change when they come to understand more about the wider implications of the tests and the uncertain meaning of the results.[8-12]

The ground is shifting almost from week to week. Physicians need to recognize the limitations of the new information and the commercial pressures behind the speed with which preliminary scientific data are being turned into tests. They should also understand the risks to patients of being stigmatized as "susceptible" by insurers or employers, as well as the psychological and social risks patients run by putting excessive faith in predictions of an often very uncertain future.

❖ About the Authors

Ruth Hubbard, Ph.D., is Professor of Bioscience, Harvard University, Cambridge, Massachusetts.

R. C. Lewontin, Ph.D., is Professor, Museum of Comparative Zoology, Harvard University, Cambridge, Massachusetts

REFERENCES

1. Giannelli F, Green PM, High KA, et al. Haemophilia B: database of point mutations and short additions and deletions. Nucleic Acids Res 1990;18:4053-9.
2. The Cystic Fibrosis Genotype-Phenotype Consortium. Correlation between genotype and phenotype in patients with cystic fibrosis. N Engl J Med 1993;329: 1308-13.
3. Papermaster DS. Necessary but insufficient. Nat Med 1995;1:874-5.
4. Humphries P, Kenna P, Farrar GJ. On the molecular genetics of retinitis pigmentosa. Science 1992;256: 804-8.
5. Collins FS, BRCA1—lots of mutations, lots of dilemmas. N Engl J Med 1996;334:186-8.
6. Hoskins KF, Stopfer JE, Calzone KA, et al. Assessment and counseling for women with a family history of breast cancer. JAMA 1995;273:577-85.
7. Kolata G. Breaking ranks, lab offers test to assess risk of breast cancer. New York Times, April 1, 1996:A1, A15.
8. Wertz DC, Janes SR, Rosenfield JM, Erbe RW. Attitudes toward the prenatal diagnosis of cystic fibrosis: factors in decision making among affected families. Am J Hum Genet 1992;50:1077-85.
9. Babul R, Adam S, Kremer B, et al. Attitudes toward direct predictive testing for the Huntington disease gene: relevance for other adult-onset disorders. JAMA 1993;270: 2321-5.
10. Seachrist L. Testing genes: physicians wrestle with the information that genetic tests provide. Science News 1995;148:394-5.
11. Siebert C. Living with toxic knowledge. New York Times Magazine. September 17, 1995;50-7, 74, 93-4, 104.
12. Geller G, Bernhardt BA, Helzlsouer K, Holtzman NA, Stefanek M, Wilcox PM. Informed consent and BRCA1 testing. Nat Genet 1995;11:364.

❖ Chapter 5
Women's Health

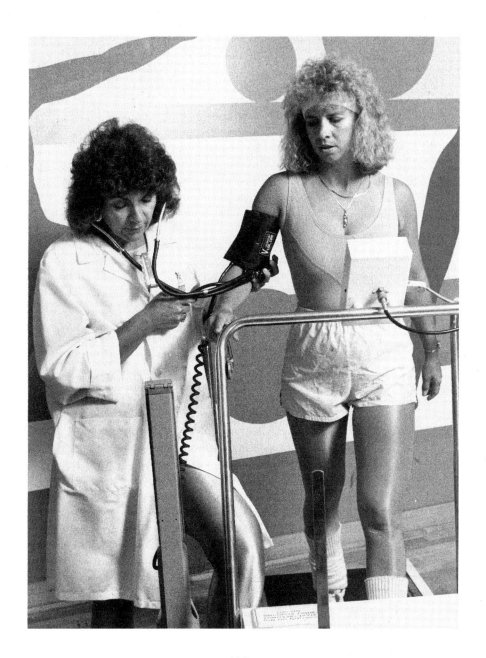

Since the last edition of this book, unprecedented progress has been achieved in the field of women's health and health care in this country. A long-neglected, substantial agenda remains to be addressed, however. Although funding in women's health research at the National Institutes of Health increased from $1.02 billion to $1.56 billion from 1991 to 1994, this amount constituted only 14.2 percent of the Institutes' research budget for 1994 (Society for the Advancement of Women's Health Research, 1996).

We include in this chapter a portion of the statement on women and health from The Beijing Declaration and The Platform for Action to highlight the internationally shared challenges facing women throughout the world. An outcome of the 1995 Fourth World Conference on Women held in Beijing, China, this statement identifies commonly held beliefs about women's rights to health care and it contains a comprehensive set of specific conditions in need of attention. The four strategic objectives for women's health worldwide are: (1) to increase women's access throughout the lifespan to appropriate, affordable, and quality health care, information, and related services; (2) to strengthen preventive programs that promote women's health, (3) to undertake gender-sensitive initiatives that address sexually transmitted diseases, HIV/AIDS, and sexual and reproductive health issues; and (4) to increase resources and monitor follow-up for women's health. Within each of these four objectives, the Action Plan specifies steps to be taken to achieve the objective.

Only relatively recently have any large-scale investigations been initiated in the United States to study and clarify health issues facing women. Three major population investigations currently in progress are the Study of Women's Health Across the Nation, the Nurses' Health Study, and the Women's Health Initiative. The Study of Women's Health Across the Nation is a descriptive, longitudinal study of women (ages 42 to 52 years) sponsored by the National Institute on Aging. It is designed to investigate and compare a broad range of physiological, psychological, psychosocial, and lifestyle influences on the experience of menopause among African-American, Hispanic, Asian-American, and Caucasian women. The Nurses' Health Study, initiated in 1976 with 120,000 women between the ages of 30 and 55, is a comprehensive longitudinal study of women's health and lifestyles. Study results have been widely published and include such notable findings as the associations between obesity and risk of gallstones and excessive sun exposure and risk of melanoma. The Women's Health Initiative (WHI) Clinical Trial and Observational Study, being conducted with 160,000 women at 40 centers around the country, is a descriptive and interventional study designed to address some of the major health concerns for postmenopausal women. It is a long-term study that tests whether specific interventions will decrease the incidence of several acute and chronic conditions suffered by older women.

Roussouw and associates at the National Institutes of Health recently published a comprehensive paper, "The Evolution of the Women's Health

Initiative: Perspectives from the NIH," which we have included in Chapter 5. This paper chronicles the evolution of the WHI from its initial antecedent meetings in the early 1980s to its funding and implementation in 1991. The authors relate details of the planning and feasibility studies conducted around the issues of hormone replacement therapy and optimal diet for postmenopausal women. Although the topic has for many years warranted thorough scientific evaluation, the project was finally legitimately launched as a result of ". . . the confluence of scientific need and capability with the social priorities to improve the health and welfare of women" (Roussow et al., 1995, p. 50). One of its important research goals is to determine if the risk of heart disease and osteoporosis are mediated by postmenopausal hormone supplementation and what potential side effects are attributable to this treatment. The evolution of this landmark research study on a uniquely female life process documents the complexity involved in socio-political processes bringing neglected women's health issues to the forefront of the national health agenda.

In the fourth edition of *The Nation's Health* (1994), we included Rodin and Ickovic's (1990) review of past research and projected future research directions regarding women's health. They identified neglected areas that would required greater research allocations, including women and AIDS, psychopharmacology, substance abuse, hormone replacement therapy, the aging of the female population, and reproductive technologies. The importance of these and other areas of medical research on women's health cannot be understated in the quest to assure personal and public health in the United States.

It is also essential for the women's health research agenda to actively include the study of public policy formulation and implementation in relation to assumptions about the familial division of labor and informal (unpaid) health and long-term care provision (Estes and Close, 1994), the influence of social structure and socioeconomic status on women's opportunities to engage in healthful behaviors and obtain health care (Estes and Rundall, 1992), and the relationship of income, social class, and long-term care insurance to access and utilization of health care and social services among older women (Estes and Close, 1994). We conclude this chapter with "Public Policy and Long Term Care" in which authors Carroll Estes and Liz Close identify salient public policy issues in long-term care and research needs particularly addressing the rapidly growing over-65 population in this country. Specific recommendations focus research attention on structural level issues influencing older women's health, informal care, and long-term health care services research.

Two important recent papers included in the Recommended Reading list address issues of significance in woman's health. The development of FDA regulation of silicone breast implants is explored by Howard Palley in his study of public regulatory policy and women's health issues. Palley (1995) raises consequential questions about medical device risk evaluation prior to unrestricted marketing and the powerful influence of the private corporate sector in the federal regulatory process. This analysis clearly highlights how women's health concerns can take a relatively low priority when the potential for profitability is present and the regulatory process is exploitable. Although recent changes have occurred in the federal regulatory process concerning some of these problems, this paper is instructive both for the study of women's health and for the study of federal regulatory process. The 1995 article by Charles Mann, "Women's Health Research Blossoms," documents the expanding involvement of women in health related research as investigators and as subjects. Unfortunately the historical omission of women subjects from a variety of clinical studies assessing the association of risk factors and disease has resulted in a paucity of information guiding appropriate and timely medical decision-making.

❖ The Beijing Declaration and The Platform for Action
Women and Health
FOURTH WORLD CONFERENCE ON WOMEN
BEIJING, CHINA
4-15 SEPTEMBER 1995

❖ C. Women and Health*

89

Women have the right to the enjoyment of the *highest attainable standard of physical and mental health*. The enjoyment of this right is vital to their life and well-being and their ability to participate in all areas of public and private life. Health is a state of complete physical, mental and social well-being and not merely the absence of disease or infirmity. Women's health involves their emotional, social and physical well-being and is determined by the *social, political* and *economic* context of their lives, as well as by *biology*. However, health and well-being elude the majority of women. A major barrier for women to the achievement of the highest attainable standard of health is inequality, both between men and women and among women in different geographical regions, social classes and indigenous and ethnic groups. In national and international forums, women have emphasized that to attain optimal health throughout the life cycle, *equality*, including the *sharing of family responsibilities, development* and *peace* are necessary conditions.

90

Women have different and unequal access to and *use of basic health resources*, including primary health services for the prevention and treatment of childhood diseases, malnutrition, anaemia, diarrhoeal diseases, communicable diseases, malaria and other tropical diseases and tuberculosis, among others. Women also have different and unequal *opportunities for the protection, promotion and maintenance of their health*. In many developing countries, the lack of emergency obstetric services is also of particular concern. Health policies and programmes often *perpetuate gender stereotypes*

---

*The Holy See expressed a general reservation on this section. The reservation is to be interpreted in terms of the statement made by the representative of the Holy See at the 4th meeting of the Main Committee, on 14 September 1995 (see chap. V of the present report, para. 11).

and fail to consider socio-economic disparities and other differences among women and may not fully take account of the lack of autonomy of women regarding their health. Women's health is also affected by *gender bias* in the health system and by the provision of inadequate and inappropriate medical services to women.

91

In many countries, especially *developing countries,* in particular the least developed countries, a *decrease in public health spending* and, in some cases, *structural adjustment,* contribute to the *deterioration of public health systems.* In addition, *privatization* of health-care systems without appropriate *guarantees of universal access* to affordable health care further reduces health-care availability. This situation not only directly affects the health of girls and women, but also places disproportionate responsibilities on women, whose multiple roles, including their roles within the family and the community, are often not acknowledged; hence they do not receive the necessary social, psychological and economic support.

92

Women's right to the enjoyment of the highest standard of health must be secured throughout the whole *life cycle* in equality with men. Women are affected by many of the same health conditions as men, but women experience them differently. The prevalence among women of poverty and economic dependence, their experience of violence, negative attitudes towards women and girls, racial and other forms of discrimination, the limited power many women have over their sexual and reproductive lives and lack of influence in decision-making are social realities which have an adverse impact on their health. Lack of food and inequitable distribution of food for girls and women in the household, inadequate access to safe water, sanitation facilities and fuel supplies, particularly in rural and poor urban areas, and deficient housing conditions, all overburden women and their families and have a negative effect on their health. Good health is essential to leading a productive and fulfilling life, and the right of all women to control all aspects of their health, in particular their own fertility, is basic to their empowerment.

93

Discrimination against girls, often resulting from son preference, in *access to nutrition* and *health-care services endangers* their current and future health and well-being. Conditions that force girls into early marriage, pregnancy and child-bearing and subject them to harmful practices, such as female genital mutilation, pose grave health risks. Adolescent girls need, but too often do not have, access to necessary health and nutrition services as they mature. *Counselling* and *access to sexual and reproductive health* information and services for adolescents are still inadequate or lacking completely, and a young woman's right to privacy, confidentiality, respect and informed consent is often not considered. Adolescent girls are both biologically and psychosocially more vulnerable than boys to sexual abuse, violence and prostitution, and to the consequences of unprotected and premature sexual relations. The trend towards early sexual experience, combined with a lack of information and services, increases the *risk of unwanted and too early pregnancy, HIV infection and other sexually transmitted diseases, as well as unsafe abortions.* Early child-bearing continues to be an impediment to improvements in the educational, economic and social status of women in all parts of the world. Overall, for young women early marriage and early motherhood can severely curtail educational and employment opportunities and are likely to have a long-term, adverse impact on the quality of their lives and the lives of their children. Young men are often not educated to respect women's self-determination and to share responsibility with women in matters of sexuality and reproduction.

94

Reproductive health is a state of complete physical, mental and social well-being and not merely the absence of disease or infirmity, in all matters relating to the reproductive system and to its functions and processes. Reproductive health therefore implies that people are able to have a satisfying and safe sex life and that they have the capability to reproduce and the freedom to decide if, when and how often to do so. Implicit in this last condition are the right of men and women to be informed and to have access to safe, effective, affordable and acceptable methods of family planning of their choice, as well as other methods of their choice for regulation of fertility which are not against the law, and the right of access to appropriate health-care services that will enable women to go safely through pregnancy and childbirth and provide couples with the best chance of having a healthy infant. In line with the above definition of reproductive health, reproductive health care is defined as the constellation of methods, techniques and services that contribute to reproductive health and well-being by preventing and solving reproductive health problems. It also includes sexual health, the purpose of which is the enhancement of life and personal relations, and not merely counselling and care related to reproduction and sexually transmitted diseases.

95

Bearing in mind the above definition, reproductive rights embrace certain human rights that are already recognized in national laws, international human rights documents and other consensus documents. These rights rest on the recognition of the basic right of all couples and individuals to decide freely and responsibly the number, spacing and timing of their children and to have the information and means to do so, and the right to attain the highest standard of sexual and reproductive health. It also includes their right to make decisions concerning reproduction free of discrimination, coercion and violence, as expressed in human rights documents. In the exercise of this right, they should take into account the needs of their living and future children and their responsibilities towards the community. The promotion of the responsible exercise of these rights for all people should be the fundamental basis for government- and community-supported policies and programmes in the area of reproductive health, including family planning. As part of their commitment, full attention should be given to the promotion of mutually respectful and equitable gender relations and particularly to meeting the educational and service needs of adolescents to enable them to deal in a positive and responsible way with their sexuality. Reproductive health eludes many of the world's people because of such factors as: inadequate levels of knowledge about human sexuality and inappropriate or poor-quality reproductive health information and services; the prevalence of high-risk sexual behaviour; discriminatory social practices; negative attitudes towards women and girls; and the limited power many women and girls have over their sexual and reproductive lives. Adolescents are particularly vulnerable because of their lack of information and access to relevant services in most countries. Older women and men have distinct reproductive and sexual health issues which are often inadequately addressed.

96

The human rights of women include their right to have control over and decide freely and responsibly on matters related to their sexuality, including sexual and reproductive health, free of coercion, discrimination and violence. Equal relationships between women and men in matters of sexual relations and reproduction, including full respect for the integrity of the person, require mutual respect, consent and shared responsibility for sexual behaviour and its consequences.

97

Further, women are subject to particular health risks due to inadequate responsiveness and lack of services to meet health needs related to sexuality and reproduction. Complications related to pregnancy and childbirth are among the leading causes of mortality and morbidity of women of reproductive age in many parts of the developing world. Similar problems exist to a certain degree in some countries with economies in transition. Unsafe abortions threaten the lives of a large number of women, representing a grave public health problem as it is primarily the poorest and youngest who take the highest risk. Most of these deaths, health problems and injuries are preventable through improved access to adequate health-care services, including safe and effective family planning methods and emergency obstetric care, recognizing the right of women and men to be informed and to have access to safe, effective, affordable and acceptable methods of family planning of their choice, as well as other methods of their choice for regulation of fertility which are not against the law, and the right of access to appropriate health-care services that will enable women to go safely through pregnancy and childbirth and provide couples with the best chance of having a healthy infant. These problems and means should be addressed on the basis of the report of the International Conference on Population and Development, with particular reference to relevant paragraphs of the Programme of Action of the Conference.[14] In most countries, the neglect of women's reproductive rights severely limits their opportunities in public and private life, including opportunities for education and economic and political empowerment. The ability of women to control their own fertility forms an important basis for the enjoyment of other rights. Shared responsibility between women and men in matters related to sexual and reproductive behaviour is also essential to improving women's health.

98

HIV/AIDS and other sexually transmitted diseases, the transmission of which is sometimes a consequence of sexual violence, are having a devastating effect on women's health, particularly the health of adolescent girls and young women. They often do not have the power to insist on safe and responsible sex practices and have little access to information and services for prevention and treatment. Women, who represent half of all adults newly infected with HIV/AIDS and other sexually transmitted diseases, have emphasized that social vulnerability and the unequal power relationships between women and men are obstacles to safe sex, in their efforts to control the spread of sexually transmitted diseases. The consequences of HIV/AIDS reach beyond women's health to their role as mothers and caregivers and their contribution to the economic support of their families. The social, developmental and health consequences of HIV/AIDS and other sexually transmitted diseases need to be seen from a gender perspective.

99

Sexual and gender-based violence, including physical and psychological abuse, trafficking in women and girls, and other forms of abuse and sexual exploitation place girls and women at high risk of physical and mental trauma, disease and unwanted pregnancy. Such situations often deter women from using health and other services.

100

Mental disorders related to marginalization, powerlessness and poverty, along with overwork and stress and the growing incidence of domestic violence as well as substance abuse, are among other health issues of growing concern to women. Women throughout the world, especially young women, are increasing their use of tobacco with serious effects on their health and that of their children. Occupational health issues are also growing in importance, as a large number of women work in low-paid jobs in either the formal or the informal labour market under tedious and unhealthy conditions, and the number is rising. Cancers of the breast and cervix and other cancers of the reproductive system, as well as infertility, affect growing numbers of women and may be preventable, or curable, if detected early.

101

With the increase in life expectancy and the growing number of older women, their health concerns require particular attention. The long-term health prospects of women are influenced by changes at menopause, which, in combination with lifelong conditions and other factors, such as poor nutrition and lack of physical activity, may increase the risk of cardiovascular disease and osteoporosis. Other diseases of ageing and the interrelationships of ageing and disability among women also need particular attention.

102

Women, like men, particularly in rural areas and poor urban areas, are increasingly exposed to environmental health hazards owing to environmental catastrophes and degradation. Women have a different susceptibility to various environmental hazards, contaminants and substances and they suffer different consequences from exposure to them.

103

The quality of women's health care is often deficient in various ways, depending on local circumstances. Women are frequently not treated with respect, nor are they guaranteed privacy and confidentiality, nor do they always receive full information about the options and services available. Furthermore, in some countries, women's life events are often treated as medical problems, leading to unnecessary surgical intervention and inappropriate medication.

104

Statistical data on health are often not systematically collected, disaggregated and analyzed by age, sex and socio-economic status and by established demographic criteria used to serve the interests and solve the problems of subgroups, with particular emphasis on the vulnerable and marginalized and other relevant variables. Recent and reliable data on the mortality and morbidity of women and conditions and diseases particularly affecting women are not available in many countries. Relatively little is known about how social and economic factors affect the health of girls and women of all ages, about the provision of health services to girls and women and the patterns of their use of such services, and about the value of disease prevention and health promotion programmes for women. Subjects of importance to women's health have not been adequately researched and women's health research often lacks funding. Medical research, on heart disease, for example, and epidemiological studies in many countries are often based solely on men; they are not gender specific. Clinical trials involving women to establish basic information about dosage, side-effects and effectiveness of drugs, including contraceptives, are noticeably absent and do not always conform to ethical standards for research and testing. Many drug therapy protocols and other medical treatments and interventions administered to women are based on research on men without any investigation and adjustment for gender differences.

105

In addressing inequalities in health status and unequal access to and inadequate health-care services between women and men. Governments and other actors should promote an active and visible policy of mainstreaming a gender perspective in all policies and programmes, so that, before decisions are taken, an analysis is made of the effects for women and men, respectively.

❖ About the Author

"Women and Health" is one of 12 "critical areas of concern" considered to represent the main obstacles to women's advancement throughout the world as identified at the Fourth World Conference on Women (4-15 September 1995) sponsored by the United Nations. It is part of The Beijing Declaration and Platform for Action, adopted unanimously at the conference by representatives from 189 countries, and reflects a new international commitment to the goals of equality, development and peace for all women everywhere.

❖ The Evolution of the Women's Health Initiative: Perspectives from the NIH

Jacques E. Rossouw, Loretta P. Finnegan, William R. Harlan, Vivian W. Pinn, Carolyn Clifford, Joan A. McGowan.

Coronary heart disease is the leading cause of death in women, accounting for about 250,000 deaths every year; women suffer about twice that number of coronary events annually.[1] Breast cancer is the cancer with the greatest incidence and the one with the second highest mortality, after lung cancer. In 1991, approximately 175,000 cases of breast cancer were diagnosed and about 45,000 deaths were attributed to this disease.[1] Colorectal cancer is the third leading cause of cancer deaths among women, with approximately 78,000 new cases diagnosed and about 31,000 deaths reported in 1991.[1] Osteoporotic fractures, while not being a leading cause of mortality, account for much disability and decreased quality of life in older women. It has been estimated that a 50-year-old woman has a 15% chance of suffering a hip fracture during the remainder of her life.[2]

Because of increasing incidence with age, by far the greatest disease burden is borne by women age 50 or more. Postmenopausal estrogen deficiency may contribute to at least two of these conditions, namely coronary heart disease and osteoporosis-related fractures. Reductions in morbidity from these common diseases may translate into substantial improvements in the quality of life of postmenopausal women, and result in major societal benefits if successful treatments are widely adopted by American women. As judged from a range of observational epidemiologic studies, these diseases may be forestalled or ameliorated by dietary, behavioral, and drug interventions. These interventions require testing through clinical trials before the full range of any benefits and risks can be assessed or credible public health recommendations made.

During the 1980s, it became apparent that past research had disproportionately focused on white men, and that less attention had been paid to preventing and treating diseases that are unique to or more common in women. In order to rectify this situation, the National Institutes of Health (NIH) established the Office of Research on Women's Health (ORWH) in 1990.[3] The perception of relative neglect of studies in women set the stage for the announcement of the Women's Health Initiative (WHI), which addresses the prevention of many of the diseases of importance to women, especially postmenopausal women.[4]

The WHI, the largest US prevention study of its kind, has three major components: a cluster of randomized controlled clinical trials of promising but unproven approaches to prevention; an observational study to identify predictors of disease; and a study of community approaches to encourage the development of healthful behaviors. This article will outline the developmental stages of the clinical trial and observational study from an NIH perspective. It will not address in detail the scientific rationale and design of the clinical trial and observational study (manuscript in preparation), but will describe the antecedent research development and planning that led to the adoption of the major design features. The community prevention study, which will test approaches to the implementation of healthful behaviors, is not addressed here as it is still under development.

❖ Antecedents to the WHI

The NIH has been examining the desirability and feasibility of clinical trials to prevent heart disease and breast cancer in women for at least a decade. Preliminary planning for the WHI was conducted over many years in individual NIH institutes and involved institute staff and outside scientists (see Figure). The growing scientific interest in studies of women coincided with an increasing societal awareness of the need to enhance research of health problems unique to women (see Table 1). It was this conjunction of scientific interest and changing societal priorities that, by 1991, made the launching of the WHI both desirable and possible.

Hormone Replacement Therapy to Prevent Coronary Heart Disease

Starting in the mid-1980s, the National Heart, Lung, and Blood Institute (NHLBI) hosted a number of meetings to consider a trial of hormone replacement therapy (HRT) for prevention of coronary heart disease (CHD). In 1986, a Trans-NIH Working Group concluded that there was not enough information to make a realistic assessment of the long-term risks and benefits of HRT, but that the epidemiologic data were sufficiently promising to justify a clinical trial of HRT's ability to prevent cardiovascular events and fractures. The Working Group concluded that to be truly valuable, a large-scale multicenter trial should have clinical outcomes as the goal rather than intermediate physiologic or morphologic outcomes, such as lipid changes or tissue dysplasia.

However, the Working Group was uncertain about how to recruit and retain women for such a study; the selection of drugs to be tested; the use or nonuse of progestins; the dosage, pattern, and route of administration; and mechanisms of action. In addition, there was concern about cost. Therefore, it was the general consensus of the Working Group that the NIH should support a feasibility study to evaluate and compare various approaches to estrogen (ERT) and estrogen in combination with progestins (PERT).

Hormone Replacement Therapy

1986	Trans-NIH Working Group recommends feasibility study of HRT
1987	Postmenopausal Estrogen/Progestin Intervention (PEPI) funded
1989	PEPI recruitment commences
1990	NHLBI Working Group on Estrogen Replacement/CHD trials recommends primary prevention trial
	NHLBI develops contract proposal for primary/secondary prevention trial
1991	Investigator-initiated grant application for secondary prevention trial not funded by NHLBI, but is subsequently funded by pharmaceutical company as Heart and Estrogen/ Progestin Replacement Study (HERS)

Dietary Modification

1984	NCI funds Feasibility Phase of Women's Health Trial (WHT)
1988	NCI makes decision not to proceed to full scale WHT
1989	Investigator-initiated grant application for DIET-FIT not funded by NCI
1990	NCI/NHLBI workshop recommends full scale diet trial
	NCI decides more feasibility studies needed
1991	Women's Health Trial-Feasibility Studies in Minority Populations (WHT-FSMP) funded as contract

Development of WHI

1991	Dr. Bernadine Healy announces Women's Health Initiative, to incorporate hormone and dietary studies
	Trans-NIH Working Groups formed to plan WHI studies
	Concept WHI CT/OS presented to public hearings, modifications made
	WHI Program Office established
1992	Concept approval of WHI CT/OS by non-NIH panel
	Request for Proposals issued for CCC and VCCs
	CCC funded
1993	VCCs (16) funded
	Recruitment commences
	IOM report
1994	Resolution of IOM concerns
	Additional clinical centers (24) funded

Timeline for scientific planning of WHI

This latter recommendation led to NIH funding of the Postmenopausal Estrogen/Progestin Intervention (PEPI) study in 1987. PEPI was designed to test the effects of estrogen alone and estrogen in combination with one of three progestin regimens on blood lipids, clotting factors, blood pressure, glucose homeostasis, and an array of additional physiologic and morphologic outcomes in 875 women over a period of three years. Recruitment commenced in 1989, and the results were announced in November 1994. Even before the results were made known, the PEPI experience was invaluable to the planning and execution of WHI. PEPI demonstrated that it is feasible to recruit and retain women in a clinical trial of HRT; many (but

TABLE 1 Timeline of Societal Priorities for Women's Health Research

1983	Public Health Service Task Force on Women's Health Issues established
1985	Task Force recommends expansion of research on women's health
1986	NIH establishes policy to encourage inclusion of women in research studies
1990	General Accounting Office report that NIH policy was not being fully implemented
	Congressional hearings on women's health research
	NIH Office of Research on Women's Health established
1991	NIH strengthens inclusion of women in research
1993	Congress mandates ORWH and legislates the inclusion of women and minorities in clinical research
1994	NIH issues new guidelines for the inclusion of women and minorities in clinical research

not all) of the PEPI operational procedures have been adopted in WHI. Two of the PEPI regimens have also been adopted in WHI: conjugated equine estrogen 0.625 mg daily alone and conjugated equine estrogen 0.625 mg daily plus medroxyprogesterone 2.5 mg daily.

By 1990, interest in a clinical outcome trial had grown even more intense. In June 1990, the Food and Drug Administration declined to approve estrogen for the prevention of heart disease, primarily because of the lack of evidence from clinical trials. On August 17, 1990, a Working Group on Estrogen Replacement/CHD trials was convened by the NHLBI. The Working Group included leading non-NIH scientists and was chaired by Bernadine Healy, MD, (from the Cleveland Clinic at the time). The Working Group believed it was time to move forward with a clinical outcome trial. The highest level of enthusiasm was for a widely generalizable primary prevention trial in older women from the general population (as opposed to high-risk women). The next levels of enthusiasm were for a secondary prevention trial with clinical outcomes and for trials using angiographic outcomes.

Given this encouragement from the scientific community, during the latter part of 1990 and early 1991, the NHLBI prepared a proposal to commence a trial of ERT and PERT in older women from the general population (the HRT-CVD Trial). While still having a primary prevention focus, the proposed study extended the generalizability by including women with prevalent cardiovascular disease. This proposal had been approved at all levels of review but was put on hold when, on April 9, 1991, Dr. Bernadine Healy took office as NIH director and shortly thereafter (April 19, 1991), introduced her plans for a Women's Health Initiative to legislators on Capitol Hill. Her plan included a study of the effects of HRT in postmenopausal women. The HRT-CVD trial design with some modifications has been integrated into the WHI as the HRT component.

Between the meeting of the Working Group and the announcement of WHI, an investigator-initiated proposal for a secondary prevention trial of HRT was submitted to the NHLBI. This proposal did not receive a fundable score at primary peer review in February 1991, but with modification was subsequently funded by a pharmaceutical company (Wyeth-Ayerst) as the Heart and Estrogen/Progestin Replacement Study (HERS). HERS randomized 2,763 women with established coronary disease to either combined estrogen (conjugated equine estrogen 0.625 mg daily) and progestin (medroxyprogesterone 2.5 mg daily) or placebo.

Low-fat Dietary Pattern to Prevent Breast Cancer

In 1984, the National Cancer Institute (NCI) made five awards for a feasibility phase of the Women's Health Trial (WHT) of low-fat dietary pattern to prevent breast cancer. The study of 303 women demonstrated that women could be recruited into the trial and that compliance with the low-fat dietary pattern over two years appeared to be good. Beginning in 1986, an initial 1,761 women were randomized into the full-scale trial. Early in 1988, however, the NCI, acting on the recommendations of the Division of Cancer Prevention and Control Board of Scientific Counselors (DCPC-BSC) and the National Cancer Advisory Board (NCAB), decided not to go forward with the full-scale trial. The reasons given for this decision included doubts about the strength of the rationale, the ability of the study to test the hypothesis, the actual as opposed to self-reported compliance with the dietary intervention, and the lack of biochemical markers for dietary compliance.

Two years later, in 1990, an investigator-initiated grant application by the WHT investigators for a full-scale trial received a borderline fundable score on peer review, but was not funded by NCI, primarily because of the high cost. NCI was acting on the advice of its DCPC-BSC and NCAB. The proposed study (Dietary Fat Intervention Trial for Disease Prevention in Women, or DIET-FIT) would have tested the effect of low-fat dietary pattern on a combination of cancer outcomes (breast, colon, rectum, ovary, endometrium), as well as on CHD and total mortality. The proposal called for 24,000 women to be randomized to dietary intervention or to current diet. The combined outcome decreased the sample size required and hence the cost of the trial, in comparison to the much larger sample size required to test the effect of dietary pattern on breast or colorectal cancer individually.

In July 1990, a workshop convened jointly by the NCI and the NHLBI concluded that a full-scale dietary intervention trial aimed at cancer and cardiovascular disease prevention in women was feasible and of high priority. The workshop endorsed the concept of testing a dietary pattern (low fat, high fruit and vegetables, high grains and cereals) that might have benefits for prevention of both cancer and cardiovascular disease. Accordingly, in collaboration with NHLBI, the NCI prepared a concept contract proposal for a full-scale trial that was subsequently approved by the DCPC-BSC. However, in an unusual development, the NCAB overturned the decision of the DCPC-BSC. In doing so, the NCAB noted concerns about cost, control group drift, and the ability of elderly women to keep records. It also noted more information was needed on the feasibility of the dietary intervention in minority women and recommended that another feasibility study be undertaken. NCI staff took up the challenge to test the generalizability of the dietary intervention and in 1991 launched the WHT-Feasibility Study in Minority Populations (WHT-FSMP) in three clinical centers. This study will present its findings in 1995, but preliminary data indicate that it is possible to recruit and retain black and Hispanic women in a trial of a low-fat dietary pattern. The dietary modification program developed in the original WHT and refined in WHT-FSMP has been adopted, with minor modifications, as the current WHI dietary modification program.

Societal Priorities for Women's Health Research

Over the same time frame as the events described above, other events led to placing an increasingly higher priority on women's health research within NIH. In 1983, the Public Health Service Task Force on Women's Health Issues was established, and in 1985 its report recommended that biomedical and behavioral research should be expanded to ensure emphasis on conditions and diseases unique to or more prevalent in women of all age groups. In 1986, the NIH adopted a policy to encourage investigators to include women in research studies.

A request by the Congressional Caucus on Women's Issues to the General Accounting Office led to a report asserting that NIH policy was not being fully or uniformly implemented by grant applicants and NIH staff. During 1990, a number of Congressional hearings on research in women's health were held, and the process culminated in a strengthening of NIH guidelines such that, since 1991, all grant applications and contract proposals for clinical research have had to include women, whenever appropriate, in order to be considered for funding. The hearings also led to the establishment of the ORWH at NIH in September 1990. The ORWH is charged with strengthening and enhancing research related to diseases, disorders, and conditions that affect women and ensuring the inclusion of women in clinical studies.[3] Ruth Kirschstein, MD, then director of the National Institute of General Medical Sciences, had a principal leadership role for NIH in these early efforts and was named acting director of the ORWH until Vivian Pinn, MD, was named director in November 1991. As deputy director of NIH, Dr. Kirschstein has continued her advocacy for and involvement in women's health issues.

Continuing legislative and public concerns led to language in the NIH Revitalization Act of 1993 mandating the ORWH and legislating the inclusion of women and minorities in clinical studies. This Act specified that in future Phase III clinical trials funded by NIH, women and minorities must be included in numbers adequate to allow for valid analyses of differences in intervention effect.[3] Strengthened NIH inclusion guidelines were published in 1994 and apply to fiscal year 1995 grants and contracts. Strong support for research on women from the Congressional Caucus on Women's Issues has continued, and this supportive climate improved the feasibility of obtaining funding for large-scale studies on women's health.

❖ Specific Planning for WHI CT/OS

The specific planning for what was to become the WHI CT/OS started in 1991 with the appointment of Dr. Bernadine Healy as director of NIH. On April 19, 1991, she announced her plan for the "Women's Health Initiative." To assure that the study would not detract support from existing studies related to women's health and to encourage cross-institute collaboration, discrete funding was requested through the Office of the Director, rather than from specific institutes. Her proposal was well received, and from 1992 onward, funding for the program has been obtained from Congress as a separate line item.

A period of intense activity followed Dr. Healy's announcement. On April 26, 1991, she established a WHI Executive Committee to advise her. The committee was co-chaired by William Raub, MD, (Office of the Director, NIH) and Dr. Ruth Kirschstein (acting director, ORWH), with the directors of ten NIH institutes/centers as members. The scientific planning was assigned to William Harlan, MD, of NHLBI and Peter Greenwald, MD, of NCI as co-chairs of the Technical and Scientific Working Groups. In August 1991, Dr. Harlan moved from NHLBI to the Office of the Director (as associate director for disease prevention) and the planning and operational focus shifted to the Office of the Director.

Working groups for the CT and the OS were formed including the NIH staff who originally planned the NHLBI HRT-CVD study and the NCI WHT, as well as experts in clinical trials, epidemiology, statistics, gynecology, nutrition, geriatrics, cardiology, and bone metabolism from ten NIH institutes and centers. The working group met on a weekly basis from April to September 1991 and prepared first the concept and then the detailed plans for clinical trials of HRT and of low-fat diet (dietary modification, or DM).

The group proposed a partial factorial design as the most cost-efficient means of studying both these interventions. The cost efficiency arises out of the fact that a proportion of women would participate in both trials, thus reducing the overall number of participants and the number of clinical centers. Major cost savings were derived from having one (smaller) set of clinics engaged in two trials, as the fixed costs of setting up and maintaining clinics are often responsible for 30% of the overall costs. The trial of calcium and vitamin D to prevent osteoporotic fractures was added as a third intervention in the same participants, as it would yield valuable additional information at a very low incremental cost.

A trial of antioxidants (rather than calcium and vitamin D) was considered but rejected because other NIH- and industry-sponsored trials of antioxidants had already been launched or were in the planning stage. The working group for the observational study, meeting over the same time frame, prepared detailed proposals for biomarker studies to predict future disease in women. During the planning process, outside expert groups were consulted on specific design issues for each component of the study.

During the latter part of this intensive planning period, the working groups (with input from outside epidemiology consultants) recommended that the CT and OS be integrated. Women screened for but not enrolled in the CT by reason of ineligibility or unwillingness would be offered participation in the OS. On October 17, 1991, the NIH Executive Committee of the WHI reviewed the design plan and cost estimates and recommended that the design be finalized and that preparations to issue the request for proposals (RFP) proceed.

On October 28-29, 1991, the rationale and concept design (the prospectus) for the CT/OS were presented at a public hearing. A number of changes were made to the study plan as a result of the comments collected from scientists and women's health advocates at the public hearing. For example, concerns about feasibility were addressed by introducing the concept of a vanguard phase during which a smaller number of experienced clinics would test and refine the study plan and by decreasing the sample size needed for the DM component (by screening out subjects who were already consuming less fat at baseline). The behavioral/health quality of life component was expanded. Inclusion of diverse populations would be assured by a plan to allocate a proportion of the contracts to centers that would recruit mainly minorities.

Concept review of the study prospectus was conducted by a group of ten non-NIH experts on January 15, 1992. The panel reviewed the revised concept proposal (including detailed statistical power calculations), a set of four consultant reports, and a synopsis of comments from the public hearing of October 28-29, 1991. The panel recommended some changes in details and gave concept approval for the overall proposed CT/OS study plan. From this point on, the working group prepared a detailed draft protocol that was to form the basis for the development of the eventual RFP.

❖ Implementation

By the end of 1991, the WHI Program Office had been set up in the Office of Disease Prevention and a project officer for the CT/OS had been appointed. The project officer prepared a request for contracts for the WHI Central Coordinating Center (CCC), which had passed through all the relevant NIH reviews by late February 1992. The RFP was issued on March 17, 1992, and by late September 1992, the Fred Hutchinson Cancer Research Center had been awarded the CCC contract. The RFP for the Vanguard Clinical Centers (VCC) was issued on April 29, 1992, and the initial 16 VCC contracts were awarded in March 1993. Further modifications of the draft protocol were jointly made by the CCC and Program Office between September 1992 and March 1993. These modifications included, with permission, those suggested during the selection process by a majority of the potential VCC investigators. They included decisions to introduce the calcium-vitamin D component to women one year after initial enrollment in either the HRT or DM components, and to randomize women who had had hysterectomies to ERT or placebo only (no PERT), while maintaining the three-way randomization to ERT, PERT, or placebo in women with an intact uterus. Recruitment of participants started on schedule in September 1993.

The WHI Program Advisory Committee (WHIPAC) met for the first time on April 28, 1993, and the WHI Data and Safety Monitoring Board (DSMB) on June 16, 1993. The memberships of both these bodies were drawn from outside NIH. WHIPAC advises the NIH director on public perceptions and concerns about WHI, while the DSMB advises on protocol issues, study integrity, plans to monitor the study, participant safety, and makes recommendations for stopping.

Congressional concerns that the cost of the program would escalate beyond that initially projected led to a directive dated July 23, 1992 that NIH contract with the Institute of Medicine (IOM) to make an assessment of the cost of WHI and the reliability of the results likely to be obtained. In October 1993, the IOM committee recommended that the study could continue, but at the same time noted concerns about breast cancer as the primary outcome for the DM component, the duration of the overall study, the informed consent for the HRT component, and the adequacy of the estimated budget.[5]

A position document responding to these concerns was prepared by the NIH and the WHI investigators and endorsed by WHIPAC and the DSMB. A series of briefings by NIH staff, IOM staff, and WHI investigators was held with Congressional staff to discuss the IOM concerns. A final meeting was held on February 11, 1994 to brief the new director of NIH, Harold Varmus, MD, on the IOM concerns and the proposed NIH response. At that meeting, key IOM committee members and key WHI investigators reached agreement that the concerns regarding study duration, informed consent, and cost had been addressed. The IOM committee members and the WHI investigators did not agree on whether breast cancer or coronary heart disease should be the primary outcome of the DM component. After considering the meeting summary and the recommendations of the various participants, Dr. Varmus, in testimony to Congress, endorsed the continuation of WHI as designed. The final outcome was that Congress endorsed continuation of the WHI CT/OS as designed.

❖ Summary of WHI CT/OS

The randomized controlled clinical trial component of the WHI will enroll approximately 63,000 postmenopausal women 50 to 79 years of age. This trial has three interventions, and women may enroll in one or more of the intervention components. The essential features of the design are shown in Table 2.

The first intervention component will evaluate the effect of a low-fat dietary pattern on prevention of breast and colorectal cancer and coronary heart disease (n=48,000 women). The second will examine the effect of HRT (ERT and PERT) on the prevention of coronary heart disease and osteoporotic fractures (n=25,000 women). The third will evaluate the effect of calcium and vitamin D supplementation on the prevention of osteoporotic fractures and colorectal cancer (n=45,000 women).

The trial is scheduled to entail a four-year period for protocol development and recruitment, nine years of follow-up to achieve the goals, and two years for data analysis. Women who are ineligible or unwilling to participate in the trial will be offered the opportunity to enroll in the concurrent OS that delineates new risk factors and biological markers for diseases in women. It is expected that 100,000 women will join this part of the study. Thus, a total of approximately 163,000 women will be studied over time.

The CT and OS will be performed at 40 WHI clinical centers located throughout the United States, with a single clinical coordinating center to manage data collection and analysis. The broad geographic distribution of

TABLE 2   Design of Women's Health Initiative Clinical Trial and Observational Study

Component	Primary Outcome(s)	Secondary Outcomes	Number of Participants
Hormone Replacement Therapy	coronary heart disease	combined fractures	25,000*
Dietary Modification	breast cancer colorectal cancer	coronary heart disease	48,000*
Calcium and Vitamin D	hip fractures	combined fractures colorectal cancer	45,000*
Observational Study	various	various	100,000

*Women may be eligible for both the HRT and DM trials. Assuming a 16% overlap, the total number of participants is estimated to be 63,000. It is assumed that ±5% of the women enrolled in one of the above trials will subsequently be enrolled in the Calcium and Vitamin D trial.

the clinical centers allows for recruitment in medically undeserved areas and targets minority populations across the country, in order to obtain a cross-section of the US population. Ten of the clinical centers will recruit primarily minority populations—African-Americans, Hispanics, Asian-Americans/Pacific Islanders, and Native Americans. Women from all racial/ethnic groups are encouraged to participate in the study.

❖ Current Status

By the end of September 1994, the experience gained during the vanguard phase and the input from investigators had allowed the WHI protocol and the manual of operating procedures to be finalized. By the end of December 1994, the 16 VCCs had performed more than 78,000 clinic visits and had randomized more than 7,3000 participants. Studywide, DM recruitment was at 88% of cumulative goal and catch up was occurring at about 3% per month, and HRT recruitment was at 72% with similar rates of catch up. At current catch-up rates, the VCC recruitment is conservatively projected to be at 100% by September 1995, with more than one year of recruitment still remaining (three-year total recruitment).

In September 1994, the final set of 24 clinical centers was added; these clinical centers commenced recruitment in February 1995, to continue through January 1998. Recruitment for the OS was delayed until September 1994, awaiting approval of study questionnaires from the Office of Management and Budget. The calcium-vitamin D component commenced in December 1994 (one year after initial randomization into either the DM or HRT components). A regional management system has been developed to manage the study in a most efficient manner. The new clinical centers will be mentored by the existing clinics though participation in the regional meetings and a "buddy system" by which each new center is aligned with one of the nearby VCCs.

❖ Discussion

The experience gained thus far has demonstrated that the overall plan for the WHI CT is feasible and that women are interested in joining a clinical trial of DM and/or HRT. The trial is proceeding on time and on budget.

There are many potential reasons for the relatively smooth start-up of this large and complex study, only some of which are apparent at this early juncture. However, these reasons have to include the extensive preliminary planning, followed by one year of intensive focused planning by a committed group of trans-NIH staff, input from the research community, the experience gained from feasibility studies for both the DM and HRT components, and the wealth of talent and experience brought into the study implementation by the WHI investigators. Finally, it is clear that older women are very enthusiastic about this study, so that early concerns about recruitment have not been realized.

Many of the design features of the final protocol had been anticipated by the working groups, which met from the mid-1980s on. For example, testing both ERT and PERT; recruitment from the general population to maximize generalizability; treatment duration of about ten years to test prolonged exposure; a factorial design allowing the testing of other interventions in the same study population; measurement of multiple outcomes including disease and biobehavioral outcomes; evaluating the overall benefit and risk of an intervention; and use of the screens for the trial as an observational cohort. Also, the choice of HRT interventions and monitoring procedures in WHI were influenced by the PEPI protocol, while the DM intervention is directly descended from the WHT. The WHI study plan will continue to be refined as new knowledge becomes available. For example, following publication of the PEPI results, the protocol was changed so that women with intact uterus would no longer be randomized to unopposed ERT.

In summary, WHI is the culmination of many years of scientific planning and preparation. This was a time during which the science matured and confidence in the ability to perform large and complex studies grew. The components of WHI were about to be tested, or were likely to be tested in the near future. At the same time, WHI had the benefit of a growing societal interest in resolving issues of women's health. The convergence of the scientific and societal momentum, together with the catalytic appointment of Dr. Healy as NIH director, led to an integration of the component studies and an accelerated timeline for implementation. The results of these studies will answer important questions affecting the lives of millions of women and will yield a rich harvest of information and ideas beyond those that can be imagined at present. The answers to the primary design questions will be available by the year 2007. That may seem a long time to wait; however, these are questions relevant to the entire life-span of older women. It is likely that this study will only be done once, and all concerned with WHI are determined that it be done right.

❖ About the Author

All of the authors are with NIH. Dr. Roussow is a project officer with the Women's Health Initiative Clinical Trial and Observational Study and Dr. Finnegan is director of the WHI. Dr. Harlan is director of the Office of Disease Prevention, Dr. Pinn is director of the Office of Research on Women's Health, Dr. Clifford is chief of the Diet and Cancer Branch, Division of Cancer Prevention and Control, National Cancer Institute, and Dr. McGowan is director of Bone Biology and Bone Diseases Branch of the National Institute of Arthritis and Musculoskeletal and Skin Diseases.

REFERENCES

1. National Center for Health Statistics: *Vital Statistics of the United States,* vol II, Part B. DHSS Public Health Service publication No. (PHS) 90-1102. Washington, DC: US Government Printing Officer; 1990.

2. Black DM, Cummings SR, Genant K, et al: Axial and appendicular bone mineral and a woman's life time risk of hip fracture. *J Bone Min Res* 1992;7:633-638.

3. Pinn VW: The role of the NIH's Office of Research on Women's Health. *Acad Med* 1994;69:698-702.

4. Healy proposes historical Women's Health Initiative. *The NIH Record.* May 14, 1991; p4.

5. Thaul S, Hocra D: *An Assessment of the NIH Women's Health Initiative: Institute of Medicine.* Washington, DC: National Academy Press; 1993.

❖ Public Policy and Long-Term Care

CARROLL L. ESTES AND LIZ CLOSE

The research agenda concerning health status, health promotion, and disease prevention in the elderly is well documented (IOM, 1991). In contrast, there is a dearth of empirical work on the effects on older and disabled persons of public policy concerning the organization, financing, and delivery of long-term care (LTC). The growing health care burden of the disabled and socially dependent older population (Kunkel & Applebaum, 1992; Manton & Suzman, 1992) emphasizes the urgency of addressing this issue despite the recent finding that the magnitude of disability rates among the elderly decreased slightly in the last decade (Manton, Corder, & Stallard, 1993).

Within the existing social structure, inequities in access to health care occur across the lifespan (Estes & Rundall, 1992). The complex and dynamic relationships between the need for and utilization of formal and informal long-term care are not yet clearly explicated. It has been argued that public policy tends to reflect and preserve existing inequalities in the social structure, particularly the relative positions of advantage and disadvantage that are structured along racial, ethnic, gender, and class lines (Estes, 1979). The existence and effects of such potential policy bias will neither be illuminated by research, nor eliminated by social policy unless scientific inquiry focuses sharply on understanding the social structures and social processes that impede access to a quality life.

Science continues to identify, analyze, and suggest remedies for specific organic diseases as well as some behavioral ills. Much less research attention, however, has been given to explicating the societal mechanisms and sociocultural forces that might explain the origin, manifestation, acceleration, and prevention of specific diseases and chronic conditions endemic to certain population groups. Many of these "individual" diseases and chronic conditions may be mediated more by life course experience associated with sociostructural location than by genetic, biological, or even behavioral factors. Thus the capacity of science to inform public policy is contingent on well-designed research that explicitly addresses the sociostructural dimensions of health and the effects of differential access to resources (including health and long-term care) across the life course.

This chapter briefly reviews the interplay of major societal forces shaping public policy and long-term care, highlights current knowledge about selected social issues, and suggests specific knowledge that is needed to assist in the design of long-term care policy with special focus on a research agenda that will address policy considerations attentive to racial, ethnic, gender, and social class differences.

❖ Societal Forces Shaping Public Policy

Public policy and long-term care are shaped by the confluence of four societal forces: sociodemographic changes, the biomedicalization of aging, unresolved problems concerning health care access and costs, and dependency (Estes, Swan, & Associates, 1993).

Demographic changes reviewed in earlier chapters indicate several trends relevant to the influences of population dynamics on policy decisions concerning long-term care in the United States. By the mid-twenty-first century, as a result of the rapidly increasing over-65 (and particularly over-85) population group, the need for long-term care (for both home care and nursing home care) will at least triple and associated costs will increase tenfold (Rice, 1986; Taeuber, 1992). There will no doubt be absolute increases in the need for long-term care since even the most optimistic declines in disability rates "do not wholly compensate for population aging" (Manton et al., 1993, p. 5164). Notably, increasing "population frailty" (Verbrugge, 1989) and increasing life expectancy but worsening health (Brody, Brock, & Williams, 1987; McKinlay, McKinlay, & Beaglehole, 1989; Verbrugge, 1991) combine to place an extraordinary demand on the long-term care system in the future. Regardless of the specific forecasting model used, the predicted increase in the elderly population raises ominous issues (Kunkel & Applebaum, 1992).

The biomedicalization of aging has significantly influenced research and the development of a knowledge base in the field of aging (Estes, 1979; Estes & Binney, 1989; Estes et al., 1993). The tendency to focus on individual organic pathology amenable to medical intervention has resulted in the conceptualization of old age as a disease, aging as a medical problem, and palliation of the aging process as a venerable goal.

The unrelenting issues of health care costs and access—compounded by gaps in private insurance protection and negligible long-term care insurance coverage—render quality of life for elderly in the future increasingly problematic (Estes et al., 1993). Out-of-pocket expenses for health care consume increasingly larger proportions of the elderly's disposable retirement income because Medicare currently covers less than one-half of the cost of their health care. Recent Congressional budget agreements add more than $10 billion to out-of-pocket Medicare beneficiary costs by 1996 (U.S. Senate Special Committee on Aging, 1991). Health care costs have become particularly burdensome to older women who pay as much as 42% of their annual income for medical expenses not covered by Medicare (Families, USA, 1992; ICF, 1985).

The life chances of elders (mortality, disability, chronic illness, and self-reported health) are strongly influenced by gender, race, ethnic status, and social class (Estes & Rundall, 1992). Recent research indicates that age related-disease and disability among the elderly is related to cumulative exposure to risk rather than simply to aging per se (Manton & Suzman, 1992). Long-term care policy and associated research should be informed by and attentive to the nature, extent, and effects of persistent risk exposure associated with the sociostructural characteristics of populations. Dependency and the contribution of social policy and practice (e.g., age discrimination) induce more dependency, which reflects a major potential problem. The medical and high-tech approach to care of older persons, as well as declining access to health care, further exacerbate the sense of loss of personal control and elder dependency.

As a result of multiple changes occurring in the past decade, the system of community-based services has been challenged, weakened, and transformed (Estes et al., 1993). Public policy simultaneously financed the medicalization of care (Estes & Binney, 1989), challenged the charitable impulse in nonprofit service delivery through cost containment and competition, and indirectly fostered the dependency of elders through its major long-term care policy—the impoverishment and institutionalization of elders who need extensive long-term care and are not covered for it under Medicare.

The research agenda in public policy and long-term care calls for investigation of the continuing interplay of various societal forces in the social production of a dependent elderly population and the attendant challenges to traditional structures of long-term care. The process by which older persons are empowered in their own care involves active participation in decisions concerning their care and the accumulation of knowledge and skills to make informed choices (Estes et al., 1993). Governmental, organizational, and professional structures, as well as societal norms, that facilitate or impede progress toward the goal of empowerment need to be thoroughly explicated. Kunkel and Applebaum (1992) urge a research focus that examines new structural models for the delivery of long-term care; the priority research areas presented in this chapter support and resound this recommendation.

❖ Illustrative Research Problems Related to LTC and Aging

One difficulty for research is that projections of long-term care (LTC) needs in the U.S. are largely based on current patterns of availability and utilization of existing LTC resources. Problems arise from projecting need based on the present service delivery system rather than on theoretically and empirically derived hypothetical models of alternative policies. Examples of problematic assumptions that need to be examined in future research are that the family is the appropriate (and most desirable)

LTC provider in the community; that women's labor force participation does not interfere with the informal LTC that women provide; that there will be no erosion in the need for long-term care regardless of scientific advances in aging; and that public opinion is likely to remain stable regardless of the mismatch between chronic care needs and acute care policy. Priority areas of inquiry address these interrelated assumptions and include: research on older women and their health across the lifespan, informal care system costs and benefits, factors determining the need for and utilization of long-term care services, and the effects and effectiveness of various long-term care policy options. Research on the effects of policy intervention needs to investigate questions regarding the role of social policies in alleviating, as well as creating, dependency.

Older Women and Health

Although females are the majority of persons 65 years of age and older and they are the great majority of persons over 85, research on older women and their health issues is underdeveloped. The fact that most research on health has been on males is acknowledged in the recent establishment of the National Institute of Health (NIH) Office of Research on Women's Health (Kirschstein, 1991). Older women are a vulnerable population about whom relatively little is known. For example, little is known about how risk factors vary for older women or how gender roles and life experiences of men and women are associated with different health effects. Rodin and Ickovics (1990) have identified several factors that are likely to differentially affect men's and women's health in old age including sociostructural conditions that promote continuing imbalances in role expectations related to work and family and concomitantly in power, equality, and control. Key issues also pertain to women's patterns of health care access and utilization. These include observations that women account for 70% of all psychoactive drug prescriptions (Lipton & Lee, 1989); two-thirds of all surgical procedures (Travis, 1988); limited use of certain kinds of medical technologies (e.g., cardiac catheterization), yet the high use of others (e.g., reproductive technologies); and relatively restricted access to health insurance (Rodin & Ickovics, 1990).

The differing sociodemographic profiles of older women and men raise additional questions about both health status and access to health care that are extremely important for the formulation of public policy and long-term care. Although women in the United States live an average of 8 years longer than men, evidence strongly suggests they live those years in poorer health due to the high incidence of disability associated with chronic conditions and the higher incidence and prevalence of acute fatal diseases among men (Verbrugge, 1991). Older women also have higher rates of institutionalization than older men. These gender differences become greater after age 75 (Minkler & Stone, 1983; NCHS, 1991; U.S. Senate, 1988). Rodin and

Ickovics (1990) observe that these differences are theorized to emanate from biological and social (life-style) explanations. Stress and sociodemographic factors have emerged as important explanatory variables to account for gender differences in physical health. The relationship between social class and health is well established. Older women's vulnerable economic status is also demonstrated. For example, older women have lower incomes from every source including pensions and social security, and three-fourths of elder poverty is female (O'Rand, 1988; Sofaer & Abel, 1990). Much more needs to be understood about the intersection of these gender and social class differences with health in old age.

Gender differences in access to health insurance are well documented, with women generally having more limited access to care. Older women spend a substantial portion of their income on out-of-pocket health care expenses, with Medicare covering on average about one-third of their expenses. Particularly for single older women, the costs exceed one-third of their annual income (ICF, 1985; U.S. House of Representatives, 1990). It is significant that, as a consequence of their socioeconomic status including poverty, widowhood, and care-giving responsibilities, older women are more affected than men by governmental policy changes and particularly program cutbacks (Rodin & Ickovics, 1990).

The research agenda in older women's health is not only large; the research must go beyond simply using gender as a predictor variable, to embrace "gender as a dynamic construct that itself varies across ethnic groups and social classes and works in complex interactions with other psychological and social factors" (Russo, 1987, p. 54).

Informal Care

It is well established that women are the major providers of informal unpaid long-term care for the 80% of LTC given to impaired older persons. Controversy about the relative proportions of women "sandwiched" by caregiving for both younger and older family members (OWL, 1989; Rosenthal, Matthews, & Marshall, 1989; Stone & Kemper, 1989) indicates a continuing need for explication of this contemporary phenomenon. Much more research is needed to further specify the subgroups of older women "in the middle" and to understand associated cohort health and economic risks. In addition, the effects of contending with informal care provision and workplace responsibilities has potentially tremendous influence on both the individual lives of women and the economic well-being of the labor force. Research in this area is challenging in part due to ambiguous definitions of formal and informal care (NRC, 1988), underdeveloped measures of workforce disruption, and minimal knowledge of the long-term health effects of caregiver burden.

Increasing longevity means that caregiving spouses will be older themselves. Adult female children of older persons are likely to be less available as future caretakers as a result of changes in family size, increasing employment among middle-aged women, and physical distance from elderly parents (NRC, 1988). Pressures on the informal caregiving system will grow as caregivers of the future will have informal care responsibilities for not just one, but two, disabled parents. Assuming continuing birthrates, there will be fewer adult children to care for their older parents (Stone & Kemper, 1989). How these changes will ultimately increase the demand for formal health and personal care services has not been investigated.

The movement toward services and systems that promote independent living and support informal caregivers for the elderly cite the preference of most individuals to remain at home as evidence that nursing homes should be an approach of last resort for care delivery to disabled older persons (Harrington et al., 1991). The fact that elders are believed to prefer to live at home does not necessarily mean that their care, by definition, should be provided by family, friends, and other informal caregivers, with or without subsidy.

Knowledge about the use of formal care services to supplement or substitute for informal care is growing. Formal care provision does not appear to substitute for informal care (Tennstedt & McKinlay, 1989) and recent evidence strongly suggests that increases in paid home care will not deter current levels of informal support (Hanley, Wiener, & Harris, 1991). The exclusive use of formal care services is rare among older impaired persons (Commonwealth Fund Commission on Elderly People Living Alone, 1989) and the relationship between formal and informal care appears to be more one of complementarity rather than substitutability (DeFriese & Woomert, 1992). There is also some research indicating that use of formal services to augment in-home care does not reduce or mediate the negative effects of caregiving. It has been suggested that much of the stress suffered by primary informal caregivers involves frustrations related to negotiating home care coordination among a plethora of agencies, regulations, and negatively oriented service providers (McKinlay, Crawford, & Tennstedt, 1993).

On the policy level, the cumulative data on informal care point, rather menacingly, to a significant and potentially unstable (even volatile) "non-system" of informal long-term care, staffed to a major degree by economically poor, stressed older women with limited access to resources—many of whom will, themselves, constitute the largest group of LTC consumers in the nation by the year 2020. This situation raises the salience of a research agenda that is attentive to the social policy consequences and effects of informal care, but it must be one that addresses both the caregiver *and* the care recipient perspectives (Barer & Johnson, 1990); the design of systems to effectively link informal and formal care services provided to frail older persons; the economic and environmental realities of informal and formal care patterns across ethnic, racial, gender, and socioeconomic variables; and the questionable stance of public policy promoting informal care by embracing kinship obligation (Collins, 1991; Finch, 1989) as an appropriate social contract for provision of health and social services to older persons (Estes & Rundall, 1992; Phillipson, 1992).

❖ Long-Term Care

Health services research is a relatively new field that has been empirically, rather than theoretically driven. Because the knowledge base is just now emerging, policymakers have had to cope with extremely complex health policy questions without a coherent cumulative body of knowledge elucidating the social behavior of the health field. Although health services research must be responsive to present and future policy needs, the constant pressure to achieve immediate results poses a serious problem for the scientific development of the field. These urgent demands present difficulties in attaining an environment that is committed to the long view that will support the required period of conceptualization and specification, methodological and data-base development, and the rigorous, yet tedious, research process on which the accretion of scientific knowledge must be built.

There is an ever-mounting impatience with health services research because of increasing concern about high and rising costs and deepening problems of access. In addition, the proliferation of new technologies appears to add to health care costs rather than to contain them, in many cases, without improving either quality or outcomes of care (McKinlay et al., 1989). Based on the agenda setting work of several authors and institutions (Greenlick, 1989; IOM, 1991; Rodin & Ickovics, 1990) important issues in long-term care relate to broader social policy questions yet to be well defined and analyzed.

Medical, Functional, and Social Needs in the LTC Population

It is now well established that there are complex relationships between medical conditions and the use of acute care services on the one side, and chronic disabilities and the use of LTC services on the other. The users of LTC services are also high users of acute care services, and many elders' first need for LTC results from an acute care incident. Cross-sectional studies that have been used to date to explore these dynamics are substantially limited. Research is needed to explore the dynamic relationships over time between the need for medical care and the need for long-term care and the variety of environments in which care is provided (Capitman, 1989; Kane & Kane, 1989; Ory & Duncker, 1992; Weissert, 1991; Weissert, Pawlecek, & Creary, 1988).

Need and Utilization of Formal LTC Service

Caution should be used in interpreting current patterns of LTC utilization as valid indicators of the future need for LTC. Low income among the disabled elderly and the lack of community services in many states and localities retard and distort the extent to which needs are met through the formal service system. Because of these distortions by wealth, service availability, and third party coverage and reimbursement policies, care must be exercised in interpreting utilization data as adequate or accurate measures of need. Factors such as living arrangements, income, preferences, and professional values should be considered in any attempt to predict future needs.

Efficiency and Effectiveness of Services

Knowledge of how to deliver community LTC is less developed than either medical or nursing home care. Because of continuing government and consumer interest in expanded public and private funding for services, this area should be a primary focus of research and demonstration. In addition to traditional organizational efficiency measures such as productivity, longitudinal studies should employ multiple measures to explicate characteristics and health outcomes associated with various components of the service delivery system. Policy research needs to consider the impact of policy (e.g., OBRA 1987, U.S. Congress, House of Representatives) on the quality, outcomes, and costs of analogous care in different care settings.

Financing Arrangements

The role of health insurance in reducing or exacerbating financial barriers to all types of care for older persons has not been sufficiently explored. Even with Medicare one can not assume that there is uniformity of health insurance coverage and risk protection among beneficiaries (PPRC, 1988). In addressing the problem of financial risks of illness and injury, an important and understudied area is the determinants of patterns of public and private health insurance arrangements in the elderly population. Policy discussions about health service financing for the elderly do not often consider the differential effects of proposed changes or alternatives on men and women, although the effects may be different because insurance coverage, income and assets, availability of caregivers, and other variables are mediated over many years by factors that tend to vary by gender. Gender also is important because of the relationship of women's ability to pay to husband's pensions and health insurance entitlements and gender-typed jobs in previous work history, and because of the significance of personal economic resources that could compensate for lower levels of functional capacity.

Financing Disease Prevention and Health Promotion

Medicare and Medicaid are *disease* insurance programs; they pay for services and treatment of medically diagnosed conditions. Preventive services such as health screening and health promotion are generally not covered and must be financed by each beneficiary. A fundamental question for research and policy is whether omission of health screening and preventive services financing leads to underconsumption with consequent increased morbidity, mortality, and health care expenses.

Financing Long-Term Care and Mental Health Services

Financing of LTC services represents a crucial problem in supplying appropriate incentives for providers. Without adequate adjustment for case mix (risk), providers often skim off the lightest care patients, leaving the heavier care patients with substantial barriers to access. Current payment mechanisms do not provide appropriate dynamic incentives. Providers are paid to maintain patients at current or higher levels of dependency and there is little research on the resources required to rehabilitate patients to improve functional levels. Various models of financing health care system elements need to be theoretically and empirically investigated to determine financing mechanisms that support higher levels of independence among care recipients and the associated cost outcomes for LTC and mental health care providers. Scholarly debate (Cohen, Kumar, McGuire, & Wallack, 1992; Harrington et al., 1991) facilitates the conceptualization of these challenges.

Effects of Financial Barriers on Access, Use, and Health Outcomes

The sources of financing of health services for the aged are many and varied, including third-party payments and out-of-pocket payments. The latter include payments for premiums, co-insurance, balance billing, deductibles, uncovered services, and unclaimed coverage. The sources of funds to meet these out-of-pocket liabilities are multiple as well, including current income, savings, gifts from relatives, charity, loans, and debt forgiveness by providers. With the elderly spending 4.3 months of their average annual Social Security checks (18% of their incomes) on

TABLE 1 Priority Areas for Research on Public Policy and Long-Term Care

---

Older Women and Health

- the link between social and economic conditions of women and multiple epidemiological dimensions of health and illness across the life span
- the effects on older women of public policy, including policy that directly or indirectly affects labor force participation, retirement, income, and long-term care
- conditions that uniquely or disproportionately affect older women (eg., osteoporosis, breast cancer)
- mechanisms by which racial and ethnic status and social class influence older women's health

---

Informal Care

- the economic and psycho-social consequences for older caregivers and the relation of these to health and illness and to social policy
- the relationships between the formal and informal provision of care, caregiver and care recipient burden, and socioeconomic class, gender, race, and ethnic status
- documentation of total support process in older life as basis for designing systems which effectively inter-relate formal and informal care systems
- relationship between informal and formal care including outcomes of untargeted formal services

---

Long-Term Care (Health Services Research)

- longitudinal studies that trace changes in needs, access, and utilization patterns that accompany transitions between acute and chronic care, between forms of acute care, and between forms of chronic care
- the equity, effects, and effectiveness of long-term care policy per se to differentiate LTC policies that exacerbate or create dependency from those that do not
- the determinants of health insurance arrangements by older persons and the relationship of health insurance coverage to health care access and utilization
- cost-effectiveness and net benefits of alternative disease prevention and health promotion strategies and services targeted to aging populations
- determinants of risk of LTC and mental health care expense and the efficacy of innovative rehabilitation strategies for frail and chronically dependent older persons
- relationship of income, social class, and LTC insurance to access and utilization of health care and social services

---

medical care, financial barriers remain a real and substantial obstacle for many aged persons, despite Medicare and Medigap coverage. Such barriers are associated with hesitance to seek timely care (PPRC, 1988), which may negatively affect health outcomes. Evaluation is needed in the area of income and price elasticities of demand for health care services by aging populations and effects of financial barriers on access, use, and health status of older persons and their standards of living.

❖ Priority Areas of Research

Principles guiding the design and implementation of and research on public policy and long-term care include attention to: (1) the possibility that specific interventions may generate more rather than less dependency; (2) the multiple levels of intervention needed to promote empowerment, including interventions that deal with everyday lives, professional practice and organization, and social structure (Riley & Riley, 1989); and (3) maximizing personal control, sense of self-efficacy and competence, and control of the elder's environment (Rodin, 1989). The challenge on all three levels is to break the link between aging and dependency (Phillipson & Walker, 1986). Research is a vital and essential element of meeting this challenge.

Priority areas for research on public policy and long-term care based on the three illustrative issues reviewed in this chapter are presented in Table 1.

❖ Conclusion

Social, behavioral, and health services research hold great promise for informing policymakers about crucial elements of public policy and long-term care. Without serious, sustained efforts, the development and implementation of policies to maximize active life expectancy will not be realized, however (Estes & Rundall, 1992; Katz et al., 1983)

To succeed, social policy and the research on it must attend to an understanding of how health in old age is linked to social factors that shape the entire life course. Health status at age 65 does not come "out of nowhere". Location in the social structure (e.g., gender, social class, racial/ethnic group) mediates lifelong opportunities to engage in healthful behaviors and obtain health care (Estes & Rundall, 1992) as well as to live in health-enhancing environments. The import of adequate income and social opportunities throughout the lifecourse including access to prenatal, primary, and preventive care, should not be underestimated nor continue relatively uninvestigated. Much work remains to be done to understand these relationships and to document the impact of social policy on health and health care in old age.

Social structural change in the direction of universal life course entitlement (Estes & Binney, 1988) would promote the abatement of inequities based on age, gender, race, and class (Estes et al., 1993). The "plasticity" of the aging process represents more than mind-body phenomena—our individual and collective perceptions of the process influence its malleability (Estes, et al., 1993). As scholars we must give as much research attention to the concepts of empowerment and equity as we do to those of efficiency and cost. Research knowledge does not yet exist that would permit the design of long-term care policy that would promote healthy aging throughout the life course for Americans irrespective of racial, ethnic, gender, or social class origins. The health and quality of life of future generations of elders depends on our commitment to the development of research that investigates present gaps and extends our knowledge of the multifaceted experience of aging under defined social structural conditions.

Public policy reform including the elimination of economic obstacles that block access to health care is high on the current federal agenda. The Clinton administration's commitment to health care reform constitutes a signpost announcing that change in the health care system is no longer debatable. Rather, the exact nature and extent of that reform now constitute the discussion. Although costs are a central concern, issues of access to care have been restored to the dialogue on health care. It is expected that there will be universal access to uniform benefits without discrimination with regard to preconditions or preselection screening. Long-term care is a unifying force; it is an issue that binds families and generations through the universality of caregiving, women's roles, and the children's stake. A long-term care system, however designed and financed, relies heavily on the body of scientific knowledge generated in the social and behavioral sciences to adequately address the structural conditions necessary to ensure a high quality of life for older and disabled persons.

❖ About the Authors

Carroll L. Estes, Ph.D., is Director, Institute for Health & Aging and Professor of Sociology, Department of Social and Behavioral Sciences, School of Nursing, University of California, San Francisco.

Liz Close, Ph.D., R.N., is Professor and Chair, Department of Nursing, School of Natural Sciences, Sonoma State University, Rohnert Park, California.

REFERENCES

Barer, B. M., & Johnson, C. L. (1990). A critique of the caregiving literature. *The Gerontologist, 30,* 26–29.

Brody, J. A., Brock, D. B., & Williams, T. F. (1987). Trends in the health of the elderly population. In J. E. Fielding & L. B. Lave (Eds.), *Annual review of public health,* Vol. 8 (pp. 211–234). Palo Alto, CA: Annual Reviews.

Capitman, J. A. (1989). Policy and program options in community-based long-term care. *Annual Review of Gerontology and Geriatrics, 9,* 357–388.

Cohen, M. A., Kumar, N., McGuire, T., & Wallack, S. S. (1992). Financing long-term care: A practical mix of public and private. *Journal of Health, Politics, Policy and Law, 17*(3), 403–423.

Collins, J. (1991). Power and local community activity. *Journal of Aging Studies, 5*(2), 209–218.

Commonwealth Fund Commission on Elderly People Living Alone. (1989). *Help at home: Long-term care assistance for impaired elderly people.* Report prepared by Diane Rowland. Baltimore, MD.

DeFriese, G. H., & Woomert, A. (1992). Informal and formal health care systems serving older persons. In M. G. Ory, R. P. Abeles, and P. D. Lipman, (Eds.) *Aging, health, and behavior* (pp. 57–82). Newbury Park, CA: Sage.

Estes, C. L. (1979). *The aging enterprise.* San Francisco, CA: Jossey-Bass.

Estes, C. L., & Binney, E. A. (1989). The biomedicalization of aging: Dangers and dilemmas. *The Gerontologist, 29*(5), 587–596.

Estes, C. L., & Rundall, T. G. (1992). Social characteristics, social structure, and health in the aging population. In M. G. Ory, R. P. Abeles, & P. D. Lipman (Eds.), *Aging, health, and behavior* (pp. 299–326). Newbury Park, CA: Sage.

Estes, C.E., Swan, J.H., & Associates. (1993). *The long-term care crisis: Elders trapped in the no care zone.* Newbury Park, CA: Sage.

Families USA Foundation. (1992). *The health cost squeeze of older Americans.* Washington, DC: Families USA Foundation.

Finch, J. (1989). *Family obligations and social change.* London: Polity Press and Basil Blackwell.

Greenlick, M. R. (1989). *Health services research on aging.* Draft report. Liaison Team for Health Services Delivery Research, Institute of Medicine Committee on a National Research Agenda on Aging.

Hanley, R. J., Wiener, J. M., & Harris, K. M. (1991). Will paid care erode informal support? *Journal of Health Politics, Policy, and Law, 16*(3), 507–521.

Harrington, C., Cassell, C., Estes, C. L., Woolhandler, S., Himmelstein, D. U., & The Working Group on Long-Term Care Program Design, Physicians for a National Health Program.

(1991). A national long-term care program for the United States: A caring vision. *Journal of the American Medical Association, 266*(21), 3023–3029.

ICF, Inc. (1985). *Medicare's role in financing the health care of older women.* Paper submitted to the American Association of Retired Persons (AARP). Washington, DC: ICF.

Institute of Medicine (IOM). E. T. Lonergan (Ed.) (1991). *Extending life, enhancing life: National research agenda on aging.* Washington, DC: National Academy Press.

Kane, R. A., & Kane, R. L. (1989). Transitions in long-term care. In M. G. Ory & K. Bond (Eds.), *Aging and health care: Social science and policy perspectives* (pp. 217–243). London: Routledge.

Katz, S., Branch, L., Bronson, M., Papsidero, J., Beck, J. & Greer, D. (1983). Active life expectancy. *New England Journal of Medicine, 309*(20), 1218–1224.

Kirchstein, R. L. (1991). Research on women's health. *American Journal of Public Health, 81,* 291–293.

Kunkel, S. R., & Applebaum, R. A. (1992). Estimating the prevalence of long-term disability for an aging society. *The Journal of Gerontology: Social Sciences, 47,* s253–s260.

Lipton, H. P., & Lee, P. R. (1988). *Drugs and the elderly: Clinical, social, and policy perspectives.* Stanford, CA: Stanford University Press.

Manton, K.G., Corder, L.S., & Stallard, E. (1993). Estimates of change in chronic disability and institutional incidence and prevalence rates in the U.S. elderly population from the 1982, 1984, and 1989 National Long-term Care Survey. *Journal of Gerontology: Social Sciences, 48*(4), S153–S166.

Manton, K. G., & Suzman, R. (1992). Forecasting health and functioning in aging societies: Implications for health care and staffing needs. In M. G. Ory, R. P. Abeles, & P. D. Lipman (Eds.), *Aging, health, and behavior* (pp. 327–357). Newbury Park, CA: Sage.

McKinaly, J. B., Crawford, S., & Tennstedt, S. (1993). Everyday social and physical impact of providing informal care to dependent elders. *Milbank Memorial Fund Quarterly*.

McKinlay, J. B., McKinlay, S. M., & Beaglehole, R. (1989). Trends in death and disease and the contribution of medical measures. In H. E. Freeman & S. Levine (Eds.), *The Handbook of Medical Sociology*, (pp. 14–45). Englewood Cliffs, NJ: Prentice Hall.

Minckler, M., & Stone, R. I. (1983). The feminization of poverty. *The Gerontologist*, 25, 351–357.

National Center for Health Statistics (NCHS). (1991). *Health, United States, 1990*. Hyattsville, MD: U.S. Public Health Service.

National Research Council (NRC). (1988). *The aging population in the 21st century*. Washington, DC: National Academy Press.

Older Women's League (OWL). (1989). *Failing America's caregivers: A status report on women who care*. Washington, DC: OWL.

O'Rand, A. (1988). Convergence, institutionalization and bifurcation: Gender and the pension acquisition review. In G. Maddox & P. Lawton (Eds.) *Varieties of aging: Annual review of gerontology and geriatrics*, Vol. 8 (pp. 132–155). New York: Springer Publishing Co.

Ory, M. G., & Duncker, A. P. (1992). Introduction: The home care challenge. In M. G. Ory & A. P. Duncker (Eds.), *In-home care for older people: Health and supportive services*, pp. 1–8. Newbury Park, CA: Sage Publications.

Phillipson, C. (1992). Challenging "the spectre of old age": Community care for older people in the 1990s. In W. Manning and R. Page (Eds.), *Social Policy Yearbook* (pp. 1–22). London: Social Policy Association.

Phillipson, C., & Walker, A. (1986). Conclusion: Alternative forms of policy and practice. In C. Phillipson & A. Walker (Eds.), *Ageing and social policy: A critical assessment*, (pp. 280–281). England: Glower.

Physician Payment Review Commission (PPRC). (1988). *Survey of Medicare beneficiaries*. Washington, DC: Physician Payment Review Commission.

Rice, D. P. (1986). Living longer in the U.S.: Social and economic implications. *Journal of Medical Practice Management*, 1(3), 162–169.

Riley, M. W., & Riley, J. W. (1989). The lives of older people and changing social roles. *Annals of the American Academy of Political and Social Science*, 503, 14–28.

Rodin, J. (1989). Sense of control: Potentials for intervention. *Annals of the American Academy of Political and Social Science*, 503, 29–42.

Rodin, J., & Ickovics, J. R. (1990). Women's health: Review and research agenda as we enter the 21st century. *American Psychologist*, 45(9), 1018–1034.

Rosenthal, C. J., Matthews, S. H., & Marshall, V. W. (1989). Is parent care normal? The experiences of a sample of middle-aged women. *Research on Aging*, 11, 244–260.

Russo, N. F. (1987). Position paper. In A. Eichler and D. L. Parron (Eds.), *Women's mental health: Agenda for research* (pp. 42–56). Rockville, MD: National Institute for Mental Health.

Sofaer, S., & Abel, E. (1990). Older women's health and financial vulnerability: Implications of the Medicare benefit structure. *Women and Health*, 16(3–4), 47–67.

Stone, R., & Kemper, P. (1989). Spouses and children of disabled elders: How large a constituency for long-term care reform? *Milbank Memorial Quarterly*, 67, 485–506.

Taeuber, C. M. (1992). *Sixty-five plus in America*. Washington, DC: U.S. Bureau of the Census.

Tennstedt, S., & McKinlay, J. B. (1989). Informal care for frail older persons. In M. G. Ory & K. Bond (Eds.), *Aging and health care: Social science and policy perspectives* (pp. 145–166). London: Routledge.

Travis, C. B. (1988). *Women and health psychology: Biomedical issues*. Hillsdale, NJ: Erlbaum.

U. S. House of Representatives (Select Committee on Aging). (1990). *Emptying the elderly's pocketbook: Growing impact of rising health care costs.* A Report by the Chairman. Washington, DC: U. S. Government Printing Office.

U. S. Senate (Special Committee on Aging). (1991). *Developments in aging: 1990,* Vol. 1. Washington, DC: U. S. Government Printing Office.

U. S. Senate (Special Committee on Aging), American Association for Retired People, Federal Council on Aging, & U. S. Administration of Aging. (1988). *Aging America: Trends and projections.* Washington, DC: U. S. Department of Health and Human Services.

Verbrugge, L. M. (1989). Recent, present, and future health of American adults. In L. Breslow, J. E. Fielding, and L. B. Lave (Eds.), *Annual review of public health,* Vol. 10 (pp. 333–361). Palo Alto, CA: Annual Reviews, Inc.

Verbrugge, L. M. (1991). Pathways of health and death. In R. D. Apple (Ed.), *Women, health, and medicine: A history handbook* (pp. 41–79). New Brunswick, NJ: Rutgers University Press.

Weissert, W. G. (1991). Home care: Measuring success. In P. R. Katz, R. L. Kane, & M.D. Mezey (Eds.), *Advances in long-term care,* Vol. 1 (pp. 186–199). New York: Springer Publishing Co.

Weissert, W. G., Cready, C. M., & Pawelak, J. E. (1988). The past and future of community-based long-term care. *Milbank Memorial Quarterly, 66,* 309–388.

❖ PART III

Health Policy and the Politics of Health

❖ Chapter 6
The Politics of Health: Establishing Policies and Setting Priorities

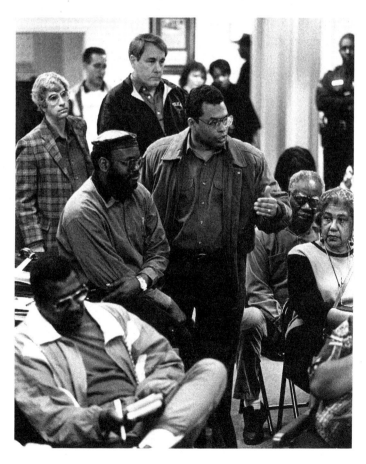

In the past, Americans have placed great trust in the professionals who provide their health care, in the insurance companies that pay for much of their care, and in the government that regulates, oversees, and, to a great extent, finances the health care system. The public had little awareness or understanding of public health. Only relatively recently has the American public begun to question the efficiency, effectiveness, and costs of the health care system in response to constant media exposure and personal experience with a system rife with increasing costs, rationing, and decreasing access. In Part III, a critical view of the underpinnings of the U.S. health care system is taken including the struggle for financial resources and interest group control of various system components. Underneath the regulation and legislation are power struggles, the outcomes of which ultimately determine the availability, cost, and quality of health care services. They determine who will care for us when, where, and how; the methods by which we will pay for care; how much we will pay; where hospitals will be located and their size and scope. The outcomes of these perpetual struggles also significantly influence health professions education and determine the scope and direction of health related research, and the investment in public health programs.

On the surface, it appears that policy decisions emanate from the government. But, in reality, policymakers take their cues for health care legislation and regulation from a variety of sources. Historically, particular special-interest groups, such as physicians and hospitals, have been able virtually to dictate health policy in specific areas. This dominant role of a limited number of special interest groups has changed in recent years as more and better organized special interest groups have appeared as proprietary organizations have proliferated and become more concentrated, as consumers have taken a more active role in securing public accountability, and as the stakes have escalated to skyhigh proportions. The four most powerful structural interests in health care are still physicians, hospitals, insurance companies, and the pharmaceutical industry. There are also lobbying groups for dentists, nurses, and many other health professions; for nursing homes; for labor and business groups; and for most other participants in the health care arena. Public health has been relatively weakly represented, although disease specific groups (e.g., HIV/AIDS) have exerted a significant influence at the federal and state levels. While some would argue that all of these groups contribute to the high-quality care we receive, they are driven to protect and promote their own interests in order to survive and thrive in an increasingly market-driven health care system.

The formulation of health policy across several levels of government and hundreds of programs is complex. Lee and Benjamin (1997) have identified four characteristics of the policy process in the United States: (1) the American character; (2) the distribution of authority and responsibility within a federal system of government; (3) pluralistic ideology as a basis

196

of politics; (4) and incrementalism as a strategy for reform. These characteristics are considered from a variety of perspectives in this chapter.

Today, policymakers and citizens continue to debate the relative efficacy of various methods to tackle the fragmentation in financing and provision of health care, crippling cost escalation, high expenditures for administration, the commercialization of medicine, the trend toward defensive
medicine, the erosion of physician authority, and the lack of access to health
care for increasing numbers of U.S. citizens and the deterioration of the
public health infrastructure particularly at the local level.

In the previous edition of *The Nation's Health* (1994) we included
"Health Policy and the Politics of Health Care" in which Philip R. Lee and
A. E. Benjamin identify and discuss the political influences on health policy
formulation over the past two hundred years. The authors' documentation
of the evolution of U.S. health policy indicates that although consensus has
emerged about the nature of the problems confronting the system, there is,
by no means, agreement on the solutions. This conclusion was reflected in
the health care reform debates of the early nineties. Last year, Lee, Benjamin, and Weber (1996) updated their earlier analysis and we include that
book chapter in our Recommended Reading list.

In "Privatization, the Welfare State, and Aging: The Reagan-Bush Legacy," Carroll Estes contends that aging and health policy serve as a major
constructed battleground on which the nation's social struggles are being
fought. She outlines the various reasons given by policymakers for refusing
to provide essential services such as long-term care and argues that their
fundamental line of reasoning presumes that such care for older Americans
should be provided by unpaid (female) caregivers. Estes also suggests that
the chronic illness "burden" associated with elderly citizens is undeserv-
edly blamed for crippling the national economy, raising the question of
whether and how the administration of President Bill Clinton will alter the
course set by Presidents Reagan and Bush.

Marion Nestle highlights the complex interplay and consequence of
special interest group politics and conflicts of interest embedded in the
government agency simultaneously responsible for advising the public on
matters of health and for the agricultural industry's market success in her
article, "Food Lobbies, The Food Pyramid, and U.S. Nutrition Policy." Dr.
Nestle raises significant questions concerning the policy development process when a single governmental agency must function in a clear conflict of
interest mode. Ultimately, the health of U.S. residents can be affected when
access to current nutrition and health care information is impeded because
of structural arrangements that promote information control battles that
protect the financial interests of proprietary organizations.

Stanton Glantz, in his "Preventing Tobacco Use—The Youth Access
Trap" reveals the subtle and very powerful message created by tobacco
industry advertising that appears to discourage young people from smok-

ing by establishing and supporting smoking as an adult ritual. The resultant shift in focus to youth undermines the broader attempts to effect a smoke-free society. We include this article in chapter 6 to illustrate how a seemingly slight shift in advertising practice can effectively disrupt the otherwise focused agenda of many powerful organizations dedicated to the health and safety of the American public.

Carroll Estes and Karen Linkins describe the new round of health politics in the devolution of federal authority to the states and budget cuts. The central question concerns the vulnerability of safety net services and whether states will "race to the bottom" via their policy choices in Medicaid, block grants, and welfare reform given the political, social, and economic forces at work.

The development and implementation of health care policy in the United States is neither straight-forward nor innocuous. The process is susceptible to the constant influence of political struggles that inevitably mitigate outcomes that may or may not promote the interests of the population in general.

❖ Privatization, the Welfare State, and Aging: The Reagan-Bush Legacy

Carroll L. Estes

President Ronald Reagan successfully shifted the focus of discourse on social policy in the United States from activism and social improvement to crisis and budget cutting. This was accomplished with the support of an ideological revolution reinstating the primacy of the economy as the driving rationale for state action and a romanticized notion of individualism and the family as a justification for shifting social responsibility to the private sector. This paper explores the Reagan-Bush legacy, lays out the paradigm shift that has occurred, examines its symbolic and material consequences, and assesses the implications for old age in the U.S. welfare state, with particular attention to health care.

The theme of crisis was a central motif resonating throughout the Reagan presidency and preparing the way for action. Aging policy was a key element of the schema of crisis definition and the resulting outcomes. Understanding the contemporary welfare state requires theoretical and empirical attention to crisis construction and crisis management by the state. The "Reagan Revolution" was a product of the tensions among the state (government and its institutions), the corporate sector, and labor in working through the crisis tendencies associated with capitalism.

Under Reagan, economic crisis has been used to justify the imposition of cost containment policies in health care that shifted costs from the state to individuals (including the elderly) and the transfer of an increasing amount of funding from public and nonprofit health provider organizations to for-profit enterprise. Furthering a process that commenced with the passage of Medicare and Medicaid in 1965, Reagan administration policies fueled the growth of the for-profit components and the costs of the medical care system. Although 40 percent of the cost of U.S. health care spending is financed by the federal government, it supports a largely private sector medical-industrial complex. The state has limited its own activities in the health and social services to those that support and complement the market through limited public financing programs of health insurance, primarily for the aged (Medicare) and the poor who cannot afford to pay for private insurance (Medicaid).

Through the regulation and financing of medical care and social services, state policy under Reagan stimulated market investment opportunities for private capital in potentially profitable service arenas (e.g., hospital and home health services) that had been traditionally controlled by nonprofit health care entities. State policy also provided productive opportunities for private capital through civil law and regulation protecting the market and proprietary health entities including the federal tax subsidy of the purchase of private health insurance. The combination of Reagan's deliberate strategies to increase privatization and competition through the promotion of medical and community care for profit and requirements for competitive contracting, and substantial public subsidies to the corporate sector through tax cuts in 1981, significantly exacerbated the fiscal problems of the state.

These state actions and policies contributed to (1) the deepening of divisions in the *de facto* rationing system of U.S. health care based on ability to pay, and (2) a largely unchecked rise in federal health care costs. Under Reagan, the state intensified the constraints on funding for social and community care services—areas of the greatest dependency by nonprofit service organizations on the government. The state-financed services that experienced the most severe cuts early in the Reagan administration were the social and supportive services that are least attractive to business investors because they tend to be less profitable due to their labor intensity, lower technological content, and general unpredictability. Each of these state actions has altered the terrain of health and aging policy, and each has generated consequences.

In the Reagan era, health and aging policy exemplify the contradictions facing the state as it is pressed to regulate and contain government costs in medical care, while simultaneously being required to deregulate and promote economic expansion and profit through a robust state-financed but privately run and extremely costly medical-industrial complex. At the same time, as the state and the private sector shift more of the costs onto the consumer, the poor and the uninsured grow, ultimately increasing welfare costs that must be borne by the state.

❖ The Reagan Legacy: An Ideological Revolution

All political regimes use ideology as the discourse with which to communicate and impose a reflection of economic and power relations. One of the most striking and significant features of the Reagan legacy is its phenomenal success in advancing neo-liberal and neo-conservative ideologies as strategies in the social construction of crisis, subsequent crisis management, and restructuring of the welfare state. The ideological legacy of the Reagan administration is profound.

As deeply held systems of beliefs, ideologies are generally unexamined as both evidential and moral truths. Ideologies frame the possible and the ethical, orienting us to what is ("reality"), who we are, and how we relate to the world. Ideologies influence what we conceive of as imaginable and as right and wrong. The production and uses of ideology are integral to three processes by which dominant power relations are sustained: (1) the successful creation of cultural images by policymakers, experts, and the media; (2) the appeal to the necessities of the economic system; and (3) the implementation of policy and the use of expertise in ways that focus attention on rational problem solving in familiar organizational structures and professions rather than the more fundamental questions and in ways that camouflage their class, gender, racial, and ethnic implications.

Reagan's ideological revolution simultaneously promoted the revival of the free market and the now-mythical patriarchal autonomous family. Two elements of the revolution are (1) neo-liberal ideology, which is distinctly oriented toward a "minimalist state" and hostile to anything that may impede the order of the market and its natural superiority; and (2) neo-conservative ideology, which appeals to authority, allegiance, tradition, and "nature." The allegiance of the citizen to the state is seen as transcendent. "A corollary . . . is that [a particular vision of] the family is central to maintaining the state." The attractiveness of this new right model is that it embraces two potentially disparate elements: "intellectual adherence to the free market and the emotional attachment to authority and imposed tradition." The New Right is committed to a view that the primary, if not only, justification for government intervention is maintaining the national defense and law and order. President Reagan successfully blurred the concepts of national security with the national economic interest.

Reagan was remarkably influential in using ideology to shape public consciousness by limiting a vision of the "possible" to inherently pro-market solutions. In health care, the vision was that the only route to universal health care is through competition and market strategies. Not surprisingly, this ideology bolstered the U.S. health care system as a pluralistically financed and essentially private delivery system dominated by a powerful medical profession and for-profit medical industries. The doubling of the cost of health care consonant with the dramatic decline in access to care for millions of Americans during the Reagan-Bush era is testimony to the inadequacy of market approaches to health care as a means either of controlling costs or ensuring access.

❖ The Health Legacy of Ronald Reagan: 1981–1988

Reagan's strategy in health care was to focus on cost containment and to advance market principles in health (competition, deregulation, and privatization). A companion strategy was to implement cuts in the Medicaid program for the poor. While Reagan's policies stimulated a revolution in the organization of health care and its corporatization and privatization, these efforts to stimulate the market had the opposite effect of what they promised for cost containment. Medical costs continued to rise at two to three times the rate of inflation.

The Reagan administration had reaffirmed the course of health policy embarked on by previous administrations. The structure of private provision and service delivery, the pluralistic methods of financing, and the orientation of the government-financed programs of Medicare and Medicaid remained essentially intact. Significantly, however, Reagan's approach also deepened and extended the nation's commitment to the commodification and "medicalization" of old age through state policy. Health care was reconceptualized as a commodity through the rhetoric and policies that established health care as a market good rather than a right. The medicalization is reflected in the construction of "aging as illness," the exclusive targeting of federal reimbursement through Medicare for medical treatment (not social supportive or even chronic illness care), the designation and slanting of federal research priorities toward biomedical problems, and the direction of medical education.

The most important effects of the Reagan legacy in health care for the aged are (1) the fueling of the commodification and medicalization of care for the aging in ways that are consistent with capitalist expansion of the medical-industrial complex; (2) the continuing refusal of the state to provide meaningful long-term care benefits to the elderly and disabled; (3) the accumulation of multiple pressures on a beleaguered network of traditionally nonprofit home and community-based health and social service providers thinly stretched by the demands of very sick and very old patients discharged from the hospital earlier than ever before; and (4) the use of policies to promote family responsibility and the informalization of care. These efforts to restore and regulate family life (and particularly the lives of women) are congruent with the deep concerns of both the state and corporate sectors to minimize state costs for the elderly, as well as the New Right for restoring patriarchal family arrangements in order to ensure a continuing supply of women's free labor for the reproduction and maintenance of the labor force.

The Reagan administration's resistance to a federal policy solution to the problem of long-term care and its unstated policy of informalization are part of a larger austerity strategy in the context of the state's need for women (regardless of their labor force participation) to continue to perform large (and increasing) amounts of unpaid servicing work, particularly in the care of the aged.

Health Care as a Market Good

The stated health policy goals of equity, access, and accountability that were hallmarks of the 1960s died in the Reagan White House. America's elders were caught between (1) the dual interests of the state and corporate sectors, each of which was attempting to constrain and reduce its own costs and neither of which was especially concerned about inequities in access to care; and (2) the tensions between the shared goals of the state and those segments of corporate capital that wanted to reduce medical care costs *versus* that part of the corporate sector in the medical-industrial complex (including hospitals and physicians) that were pressing for the expansion of a growing and profitable market in high technology medical care guaranteed by government subsidy. The result has been a more costly and deeply stratified health care system for all Americans.

❖ The Bush Legacy in Health

The Bush approach to health policy was a continuation of the Reagan strategy of privatization, competition, and deregulation, laced with the rhetoric of crisis and the urgency of cost containment. On the *ideological* front, the Bush and Reagan legacies are virtually indistinguishable: the unswerving commitment to market rhetoric, joined with images of the aborted fetus, reflect the far right's intimidation and capture of Bush and the Republican party. With it there were serious attacks on the rights of women and minorities, as well as (not so paradoxically) children. The difference between the two administrations was in the political acumen, the charisma, and media savvy of President Reagan in contrast to that of President Bush.

President Bush's capitulation to the extreme right wing was expressed in the regulation of medical practitioners through the imposition of a "gag" rule on health providers in family planning clinics and a ban on fetal tissue research that might result in a cure for such maladies as Parkinson's or Alzheimer's diseases. Family planning and "choice" with regard to pregnancy became dirty words.

The failure of both Reagan and Bush to control health costs over the 12 years of their administrations contributed to a three-fold increase, from $1,000 to $3,000 per person and from $250 to $870 billion in national health expenditures during their combined terms of office. The average health payments of families rose 169 percent between 1980 and 1992, while wages increased far less than that (54 percent). During the Bush presidency, an estimated 1.8 million Americans lost their jobs due to rising employer health costs.

In spite of significant reductions in hospital lengths of stay (in excess of 22 percent) and the shift of health work to informal careers with the extension of ambulatory day surgery and the shortened hospital visits, the escalation of health costs continues. Market competition and the massive restructuring of the health industry of the 1980s have not fulfilled their promise as "the solution" to the cost crisis. Physician expenditures galloped at more than 13 percent a year, two to three times the inflation rate. In 1991, health insurance premiums comprised 10.7 percent of corporate payroll and, based on current trends, premiums will consume 22.9 percent of payroll by the year 2000. Health care expenditures represent one seventh of the entire U.S. economy.

When examined over 28 months, the number of Americans presently without health care insurance coverage part or all of the time exceeds 63 million, or 28 percent of the U.S. population. Without a change in policy, the number of Americans uninsured for health care is projected to rise from the present 37 million to well above 52 million between 1991 and the year 2000. In spite of the enormous and growing coverage gap, the implications of failing to systematically control U.S. health spending are staggering. The proportion of the gross national product (GNP) will almost double in the next decade alone, rising from 12 percent to 20 percent of GNP.

The failure of policy makers either to stem costs or to improve access is due in no small part to the U.S. politics of health. Health industry contributions from political action committees (PACs) to politicians—the "mother's milk" of politics—increased 22 percent over the last four-year election cycle alone. Since Mr. Reagan's election in 1981, representatives of the medical-industrial complex have contributed in excess of $65 million to House and Senate races, and members of the last (102nd) Congress have received $48.5 million. Additional millions are spent on Washington lobbyists. Indeed, health industry political contributions are rising faster than health care costs. Researchers for *Public Citizen* have projected a 178 percent increase in PAC contributions between 1989 and 1992. Although some 300 health care proposals were introduced in the last (102nd) congressional session, the president of *Public Citizen*, Joan Claybrook, contends, "Most of these bills could have been written on the word processors of the health industry." The Health Insurance Association of America will spend $4 million to discredit reform proposals. The Canadian model is a favorite target in view of recent poll data indicating the public support of Americans for this system.

President Bush's health proposals during the 1992 election promised no structural health reform. They contained four elements: (1) a health insurance credit or tax deduction to provide up to $3,750 annually to cover the purchase of private coverage and health care costs. (Critics note that this is far less than the $4,700 average cost of private insurance now and the $10,000 projected as early as 1996. They note, further, that Bush had no plan to regulate insurance industry pricing); (2) medical malpractice reform; (3) coordinated or managed care (which has not yet been proven to be cost effective); and (4) electronic billing to reduce administrative costs.

The cost of Bush's proposed tax breaks for all Americans and the tax subsidies for the purchase of private health insurance for his second term of office, should he have been elected, was estimated at $1 trillion (including his promised deficit reductions and new programs). Bush's proposed balanced budget amendment would have required major, if not draconian, cuts in existing programs like Medicare and Social Security for the elderly. Democrats estimated results of the Bush plan would have meant the loss of between 2.2 and 6.4 million U.S. jobs.

Without a dramatic change in health policy, the elderly will be negatively affected on multiple counts: (1) the predictable continuing health care cost escalation that is eroding government's ability to afford to provide adequate Medicare and other benefits; (2) out-of-pocket health care costs for elders that are continuing to rise (now exceeding 18% of annual income and consuming 4.3 months of the average elder's annual Social Security payments); (3) the private Medi-gap insurance policies that most (80 percent) older Americans purchase to supplement Medicare, which are becoming increasingly unaffordable to more and more elders; and (4) the continuing reluctance of policymakers to adopt a national long-term care policy. Finally, with a growing deficit and ever-escalating Medicare costs, there is the persistent danger of the intensified politicization and significant erosion of other major social programs that are crucial to elders, such as Social Security.

Probably the most profound effect of the Reagan and Bush presidencies is the enormous and mushrooming federal deficit, now approximating $3 trillion. A deficit of this magnitude was achieved through massive tax cuts and huge military spending. The goal was not simply to reduce welfare benefits; it was nothing less than "the transformation of the very tax structure that generated the revenues necessary for the welfare benefits. . . . Thus, tax policy became social welfare policy." The size and magnitude of the deficit and interest on the debt had their intended salutary effects for the conservative agenda; *they staved off new state programs unless they can be paid for by trading off other programs within a zero-sum or fixed state budget.*

A key priority of President Bush was an amendment to the U.S. Constitution requiring Congress to balance the budget annually. Due to extreme pressure from the White House, such an amendment almost passed in the last full congressional session of President Bush's presidency. The effects of a balanced budget amendment, should it pass, on the social domestic budget would be profound. No less than 20 percent cuts would be necessitated in virtually all social programs. If there were a protection clause to exempt Social Security from contributing to the deficit reduction under a balanced budget amendment, the level of cuts across all other federally funded domestic programs is expected to exceed 30 percent.

Legitimacy of the U.S. State

Meanwhile, the legitimacy problems of the U.S. state continued as economic problems stubbornly resisted the usual pre-election presidential tinkering with interest rates, unemployment statistics, and other economic indicators.

During the Reagan and Bush presidencies, the state successfully played its "class role" by restructuring and redistributing state benefits from the worker and middle class to business and the upper class rather than dismantling the state. Rhetoric to the contrary, both state funding and regulation have been redirected rather than reduced.

Under Reagan and Bush, the rhetoric of fiscal crisis and the state's mythical and pathetic cost containment efforts obfuscated the massive transfer that was underway—the transfer of health care benefits from labor, the poor, minorities, women, and small business to an increasingly concentrated, unstable, and disorganized complex of medical and other corporations, fending for their lives within a restructured capitalist world order. Health programs for the poor and for women and children were hit the hardest and with the most lasting and deleterious effects. One fifth of all of America's children today are in poverty and one third in California are expected to be on public welfare sometime during their childhood. The redistribution of resources and growing inequities extend to the declining standard of living of working and middle class Americans.

The astounding three-fold growth in expenditures for the medical-industrial complex under Reagan and Bush demonstrates the ability of the U.S. state and the nation's health and aging policies to assist in attending to crises in the capitalist system, as the state subsidy for profit making in medical care and technology expand. The attack on the nonprofit sector in health care is part of the same phenomenon: new opportunities for corporate investment capital in health are needed and the opportunities for proprietaries in the health care market are enhanced with the weakening of the nonprofit sector and the erosion of its legitimacy.

An important question is whether the increasing personal difficulties ("troubles") with health care of what is becoming literally all but the richest 1 or 2 percent of Americans will generate the necessary political heat to ignite an effective movement for broad health policy change. The high unemployment (officially 7.6 percent, but estimated more accurately at 10 percent), as well as the rising number of part-time workers without health benefits augments the potential that this will occur. There is substantial and enduring public support for the major U.S. entitlement programs such as Social Security and Medicare that form the bedrock of the U.S. welfare state—this despite White House and media assaults of more than a decade. According to public opinion, the momentum for structural change in health policy is building. The majority (61 percent) of the U.S. public would prefer the Canadian system of health insurance to the U.S. system, in which "the government pays most of the cost of care for everyone out of taxes, and the government sets all fees charged by doctors and hospitals." Support is strongest (68 percent) among those in the middle class.

❖ Crisis, Social Struggles, and the Reagan Legacy

The Reagan-Bush legacy is contained in the social struggles that characterize the 1980s and 1990s. These include generational struggles, gender struggles, racial and ethnic struggles, and class struggles. First, questions of generational equity were socially constructed and fueled as public and political issues in the 1980s by demographers, economists, and politicians. They remain salient today. Pointed questions of fairness between different age cohorts and of the inevitability of rationing choices between generations penetrate and now threaten to dominate political discourse on income and health policy for the aged. The specter of this socially constructed "intergenerational war" continues to plague the progressive policy agenda in health and aging.

Second, Reagan and Bush rekindled old gender struggles. Neo-conservative ideology increased pressures for family responsibility laws and more private responsibility for posthospital and informal care. Pressures on women are sure to increase both with the demographic changes and the "baby dearth," and they will be exacerbated to the extent that we lack a comprehensive national long-term care policy in the United States that addresses issues of gender justice in the caregiving work in our society.

Supposedly we have the highest standard of living in any country in the world. Do we, though? It depends on what one means by high standards. Certainly nowhere does it cost more to live than here in America. The cost is not only in dollars and cents but in sweat and blood, in frustration, ennui, broken homes, smashed ideals, illness and insanity. We have the most wonderful hospitals, the most gorgeous insane asylums, the most fabulous prisons, the best equipped and the highest paid army and navy, the speediest bombers, the largest stockpile of atom bombs, yet never enough of any of these items to satisfy the demand. Our manual workers are the highest paid in the world; our poets the worst. There are more automobiles than one can count. And as for drugstores, where in the world will you find the like?
—Henry Miller

Indeed, the 1980s were a period of reassessment of women's place in society. Women are needed in the labor force for both public (to fulfill service roles including temporary low paid work without benefits) and private reasons (to maintain individual standards of living); yet, women are essential in filling the nation's growing need for long-term care given that women's work comprises the bulk of the nation's long-term care. The Reagan-Bush period was one in which the contradictions in women's lives became starkly apparent and their roles in the labor market and the home were simultaneously but differentially reinforced and expanded (but not necessarily supported).

Third, Reagan policies exacerbated class divisions both in the distribution of wealth and along the health care access dimension. Not only have privatization policies failed to stem the rising costs of medical care, but also they spurred reductions in coverage by public and private insurance and the exclusion of more and more of the U.S. population from access to that coverage. Since 1980, there has been a significant roll-back in early achievements in health care access following the passage of Medicare and

Medicaid. With the reemergence of a two-tier system of health care, the present class war in health is experienced in the declining access to care by the poor, rising infant mortality, and the erosion of health insurance benefits for the working population.

Another aspect of the deterioration of access is the reversal of decades of legitimacy and privileged state support for the nonprofit provision of health and social services. As the role of for-profit enterprise in health has flourished in the 1980s, nonprofits have found themselves in a beleaguered, uncertain, and highly competitive environment that is eroding their capacity to continue providing charity services. Nonprofit health and social services have themselves been part of the restructuring of delivery that has affected virtually all aspects of the formal and informal care system, including the nature and scope of services provided, the clientele served and their access to care, the composition of the labor force, and organizational financing. With changes in the structure, type of ownership, and control of these organizations, there has been an increase in the fragmentation of service delivery and provider targeting to clients who can pay privately and to services that are profitable or reimbursable by the state or private insurance.

The Reagan-Bush legacy broke the labor, race, and gender accords that were reached between the 1940s and the 1970s. In addition to the resurgence of the ideology of patriarchy through the "family values" theme, there was a systematic attack with severe restrictions placed on the reproductive rights of women, particularly for poor women. Welfare rights and benefits also were eroded.

As Abramovitz observes, the support of the welfare state by both business and government prior to the 1980s was conditioned by the need to address and pacify the political movements that arose in labor in the 1930s and 1940s, in civil rights in the 1950s and 1960s, and in women's issues in the 1960s and 1970s.

The economic crisis of the 1970s changed the political scene. Abramovitz says "the welfare state became too competitive with capital accumulation and too supportive of empowered popular movements." What had to be achieved was the redistribution of income from the bottom to the top, the reduction of the costs of labor, and initiation of a new conservative social movement to counter the expansive welfare state. President Reagan's program contributed to undoing the labor, race, and gender accords.

❖ Conclusion

Aging and health policy represent a major battleground on which the social struggles presently engulfing the state are being fought as it attempts to address growing tensions between capitalism and democracy. The construction of the aging of the population in crisis terms has served dual ideological purposes. First, the "demographic imperative" has been a rallying point for those who argue that the elderly are living too long, consuming too many societal resources, and robbing the young—justifying rollbacks of state benefits for the aged. Additional antistatist sentiments have been expressed in the unfounded contention that state policy to provide formal care will encourage abdication of family responsibility for the aging, which, in turn, will bankrupt the state. This line of reasoning is consistent with the state's continuing refusal to provide long-term care and reinforcing the idea that such care is (and should remain) the responsibility of the informal sector and the unpaid labor of women.

Second, the projected chronic illness burden of pandemic proportions (another version of the crisis) has been used in ideological attacks on health care as a right for the elderly, particularly by those promoting the intergenerational war. The elderly are accused of crippling both the state and corporate sectors with unsupportable demands.

In anticipation of the continuation of crises in the face of the growing needs of an aging society and the difficulties manifest in the modern form of advanced capitalism in the United States, the nation appears to be set on a collision course. Two alternate scenarios are possible. The first is one in which the state takes actions that extend the direction and influence of the economic and ideological commitments of the Reagan-Bush presidencies. The second is one in which the contradictions and resulting potential for social struggles presently engaged (class, generation, gender, and race) are realized, exploding with a force and effect that cannot be turned aside. The issue ahead is whether President Clinton's proposals for health reform alter the direction and course on which the nation has been set by the Reagan-Bush legacy.

❖ About the Author

Carroll L. Estes, Ph.D., is Director, Institute for Health & Aging and Professor of Sociology, Department of Social and Behavioral Sciences, School of Nursing, University of California, San Francisco.

❖ Food Lobbies, The Food Pyramid, and U.S. Nutrition Policy

MARION NESTLE

In April 1991, the U.S. Department of Agriculture (USDA) halted publication of its *Eating Right Pyramid,* a new guide to help the public select foods that would help reduce dietary risk factors for chronic diseases. Despite official explanations that the guide required further research and testing, its withdrawal was widely viewed as having been prompted by pressure from meat and dairy lobbying groups that objected to the way its design displayed their products (1–3). The guide was finally released almost exactly one year later after its content was supported by additional research and its graphic design altered to appease industry concerns (4).

This incident was only the latest in a long series of attempts by the food industry to influence federal dietary recommendations, but it focused renewed attention on a continuing dilemma in U.S. government: the conflict created when federal agencies responsible for the protection of public interests are also responsive to the lobbying efforts of private businesses acting on their own behalf. In the case of the *Pyramid,* the right of food lobbying groups to act in their own economic self-interest came into conflict with federal activities designed to improve the nutritional health of the public. The *Pyramid* controversy also demonstrated the potential conflict of interest posed by the dual mandates assigned to the USDA by Congress to protect U.S. agricultural interests and to advise the public about food choices.

To illustrate issues related to this dilemma, and to stimulate development of ways to ensure that U.S. nutrition policies are based on science rather than politics, this article reviews examples of incidents in which meat and dairy producer lobbies have influenced—or have attempted to influence—federal dietary recommendations for chronic disease prevention.

❖ U.S. Dietary Guidance Policy

The antecedents of the current controversy can be traced to the two roles assigned to the USDA when it was established in 1862: to ensure a sufficient and reliable food supply and to provide to the public useful information on subjects related to agriculture (5). These roles were viewed as complementary. Increased consumption of U.S. agricultural products also was expected to improve the health of the public.

The USDA's first dietary recommendations for adults, issued in 1917, established principles that govern the agency's nutrition policies to this day.

The USDA recommended no specific foods or combination of foods. Instead, it grouped foods of similar nutrient content into five broad categories: fruits and vegetables, meats, cereals, sugar, and fat (6). A 1923 publication, noting that any food could contribute to wholesome and attractive diets, explicitly encouraged consumers to purchase foods from the full range of U.S. farm products (7).

This approach was supported by food and agricultural producers who were unaware that the market for their products was limited. By 1909, the U.S. food supply already provided 3,500 kilocalories per capita (8), nearly twice the amount of daily energy needed by an average female adult and a third higher than that needed by an average male (9). A choice of any one food commodity necessarily would exclude others (10).

During the next 35 years, the USDA produced many more pamphlets based on the food group approach, all emphasizing the need to consume foods from certain "protective" groups in order to prevent deficiencies of essential nutrients (11). The number of recommended food groups varied from five to 12 over the years, however, in no particular order (12).

Prevention of Deficiencies: The Basic Four

In the early 1950s, national surveys indicated that the diets of certain groups of low-income Americans were below standard for several nutrients. To help the public choose foods that would help prevent nutrient deficiencies, the USDA developed a simplified guide based on just four groups—milk, meats, vegetables and fruits, and breads and cereals—which specified, for the first time, the number and size of servings. This publication, usually referred to as the Basic Four (13), remained the basis of USDA nutrition education efforts for the next 20 years.

During preparation of the Basic Four, the agency invited leading nutrition authorities, including food industry representatives, to review it, noting that "food industry groups would have a vital interest in any food guide sponsored by the government" (14). Despite concerns about the small serving size of the meat recommendations (two portions daily of two to three ounces), the food industry supported the guide, and the National Dairy Council, capitalizing on the prominent position of the milk group, distributed its own version as a public service (15).

Chronic Disease Prevention

Food industry support for dietary recommendations waned, however, when the focus of dietary recommendations shifted from avoidance of nutrient deficiencies to prevention of chronic diseases. As nutritional deficiencies declined in importance as public health problems, they were replaced by diet-related chronic diseases such as coronary heart disease, certain cancers, diabetes, stroke, and others that had become leading causes of death and disability. Early reports on the role of dietary fat in atherosclerosis, for example, were published in the mid-1950s (16), advice to reduce caloric intake from fat in 1961 (17), and recommendations for dietary changes and public policies to reduce coronary heart disease risk factors in 1970 (18). These last recommendations called for significant reductions in overall consumption of fat (to 35 percent of calories or less), saturated fat (to 10 percent), and cholesterol (to 300 milligrams per day)—advice quite similar to that given today.

The 1977 Farm Bill (Public Law 95-113) specified that the USDA was to assume responsibility for a wide range of nutrition research and education activities, including dietary advice to the public. In 1988, in an effort to ensure that the federal government speak with "one voice" about diet and health, the House Appropriations Committee reaffirmed the USDA's lead agency responsibility for this activity (19). As dietary recommendations shifted from "eat more" to "eat less," the USDA's dual mandates to protect agricultural producers and to advise the public about diet created increasing levels of conflict.

Although this conflict was due in part to concerns about the scientific validity of diet–disease relationships, it also derived from the profound economic implications of the new dietary recommendations (20). Foods of animal origin—meat, dairy, and eggs—together provide nearly 45 percent of the total fat, 60 percent of the saturated fat, and all of the cholesterol in the U.S. food supply (21). Thus, advice to consume less fat and cholesterol necessarily translates into reduced intake of animal products. By 1977, this message was well understood by consumers (22) and was reflected in declining sales of whole milk and eggs (23). As these downward trends continued, and as beef sales also began to decline, food producer lobbies became much more actively involved in attempts to discredit, weaken, or eliminate dietary recommendations that suggested using less of their products.

❖ Lobbies and Lobbyists

Lobbying includes any legal attempt by individuals or groups to influence government policy or action; this definition specifically excludes bribery. Because attempts to control such pressures have been viewed by corporations and by legislatures as infringements of basic rights, Congress has found it difficult to draft regulations acceptable to its members and their constituencies (24). At present, lobbying is regulated entirely by an Act that was passed in 1946, amended once in 1954, and used only once—in 1959—to convict an abuser of the system (25). As a result, the Act simply requires individuals or groups who lobby members of Congress to report their identities and sources of funds (26). Virtually all authorities consider even these modest requirements to be widely ignored and incapable of being enforced (27). Nevertheless, about 8,000 individuals currently register as lobbyists; among these, perhaps 5 percent represent food companies (28).

The relationship between food lobbies, the USDA, and Congress has long been a source of concern. Prior to the 1970s, food producers, USDA officials, and members of the House and Senate Agriculture Committees were so interconnected that they were said to constitute an "agricultural establishment" constituted to guarantee that federal policies would support the interests of food producers (29). The perpetuation of this system was assured by the Congressional seniority system and the strong representation on Agriculture committees of members from farm states. Jamie Whitten (D-Miss.), for example chaired the House Agricultural Appropriations Subcommittee for so long that he was referred to as the "permanent Secretary of Agriculture" (30); his 26-term career in Congress began under President F. D. Roosevelt.

This system weakened as new constituencies demanded influence on agriculture policies. The development of these constituencies was stimulated by the increasing importance of agriculture in the U.S. economy, the expansion of the food industry to include processors and marketers as well as producers (30), and the assignment to the USDA of the additional responsibility for food assistance to the poor (31). The number and composition of food lobbying groups expanded to reflect these changes (32).

Today, food lobbies include a multiplicity of groups, businesses, and individuals attempting to influence federal decisions. Food lobbies are not equal in influence. For the most part, food producers and commodity associations are much better funded than advocacy groups, for example. Beef and dairy lobbies are especially influential; they are well funded and distributed among a great many states, each with its own representatives in the House and Senate (33).

❖ Food Lobbies and Dietary Recommendations

Dietary Goals for the United States

In the early 1970s, staff of the Senate Select Committee on Nutrition and Human Needs, chaired by George McGovern (D.-S.D.), held a series of hearings on associations between dietary factors and chronic diseases, and produced a report on diet-disease relationships (34). These efforts led to the publication in February 1977 of the staff report, *Dietary Goals for the United States*, the first dietary recommendations for chronic disease prevention produced by a federal agency (35). Consistent with the earlier American Heart Association recommendations, this report established six goals for dietary change: increase carbohydrate intake to 55 to 60 percent of calories; decrease fat to 30 percent, saturated fat to 10 percent, and sugar to 15 percent of calories; reduce cholesterol to 300 milligrams per day; and reduce salt to three grams per day. To achieve these goals, the committee advised an increase in consumption of fruits, vegetables, whole grains, poultry, and fish; a decrease in consumption of meat, eggs, butterfat, and foods high in fat; and substitution of nonfat for whole milk.

Many groups objected to one or another of these recommendations, but the advice to decrease intake of specific high-fat foods brought immediate protest from the groups most affected—cattlemen and dairy and egg farmers. Meat and egg producers demanded and obtained additional hearings to express their views. These hearings were notable for their explicit statements of self-interest.

A National Cattlemen's Association representative, for example, stated that the term "decrease" with respect to meat consumption should be considered a "bad word" (36).

Members of the Select Committee representing states with large meat, dairy, and egg producer constituencies demanded changes in the *Dietary Goals*, and Senator McGovern was quoted as saying that "he did not want to disrupt the economic situation of the meat industry and engage in a battle with that industry that we could not win" (37). Therefore, the Committee revised the report and published a second edition in which, among other changes, the original statement, "Decrease consumption of meat and increase consumption of poultry and fish" (35, p. 13) was altered to read, "Decrease consumption of animal fat, and choose meats, poultry, and fish which will reduce saturated fat intake" (38).

Despite such compromises, the *Dietary Goals* established the basis of all subsequent federal recommendations and altered the course of nutrition education in the United States. This contribution, however, was the Select Committee's last. Shortly after release of the revised report, the Committee's functions were transferred to a Nutrition Subcommittee of the newly constituted Committee on Agriculture, Nutrition, and Forestry (39). McGovern lost his bid for reelection in 1980.

Healthy People

In 1979, in response to an emerging consensus among scientists and health authorities that national health priorities should emphasize disease prevention, the Department of Health, Education, and Welfare (DHEW) issued *Healthy People*, a report announcing goals for a ten-year plan to reduce controllable health risks (40). In its section on nutrition, the report recommended diets with fewer calories; less saturated fat, cholesterol, salt, and sugar; relatively more complex carbohydrates, fish, and poultry; and less red meat. Noting that more than half the diet consisted of processed foods rather than fresh agricultural produce, the text suggested that consumers pay closer attention to the nutritional qualities of processed foods.

Although dietary advice to restrict red meat and be wary of processed foods was certain to attract notice, *Healthy People* was released without a press conference in July 1979 as one of the final official acts of Joseph Califano, who had been dismissed from his position as DHEW Secretary by President Carter the month before. Nevertheless, the report elicited a "storm of protest" from food producers. The National Cattlemen's Association complained that "the diet-fat-cholesterol-heart disease hypothesis is not scientifically valid . . . recommendations that red meat consumption be reduced are not without risk to millions of Americans." Representatives of the meat, dairy, and egg industries offered to fund research to counter what was perceived as a growing scientific threat to the economic security of their industries (41). *Healthy People* became the last federal publication to use the words "eat less" when referring to meat.

USDA's Food Book

In the late 1970s, certain USDA nutritionists judged diets that met the *Dietary Goals* to be "so disruptive to usual food patterns" (42, p. 81) that this advice would require an adult man to consume 13 slices of bread each day (43). To help consumers make more reasonable health-promoting food choices, the USDA initiated a series of publications under the generic title *Food*. The first of these publications presented a revised version of the *Basic Four* in which the food groups were displayed in a vertical column with the vegetable/fruit group on top and the bread/cereal, dairy, and meat groups in successively lower bands. This revision also included a fifth group of foods that are high in energy but contain few essential nutrients—fats/sweets/alcohol—at the very bottom. To reduce fat intake, the guide advised, "cut down on fatty meats" (44).

Food was the most requested USDA publication in 1979 (45). After the 1980 election, however, under pressure from representatives of the meat, dairy, and egg industries who objected both to the advice to reduce fat and cholesterol and to the placement of their products below fruits, vegetables, and grains, USDA officials decided to delete the chapter on fat and cholesterol from what was expected to be the second publication in the series, *Food II* (46). Ultimately, the USDA decided against proceeding with the series and, instead, gave the completed page boards to the American Dietetic Association, which published them as two separate booklets in 1982 (47). *Food* became the last federal publication to use the phrase "cut down" in reference to meat.

1980 Dietary Guidelines

In February 1980, the USDA and DHEW announced joint publication of the *Dietary Guidelines for Americans* (48). These advised: eat a variety of foods; maintain ideal weight; avoid too much fat, saturated fat, and cholesterol; eat foods with adequate starch and fiber; avoid too much sugar; avoid too much sodium; if you drink alcohol, do so in moderation.

Because this publication had replaced the unacceptable "eat less" phrases with "avoid too much," agency officials did not expect objections from food producers. Indeed, the Food Marketing Institutes issued a statement that the *Guidelines* are "simple, reasonable and offer great freedom of choice," and the American Meat Institute called them "helpful," noting that they provide "a continuing and central role for meat." Producers of meat and other foods, however, found even these mild recommendations too extreme. They lobbied Congress to end funding for the *Guidelines* and demanded—and obtained—hearings on the matter (49). These efforts succeeded. Shortly after the 1980 election, but before the Reagan administration assumed office, Congress instructed the USDA to establish a joint committee to revise the recommendations with what was by then called the Department of Health and Human Services (DHHS).

At this point, the demise of the *Dietary Guidelines* seemed virtually assured. The new USDA Secretary, John Block, had remarked during his confirmation hearings that he was "not so sure government should get into telling people what they should or shouldn't eat" (50), and one of his first acts had been to close a USDA human nutrition research unit remarkable for its linking of study results to dietary guidance policy (49).

1985 Dietary Guidelines

When the committee to revise the *Dietary Guidelines* was finally appointed, five of the six USDA nominees were closely connected to the food industry (51). To the surprise of critics, however, the joint committee eventually made only minor changes in the 1980 text, and USDA Secretary Block, joined by the National Cattlemen's Association, endorsed the new edition (52), admitting that, "all of us have changed in our thinking" (53).

This change in views was due principally to increasing consensus on the scientific basis of diet and disease relationships, as expressed in three comprehensive reviews of relevant research released in 1988 and 1989 (54–56). These reports identified reduction of fat—particularly saturated fat—as the primary dietary priority, and recommended an overall reduction in fat intake to 30 percent of calories or less. Because none of the reports elicited much critical comment, consensus on dietary recommendations appeared to have been achieved (57).

1990 Dietary Guidelines

Despite the apparent consensus on diet–disease relationships, USDA officials argued that research since 1985 established a need to reexamine the *Dietary Guidelines*. A new joint committee with DHHS was appointed, consisting of nutrition scientists and physicians with few apparent food industry connections. Of 13 groups who submitted written comments during committee deliberations, however, ten represented food producers, trade associations, or organizations allied with industry (58).

The third edition of the *Dietary Guidelines* (59) revealed that the current consensus had been achieved at a price. To address concerns that the public increasingly perceived certain foods as "bad" and unfit for inclusion in healthy diets, the committee altered the phrasing of the specific guidelines to make their tone more positive. For the phrase, "avoid too much . . . ," the committee substituted, "choose a diet low in. . . ." For the phrase "choose lean meat . . . ," it substituted, "have two or three servings of meat . . . with a daily total of about 6 ounces" (59, p. 17).

The new publication did suggest upper limits of 30 percent of calories from fat and 10 percent from saturated fat, similar to limits suggested by the American Heart Association in 1970 and the *Dietary Goals* of 1977. Lest these figures appear too restrictive, however, the new *Guidelines* emphasized that the "goals for meals apply to the diet over several days, not to a single meal or food." The text noted that "Some foods that contain fat, saturated fat, and cholesterol, such as fats, milk, cheese, and eggs, also contain high-quality protein and are our best sources of certain vitamins and minerals." Unlike the previous two editions, the *1990 Dietary Guidelines* elicited no noticeable complaints from food producers.

The Food Guide Pyramid

In the early 1980s, USDA nutritionists identified a need for a food guide that would specify the numbers and sizes of food servings needed to meet the recommendations of the *Dietary Guidelines.* They developed a preliminary version of this guide in a wheel format for use in an American Red Cross course in 1984 (60), fast food industry experts objected to the study guides prepared for the course and requested extensive changes in the text (61). For this reason, and because the wheel design did not convey new information to the public, USDA staff initiated consumer research study to identify a more useful format. This research demonstrated that consumers preferred a triangular ("pyramid") shape that displays the food groups in bands, with grains and cereals at the wide base, vegetables and fruits in the band above, then meat and dairy foods, and, finally, fats and sweets in the narrow peak. Unlike earlier graphic designs, this format clearly conveyed the message that the daily diet should include more servings of grains, fruits, and vegetables than of meats, dairy products, and fats and sweets (62).

Preparation of the *Pyramid* brochure began in 1988. During the next two years, these materials were reviewed extensively, publicized widely, and fully cleared for publication; they were sent to the printer in February 1991 (63). In April, representatives of the National Cattlemen's Association saw a *Washington Post* report on the guide (64) and joined other producer groups in protesting that the guide stigmatized their products and should be withdrawn. Two weeks later, the newly appointed USDA Secretary, Edward Madigan, announced that the *Pyramid* required further testing on children and poorly educated adults, and postponed its publication. His explanation for this decision, however, was widely disbelieved (–3, 63).

During the subsequent year, the USDA issued a new contract, reportedly at an additional cost of $855,000 (4), to test alternative designs on children and low-income adults. Eventually, this research confirmed consumer preferences for the *Pyramid* over a runner-up bowl design preferred by meat and dairy producers (62,65). One year and one day after withdrawing it from publication, the USDA finally released the revised *Food Guide Pyramid* (66). In a change that pleased food producers, the design had been modified to emphasize that two to three daily portions of meat and dairy foods were still recommended (4), just as they had been since 1958 (13). Ironically, the *Pyramid* had actually increased the upper range of the meat recommendation; its text calls for daily consumption of an amount equivalent to five to seven ounces rather than the six ounces recommended in the 1990 *Dietary Guidelines.*

❖ Policy Implications

One view of lobbying is that it is a healthy influence within the political system that keeps Congress informed about issues, stimulates public debate, and encourages participation in the political process. From this perspective, lobbyists are unlikely to have much ability to inappropriately influence public policy decisions (24).

More critical analysts view lobbying as a far less benign activity (27). The recent history of dietary guidance policy demonstrates an increasing involvement of certain food lobbies—and the incorporation of their views—into federal recommendations to reduce dietary risk factors for chronic disease. In 1956, USDA staff drafted the *Basic Four* and, as a courtesy, permitted industry representatives to review it. Since 1980, however, food industry representatives have routinely participated in the development and review of dietary guidance materials. This change in role occurred as dietary recommendations shifted in focus from prevention of nutrient deficiencies ("eat more") to prevention of chronic diseases ("eat less") and as food producers more vigorously defended their products against the new advice.

Through their connections in Congress and the USDA, food lobbies have successfully convinced government policymakers to alter advice about meat, a principal source of dietary fat, from "eat less" to "choose lean" to "have two to three servings". Yet, these policy shifts have occurred just as nutrition scientists were reaching consensus that reduced fat intake would improve the health of the public (54, 56), were admitting that the 30 percent target recommendation for energy from fat is a compromise figure based on political realities, and were beginning to recommend a level of 20 to 25 percent as more consistent with the research evidence (67, 68). Given the contradiction between the scientific consensus and federal advice, it is little wonder that Americans are failing to reduce their fat intake significantly (23) and that the need for effective strategies to implement dietary recommendations has become the paramount concern of policymakers (57).

It must be emphasized that lobbying activities are entirely legal and available to consumer groups as well as to food producers. It should be clear, however, that the playing field is not level; food producers possess far greater resources for lobbying activities than do consumers. As one commentator stated long ago, it is unfortunate that "good advice about nutrition conflicts with the interests of many big industries, each of which has more lobbying power than all the public-interest groups combined" (69).

That food lobbies employ legal methods is not sufficient to justify their use of power based on economic and political influence rather than the merit of their views. The controversy over the *Food Guide Pyramid* demonstrates that the connections between members of Congress, USDA officials, and food lobbies must continue to raise questions about the ability of federal officials to make independent policy decisions.

Individuals concerned about such issues might consider whether conflicts of interest have so impaired the USDA's ability to educate the public about diet and health that such functions should be transferred to a unit less tied to food industry groups. Also worth consideration are more forceful advocacy of consumer perspectives to Congress, reform of lobbying laws and election campaign funding practices, and public education about the extent of lobbying influence. What is at stake here is no less than the health of the public, an issue of vital importance at any time but of particular concern during this era of health care cost containment.

❖ About the Authors

Marion Nestle, Ph.D., M.P.H., is Professor, Department of Nutrition and Food Studies, New York University.

REFERENCES

1. Burros, M. U.S. delays issuing nutrition chart. *New York Times,* April 27, 1991, p. A9.

2. Combs, G. F. What's happening at USDA. *AIN Nutr. Notes* 27(3):6, 1991.

3. Sugarman, C., and Gladwell, M. Revised food chart killed. *Washington Post,* April 17, 1991, pp. A1, A7.

4. Sugarman, C. The $855,000 pyramid. *Washington Post,* April 28, 1992, pp. A1, A4.

5. *Department of Agriculture Organic Act,* 12 Stat 317, May 15, 1862.

6. Hunt, C. L., and Atwater, H. W. *How to Select Foods. I: What the Body Needs.* Farmers' Bulletin 808, U.S. Department of Agriculture, Washington, D.C., 1917.

7. Hunt, C. L. *Good Proportions in the Diet.* Farmers' Bulletin No. 1313. U.S. Department of Agriculture, Washington, D.C., 1923.

8. Human Nutrition Information Service, U.S. Department of Agriculture. *Nutrient Content of the U.S. Food Supply.* Administrative Report 299-21. Washington, D.C., 1988.

9. National Research Council. *Recommended Dietary Allowances,* Ed. 10. National Academy Press, Washington, D.C., 1989.

10. Levenstein, H. *Revolution at the Table: The Transformation of the American Diet.* Oxford University Press, New York, 1988.

11. Haughton, B., et al. An historical study of the underlying assumptions for United States food guides from 1917 through the basic four food group guide. *J. Nutr. Educ.* 19:169–175, 1987.

12. Nestle, M., and Porter, D. V. Evolution of federal dietary guidance policy: From food adequacy to chronic disease prevention. *Caduceus* 6(2):43–67, 1990.

13. U.S. Department of Agriculture. *Food for Fitness: A Daily Food Guide.* Leaflet No. 424. Washington, D.C., 1958.

14. Hill, M. M., and Cleveland, L. E. Food guides—their development and use. *USDA Nutr. Program News,* July–October 1970, p. 3.

15. National Dairy Council. *A Guide to Good Eating.* Chicago, 1958.

16. Page, I. H., et al. Atherosclerosis and the fat content of the diet. *Circulation* 16:163–178, 1957.

17. American Heart Association. Dietary fat and its relation to heart attacks and strokes. *Circulation* 23: 133–136, 1961.

18. Inter-Society Commission for Heart Disease Resources. Primary prevention of the atherosclerotic diseases. *Circulation* 42: A55–A98, 1970.

19. U.S. House of Representatives. *Rural Development, Agriculture, and Related Agencies Appropriation Bill,* *1989.* Report No. 100–690, p. 107. Washington, D.C., June 10, 1988.

20. Timmer, C. P., and Nesheim, M. C. Nutrition, product quality, and safety. In *Consensus and Conflict in U.S. Agriculture,* edited by B. L. Gardner and J. W. Richardson, pp. 155–192. Texas A & M University Press, College Station, 1979.

21. Raper, N. Nutrient content of the U.S. food supply. *FoodReview* 14(3): 13–17, 1991.

22. U.S. Senate Select Committee on Nutrition and Human Needs. *Dietary Goals for the United States— Supplemental Views.* Washington, D.C., November 1977.

23. Putnam, J. J. Food consumption, 1970–90. *FoodReview* 14(3): 2–11, 1991.

24. Milbrath, L. W. *The Washington Lobbyists.* Rand McNally, Chicago, 1963.

25. Congressional Quarterly Service. *Legislators and the Lobbyists,* Ed. 2. Washington, D.C., 1968.

26. Congressional Quarterly Service. *Legislators and the Lobbyists.* Washington, D.C., 1965.

27. U.S. Senate Committee on Governmental Affairs. *The Federal Lobbying Disclosure Laws.* Hearings before the Subcommittee on Oversight of Government Management, S-Hrg. 102-377. Washington, D.C., June 20, July 16, September 25, 1991.

28. Registered lobbyists. *Congress Rec.* 37(122): HL 287-372, August 15, 1991.

29. Paarlberg, D. *American Farm Policy: A Case Study of Centralized Decision-making.* John Wiley & Sons, New York, 1964.

30. Morgan, D. Trying to lead the USDA through a thicket of politics. *Washington Post,* July 5, 1978, p. A1.

31. Morgan, D. 'Plain, poor sister' is newly alluring. *Washington Post,* July 4, 1978, pp. A1, A8.

32. Browne, W. P. *Private Interests, Public Policy, and American Agricul-*

ture. University Press of Kansas, Lawrence, 1988.

33. Guither, H. D. *The Food Lobbyists: Behind the Scenes of Food and Agripolitics*. Lexington Books, Lexington, Mass., 1980.

34. U.S. Senate Select Committee on Nutrition and Human Needs. *Final Report*. Washington, D.C., December 1977.

35. U.S. Senate Select Committee on Nutrition and Human Needs. *Dietary Goals for the United States*. Washington, D.C., February 1977.

36. Senate Select Committee on Nutrition and Human Needs. *Diet Related to Killer Diseases, III. Hearings in Response to Dietary Goals for the United States: Re Meat*, p. 42. Washington, D.C., March 24, 1977.

37. Mottern, N. Dietary goals. *Food Monitor*, March/April 1978, p. 9.

38. U.S. Senate Select Committee on Nutrition and Human Needs. *Dietary Goals for the United States*, Ed. 2, p. 4. Washington, D.C., December 1977.

39. Hadwiger, D. G., and Browne, W. P. (eds.). *The New Politics of Food*. Lexington Books, Lexington, Mass., 1988.

40. U.S. Department of Health, Education, and Welfare. *Healthy People: The Surgeon General's Report on Health Promotion and Disease Prevention*. DHEW(PHS) 79-55071. Washington, D.C., 1979.

41. Monte, T. The U.S. finally takes a stand on diet. *Nutr. Action* 6(9): 4, 1979.

42. Wolf, I. D., and Peterkin, B. B. Dietary guidelines: The USDA perspective. *Food Technol.* 38(7): 80–86, 1984.

43. Peterkin, B. B., et al. Diets that meet the dietary goals. *J. Nutr. Educ.* 10: 15–18, 1978.

44. U.S. Department of Agriculture. *Food: The Hassle-free Guide to a Better Diet*, p. 18. Home and Garden Bulletin No. 228. Washington, D.C., 1979.

45. Foreman, C. T. Personal communication.

46. ADA may publish expurgated version of "Food Two" magazine. *CNI Weekly Rep.* 12(17): 1–2, 1982.

47. ADA to publish Food II magazine as separate booklets. *CNI Weekly Rep.* 12(33): 1–2, 1982.

48. U.S. Department of Agriculture and U.S. Department of Health, Education, and Welfare. *Nutrition and Your Health: Dietary Guidelines for Americans*. Home and Garden Bulletin No. 232. Washington, D.C., 1980.

49. Broad, W. J. Nutrition research: End of an empire. *Science* 213: 518–520, 1981.

50. Maugh, T. H. Cancer is not inevitable. *Science* 217:36–37, 1982.

51. USDA readies to carve up the dietary guidelines. *Nutr. Action* 10(2): 3–4, 1983.

52. U.S. Department of Agriculture and U.S. Department of Health and Human Services. *Nutrition and Your Health: Dietary Guidelines for Americans*, Ed. 2. Home and Garden Bulletin No. 232. Washington, D.C., 1985.

53. Reagan administration OK's dietary guidelines. *CNI Weekly Rep.*, September 26, 1985, p. 2.

54. National Research Council. *Designing Foods: Animal Product Options in the Marketplace*. National Academy Press, Washington, D.C., 1988.

55. U.S. Department of Health and Human Services. *The Surgeon General's Report on Nutrition and Health*. DHHS (PHS) Publ. No. 88-502010. Washington, D.C., 1988.

56. National Research Council. *Diet and Health: Implications for Reducing Chronic Disease Risk*. National Academy Press, Washington, D.C., 1989.

57. McGinnis, J. M., and Nestle, M. The surgeon general's report on nutrition and health: Policy implications and implementation strategies. *Am. J. Clin. Nutr.* 49: 23–28, 1989.

58. U.S. Department of Agriculture. *Report of the Dietary Guidelines Ad-*

visory Committee on the Dietary Guidelines for Americans. No. 261-463/20444. Washington, D.C., 1990.

59. U.S. Department of Agriculture and U.S. Department of Health and Human Services. *Nutrition and Your Health: Dietary Guidelines for Americans*, Ed. 3. Home and Garden Bulletin No. 232. Washington, D.C., 1990.

60. Cronin, F. J., et al. Developing a food guidance system to implement the dietary guidelines. *J. Nutr. Educ.* 19: 281–302, 1987.

61. Zuckerman, S. Killing it softly. *Nutr. Action*, January/February 1984, pp. 6–10.

62. Welsh, S., Davis, C., and Shaw, A. Development of the food guide pyramid. *Nutr. Today* 27: 12–23, November/December 1992.

63. A pyramid topples at the USDA. *Consumer Rep.* 56(10): 663–666, 1991.

64. Gladwell, M. U.S. rethinks, redraws the food groups. *Washington Post*, April 13, 1991, pp. A1, A7.

65. Burros, M. Testing of pyramid comes full circle. *New York Times*, March 25, 1992, pp. C1, C4.

66. Human Nutrition Information Service, U.S. Department of Agriculture. *USDA's Food Guide Pyramid*. Home and Garden Bulletin No. 249. Washington, D.C., April 1992.

67. Wynder, E. L., et al. Nutrition: The need to define "optimal" intake as a basis for public policy decisions. *Am. J. Public Health* 82: 346–350, 1992.

68. Are you eating right? *Consumer Rep.* 57(10): 644–652, 1992.

69. Jacobson, M. *Nutrition Scoreboard*, pp. 197–198. Avon, New York, 1974.

❖ Preventing Tobacco Use—The Youth Access Trap

STANTON A. GLANTZ

During his tenure, Surgeon General C. Everett Koop transformed the public debate over tobacco use by calling for a smoke-free society by the year 2000. He was the first major public official to articulate clearly the message that smoking need not be a part of American life. The tobacco industry went wild and aggressively attacked Koop, because his message went to the core of the tobacco issue: tobacco use in public was no longer socially acceptable. Today, that message has been eclipsed by a less potent—and probably counterproductive—one: "We don't want kids to smoke."

Pierce and Gilpin[1] estimate that teenagers who become smokers today will remain addicted for an average of 16 to 20 years. Escobedo and Peddicord[2] show that efforts to prevent tobacco use have not affected people with less than a high school education. DiFranza et al.[3] show that only 28% of vendors consistently obey laws limiting sales of tobacco to children, that the tobacco industry's "It's the Law" program has virtually no effect on the ability of kids to buy cigarettes, and that cigarette vending machine lockout devices have little practical effect.

Everyone seems to agree. The tobacco industry is running advertisements repeating its claim that it wants to stop "underage smoking" because smoking is an "adult custom"; the Food and Drug Administration (FDA)[4,5] has advanced proposals directed at children; and the health departments in the three states with major voter-mandated tobacco control programs—California, Massachusetts, and Arizona—have all been directed to concentrate on kids. There are several good reasons for this strategy from the tobacco industry's point of view.

First, it makes the industry look reasonable. While the industry must recruit kids to replace dying and quitting adults, it can never admit this.

Second, and more important, the message "we don't want *kids* to smoke" reinforces tobacco advertising. Tobacco marketing documents subpoenaed by the Federal Trade Commission[6] over a decade ago show how a cigarette company can introduce "starters" to its brand:

> For the young smoker, the cigarette is not yet an integral part of life, of day-to-day life, in spite of the fact that they try to project the image of a regular, run-of-the-mill smoker. For them, a cigarette, and the whole smoking process, is part of the illicit pleasure category . . . [a] declaration of independence and striving for self identity. . . .

Thus, an attempt to reach young smokers, starters, should be based, among others, on the following major parameters:

❖ Present the cigarette as one of the few initiations into the adult world.
❖ Present the cigarette as part of the illicit pleasure category of products and activities.
❖ In your ads create a situation taken from the day-to-day life of the young smoker, but in an elegant manner have this situation touch on the basic symbols of the growing-up, maturity process.

The message "we don't want *kids* to smoke" reinforces this message. Kids shouldn't smoke, but if you want to look and act like an adult, do it.

The current concentration on youth access is not the first time that the health community has inadvertently reinforced a tobacco industry message. One reason that kids start to smoke is the fact that they grossly overestimate smoking prevalence.[7] Ubiquitous tobacco advertising has contributed to this misimpression, but so has anti-tobacco education that says "resist your peers, don't smoke." The message should be "be like your friends, be a nonsmoker."

Third, the current concentration on keeping kids from buying tobacco products shifts the focus away from the tobacco industry to tens of thousands of convenience stores and gas stations and the same kind of failed law enforcement–based approach that has characterized the war on illegal drugs. If there is one lesson to be learned from the war on drugs, it is that law enforcement and supply controls cannot prevent people from getting addictive drugs that are profitable to sell. The ultimate misplacing of responsibility is when legislators criminalize children for possessing tobacco.[7-9] Although intensive youth access efforts can reduce the likelihood that some merchants will sell tobacco to kids,[10-13] there is no consistent evidence of a substantial effect on prevalence or consumption of tobacco among kids.

Fourth, the youth access campaign, with its focus on stings, actually teaches kids that cigarettes and other tobacco products are easy to get. While this fact may outrage public health professionals, it sends the wrong message to kids.

Finally, consider the politicians who are pressing tobacco control activities based on kids. In California, Governor Pete Wilson has been campaigning relentlessly—and successfully—to dismantle the state's effective tobacco control program mandated by the voters in Proposition 99.[14-19] California's anti-tobacco campaign once focused on discrediting the tobacco industry and educating the public about nicotine addiction and secondhand smoke (messages that appeal to both adults and kids); now it focuses on youth access. Last year the state ran "Nicotine Soundbites," an ad that turned Congressional testimony of tobacco company executives that nicotine was not addictive into a devastating ad that combined the three messages of discrediting the industry, nicotine addiction, and secondhand smoke into a potent 30-second television spot. Wilson has forbidden the use of the ad. I doubt that "if you see someone selling a kid a cigarette, call this number" has the same bite.

Next door, in Arizona, the voters enacted Proposition 200, which increased the tobacco tax and mandated an anti-tobacco education program. Arizona Governor Fife Symington has made his hostility to the program clear by appointing three tobacco lobbyists to the committee charged with advising the program. The tobacco industry's lawyers and the pro-tobacco members on the committee have loudly demanded that the health department strictly limit the program focus to children. Programs with any crossover between kids and adults have been opposed.

In Massachusetts, the tobacco industry raised a huge fuss when the health department mounted an aggressive and effective media campaign and coordinated local programs concentrating on secondhand smoke and denormalization of tobacco use. The department has backed off from the campaign to concentrate on the less controversial issue of youth access.

Does this mean that the FDA proposal[4,5] to regulate tobacco products using a strategy based on preventing kids from smoking is a mistake? Absolutely not. For the most part, the FDA proposal concentrates on proper labeling of tobacco products as nicotine delivery devices and attempting to curb the tobacco industry's predatory marketing practices. With a few adjustments, such as including the fact that nicotine is addictive in the product labeling and not having the tobacco industry run the anti-tobacco education campaign, these are well-conceived proposals that warrant support. Except for actions directed at manufacturers and distributors, however, the FDA should de-emphasize the law enforcement aspects of its proposal directed at keeping kids from buying tobacco and focus on keeping kids from *wanting* tobacco.

A better way to reduce the marketing of tobacco to kids is to create a real economic incentive for the tobacco industry to stop selling tobacco to kids. For example, rather than advocating taxes on cigarettes—and smokers—public health advocates should advocate taxing *tobacco companies* based on actual consumption of their products by children.[20] Despite what they say, the tobacco companies have a strong incentive to addict children. Not only do they make immediate sales, but, as Pierce and Gilpin[1] show, they also create customers for 16 to 20 years. The companies should be taxed at a level that keeps them from reaping these long-term benefits. If tobacco companies were taxed at a rate equal to twice the retail value of cigarettes of their brands smoked by kids, they would no longer benefit from addicting kids. (A higher multiplier would create an active economic disincentive.) Such a tax would create a situation in which the industry *really* would want to keep kids from smoking.

Finally, the public health community should realize that the best way to keep kids from smoking is to reduce tobacco consumption among everyone. The message should not be "we don't want kids to smoke"; it should be "we want a smoke-free society." As the tobacco industry knows well, kids want to be like adults, and reducing adult smoking sends a strong message to kids about social norms.

Ironically, in the rush to concentrate on kids, other, more adult-centered approaches to controlling the tobacco epidemic have been displaced by the kids' agenda. Indeed, while the public health community has mobilized aggressively in support of the FDA's proposals, the Occupational Safety and Health Administration's (OSHA) proposal[21] to make workplaces smoke-free has been ignored. Despite the evidence that creation of a smoke-free workplace is the best predictor of progress in smoking cessation[22] and the evidence that creation of a smoke-free workplace reduces smoking prevalence by around 25% and tobacco consumption among continuing smokers by about 20%,[23–30] except for the American Medical Association, not one of the major public health organizations is formally participating in the OSHA rule-making process. The tobacco industry is dominating the proceedings by default.

Public health professionals need to step back from the current preoccupation with youth and return to a more balanced and sophisticated tobacco control program. If current trends continue, we will look back on the mid 1990s as a time that the tobacco industry once again outsmarted the public health community.

ACKNOWLEDGMENT

This research was funded by National Cancer Institute grant CA-61021.

❖ About the Author

Stanton Glantz, M.D., is Professor, Department of Medicine, University of California, San Francisco.

REFERENCES

1. Pierce JP, Gilpin E. How long will today's new adolescent smoker be addicted to cigarettes? *Am J Public Health.* 1996;86:253–256.

2. Escobedo LG, Peddicord JP. Smoking prevalence in US birth cohorts: the influence of gender and education. *Am J Public Health.* 1996;86:231–236.

3. DiFranza JR, Savageau JA, Aisquith BF. Youth access to tobacco: the effects of age, gender, vending machine locks, and "It's the Law" programs. *Am J Public Health.* 1996;86:221–224.

4. Food and Drug Administration. Regulations restricting the sale and distribution of cigarettes and

smokeless tobacco products to protect children and adolescents. *Federal Register.* 1995;60(August 11):41313–41375.

5. Food and Drug Administration. Proposed rule analysis regarding FDA's jurisdiction over nicotine-containing cigarettes and smokeless tobacco products. *Federal Register.* 1995;60(August 11):41454–41787.

6. *Staff Report of the Cigarette Advertising Investigation.* Washington, DC: US Federal Trade Commission; 1981.

7. Institute of Medicine. *Growing Up Tobacco Free: Preventing Nicotine Addiction in Children and Youths.* Washington, DC: National Academy Press; 1994.

8. Carol J. It's a good idea to criminalise purchase and possession of tobacco by minors—NOT!". *Tobacco Control.* 1992;1:296–297.

9. Cismoski J. Blinded by the light: The folly of tobacco possession laws against minors. *Wis Med J.* 1994;93:591–597.

10. Jason LA, Ji PY, Anes MD, Birkhead SH. Active enforcement of cigarette control laws in the prevention of cigarette sales to minors. *JAMA.* 1991;266:3159–3161.

11. DiFranza JR, Carlson RR, Caisse REJ. Reducing youth access to tobacco. *Tobacco Control.* 1992;1:58.

12. Hinds MW. Impact of a local ordinance banning tobacco sales to minors. *Public Health Rep* 1992;107:356–358.

13. Lopez R, Tucker B, Childs R, et al. Reducing tobacco access to teens: Arizona pilot projects. In. *Abstracts, 123rd Annual Meeting of the American Public Health Association:* October 29–November 2, 1995; San Diego, Calif. Session 2277.

14. Skolnick A. Court orders governor to restore anti-smoking media campaign funding. *JAMA.* 1992;267:2721–2723.

15. Begay ME, Traynor MP, Glantz SA. The tobacco industry, state politics, and tobacco education in California. *Am J Public Health.* 1993;83:1214–1221.

16. Begay ME, Traynor MP, Glantz SA. *The Twilight of Proposition 99: Reauthorization of Tobacco Education Programs and Tobacco Industry Political Expenditures in 1993.* San Francisco, Calif: Institute for Health Policy Studies, University of California, San Francisco: 1994.

17. Skolnick A. Antitobacco advocates fight 'illegal' diversion of tobacco control money. *JAMA.* 1994;271:1387–1390.

18. Aguinaga S, Macdonald H, Traynor M, Begay M, Glantz S. *Undermining Popular Government: Tobacco Industry Political Expenditures in California, 1993–1994.* San Francisco, Calif: University of California Institute for Health Policy Studies; 1995.

19. Skolnick A. Judge rules diversion of antismoking money illegal. *JAMA.* 1995;273:610–611.

20. Glantz S. Removing the incentive to sell kids tobacco. *JAMA.* 1993;2669:793–794.

21. US Occupational Safety and Health Administration. Indoor Air Quality (Proposed Rule). *Federal Register* 1994;59(April 5). 15968–16039.

22. Pierce JP, Evans N, Farkas AJ, et al. *Tobacco Use in California: An Evaluation of the Tobacco Control Program, 1989–1993.* San Diego, Calif: University of California, San Diego; 1994.

23. Stillman F, Becker D, Swank R, et al. Ending smoking at the Johns Hopkins Medical Institutions: an evaluation of smoking prevalence and indoor pollution. *JAMA.* 1990;264:1565–1569.

24. Woodruff T, Rosebrook B, Pierce J, Glantz S. Lower levels of cigarette consumption found in smoke-free workplaces in California. *Arch Intern Med.* 1993;153:1485–1493.

25. Kinne S, Kristal AR, White E, Hunt J. Work-site smoking policies: their

population impact in Washington State. *Am J Public Health.* 1993;83: 1031–1033.

26. Brenner H, Fleischle B. Smoking regulations at the workplace and smoking behavior: a study from southern Germany. *Prev Med.* 1994;23:230–234.

27. Brigham J, Gross J, Stitzer ML, Felch LJ. Effects of a restricted work-site smoking policy on employees who smoke. *Am J Public Health.* 1994;84:773–778.

28. Jeffery RW, Kelder SH, Forster JL, et al. Restrictive smoking policies in the workplace: effects on smoking prevalence and cigarette consumption. *Prev Med.* 1994;23:78–82.

29. Borland R, Owen N. Need to smoke in the context of workplace smoking bans. *Prev Med.* 1995;24: 56–60.

30. Patten CA, Gilpin E, Cavin S, Pierce JP. Workplace smoking policy and changes in smoking behavior in California: a suggested association. *Tobacco Control.* 1995;4: 36–41.

❖ Long Term Care and the Race to the Bottom

CARROLL L. ESTES AND KAREN W. LINKINS

❖ Introduction

Health reform today is being driven by private sector market reform and the refusal of Congress to enact a policy of universal national health care. In the absence of a federal policy commitment, there is uncertainty regarding the fate of long term care (LTC) since it remains largely and increasingly the purview of the states.

During the past two decades, decentralization, devolution, and other reductions in the federal role in domestic health and human service policy have been fundamental processes shaping the structure and delivery of LTC in the United States. The 1996 Welfare Reform legislation signed by President Clinton illustrates the trend toward devolution of responsibility for policymaking from the federal to state level. This new law accords states much greater control over determining eligibility and benefit levels for welfare and de-couples the program from automatic Medicaid eligibility. In addition, the enactment of this law may signal the beginning of further cutbacks and decreased Federal support for other entitlement or safety-net programs such as Medicare and Medicaid.

❖ Role of Government

Decentralization of program and fiscal responsibility is an on-going political theme in the United States, as are efforts to reduce the federal role and responsibility for social needs. The notion of federalism that underlies the decentralization and devolution debate dates back to the country's beginning, and controversy about its form and function is heard among officials and citizens at all levels of government. Five themes concern the role of government: 1) the delineation of federal, state, and local responsibilities; 2) the capacity and structural incentives of the different governmental levels; 3) equity; 4) accountability; and 5) democratic participation and the distribution of power (Estes & Gerard, 1983).

The intensity of the current debate about the appropriate role of the government and the private sector underscores the fundamental questions of national purpose and goals, and the means by which these goals will be achieved. There is continuing dispute about whether devolution reform can in fact achieve national goals other than those related to a reduced federal role in domestic health and social policy.

The justification for the federal role is that it: 1) provides for a necessary equalization in the level of public services among states and localities; 2) provides for a level of services that the national interest requires; 3) reflects the capacity of the national government to collect taxes; and 4) involves national administration, performance and competence.

Deregulation is one instrument of devolution that is being used selectively, both legislatively and administratively, to further the goals of devolution. An example is the Unfunded Mandates Reform Act of 1995 that limits federal power to adopt future mandates for states, localities, and tribal governments without paying for them. Given that such Congressionally mandated actions have served as an important mechanism of federal control over state policy without itself incurring fiscal costs (Nathan, 1996, p48), the prohibition of unfunded mandates is an highly significant change in federal state relations.

Welfare reform and other recent proposals for domestic policy change are designed to diminish, and in some cases, abolish the federal role in health and welfare programs, with the devolution of responsibility to the states. The impact of the power shift from the nation's capitol to 50 statehouses through welfare reform is being augmented by Medicaid cuts and policy changes, managed care, and the massive restructuring of health care by the private market. Two key questions are: To what extent will this devolution of authority result in more or less responsive programs and expenditures? And, to what extent will the diminution of national standards, federal requirements and oversight promote politically-based rather than need-based policies and allocations at the state level?

There are six potential effects of decentralization for programs of long-term care and the disadvantaged: 1) decentralization supplants national policy goals and commitments with the more autonomous and variable state and local policy choices, particularly with regard to essential programs for the aging, blunting the more progressive changes that could be more easily generated at the national level rather than across 50 state jurisdictions; 2) with decentralization, the dominant structural economic and political interests operating at the federal level are not likely to be challenged by the fragmented and diverse interest groups for the poor operating at the state and local levels; 3) to the extent that there is a divestment of federal (and public sector) responsibility through deregulation and decentralization of policy goal-setting, the influence in policy making of private sector interests in contrast to public interests are likely to be increased. Public policy, especially for the chronically ill and disadvantaged elderly, is being mediated in largely unknown ways by business and provider interests; 4) with decentralized policy making, those who are well off, best funded and organized, have the most influence through their ability to mobilize across multiple and disperse geopolitical jurisdictions; 5) increased state and local responsibility for programs places human services demands on the most fiscally vulnerable and politically sensitive levels of decision-making, given that states and localities have more variable and limited taxing capacity and fiscal resources than the federal government. Thus, decisions about services for the elderly and low income, including long term care are located precisely where pressures to control social expenses are greatest and necessarily the most conservative. Problems of access are likely to increase; 6) decentralization raises important accountability issues as federal oversight and data give way to highly variable state and local data concerning these programs (Estes, 1994:221).

By 1996, the federally assured safety net of entitlement to welfare and the assurance of minimal access to health care for those disqualified by the states (e.g., legal aliens) have now become "choices" that states have the option of making. A concern is that, with devolution, there is little assurance of consistency or uniformity of policy and threats concerning equity for powerless groups across different states.

❖ Devolution and Long Term Care

State discretionary policies are a key element in determining long term care services for elders and the younger disabled. Policy choices under the domain of the states pose a challenge and dilemma for LTC for two reasons. First, the wide areas of policy discretion and attendant uncertainty permitted under decentralized policies such as welfare, Medicaid, and block grants for social services and mental health, lead to great variability and what are demonstrably large inequities between the states; and second, issues of accountability are raised under conditions of enhanced autonomy, reduced and fragmented data collection, and program variability (Estes, 1983:17-39).

At the heart of the devolution debate " . . . is a disagreement about which level of government in the federal system should be responsible for designing, implementing, and funding the nation's safety net." (Peterson, Rom & Scheve, 1995, p 3). The resulting increases in decentralized authority for priority setting and resource allocation with devolution and decategorization may be positive or negative in their impact for particular target groups or populations such as those needing LTC. The potential exists for resource increases in community based long term care as states are released from unfunded mandates and other federal requirements. Concurrently, there are escalating conflicts, trade offs, and resource losses among competing groups. It is particularly hazardous for those repressed interests (Alford, 1972) that are less organized and less powerful, as well as those that are considered "undeserving."

Devolution raises crucial questions about the future of social insurance and entitlement programs, and ultimately the future of aging and LTC policy. How will governors, mayors, and other state and local elected officials deal with the federal retrenchment and the shift of governmental responsibility to state and local governments, especially when confronted by increasingly difficult social and economic choices within and outside of their respective locations? States are in economic and political competition with each other (Peterson, Rom and Scheve, 1996; Dye, 1990; Eisinger, 1988), which hinges on attracting and retaining investment capital, business firms, and labor to enhance the state's economy and the political fortunes of its leaders. This competition can create a "race among the states"—referred to as a "race to the bottom" (Peterson, Rom and Scheve, 1996)—in which states compete with one another to decelerate their respective levels of commitment to welfare and other safety-net programs in order to achieve other economic and political goals.

Under devolution, more "generous" states are penalized particularly in those cases where a state's costs of providing higher levels of state-determined benefits are not matched or otherwise shared by the federal government. State generosity (defined as providing benefits or eligibility above the minimum level) is a liability under programs that are federally capped such as block grants, in contrast those with open ended federal matching as provided heretofore under Medicaid. The eradication of entitlements as with the Aid to Families with Dependent Children (AFDC) program and its replacement by a cash block grant provides a clear financial incentive to states to reduce or restrain their eligibility and costs. Stated another way, block grants and financially capped programs create an *economic disincentive for the states to offer anything more than the minimum level of benefits* that can be politically accommodated. As Peterson and his colleagues note, "The more control states have over policy choices, and the more they bear the costs of providing welfare or obtain savings from restricting it, the greater the incentives to race" (Peterson, Rom and Scheve, 1996:4).

❖ The Race to the Bottom and Long Term Care

Given this prior research on devolution and aging services during the 1980's (Estes, 1983) and that on the propensity for states to "race to the bottom" in welfare policy (Peterson & Rom, 1990; Peterson, Rom & Scheve, 1995), central issues are: 1) the extent to which state level discretionary policy options alter priorities, services, and other policy outcomes for community based LTC (CBLTC); 2) the existence of and extent to which a race to the bottom is occurring in LTC in the states; 3) whether LTC programs and populations are as vulnerable, or more or less vulnerable to cuts and entitlement reforms as other health or welfare programs and populations; 4) the factors that influence the nature and direction of such changes; 5) the tradeoffs in and consequences of shifting policy and funding on LTC and recipients along generational, gender, racial and ethnic, and social class lines (Estes & Gerard, 1983; Estes & Newcomer, 1983; Polivka, Dunlop & Rothman, 1996); 6) the role and effects of managed care on LTC including that on the "rest" of the nonprofit community based LTC system (e.g., adult day care, nutrition, and personal assistance); 7) the effects of devolution on the health of communities (population health); and 8) the extent and effects of political mobilization of LTC and other advocates on state and local choices (Estes & Swan, et al., 1982).

Factors that affect the answers to the above questions include the fiscal condition of the states, the rapid growth of managed care and the integration and accessibility of long term care services under these programs, and what the health outcomes, cost and quality of long term care will be under managed care compared to the fee-for-service (FFS) system or other alternatives. Long term care will continue to be dramatically affected by the climate of crisis and cutbacks.

There is a growing need for knowledge about the role and effects of managed care organizations (MCOs) on health and human services that comprise the long term care continuum of services. Significant questions concern their effects on the traditional nonprofit community based social supportive services and their potential to medicalize social services (Polivka, Dunlop, & Rothman, 1996).

❖ LTC Implications of Devolution, Medicare, Medicaid, and Managed Care

Political, economic, and socio-cultural factors challenge the future of long term care. The resources available for LTC will be shaped by the outcomes of partisan struggles in Congress and the White House concerning the fate of Medicare and Medicaid and the decisions of the governors and state houses intent on tax and budget cuts in social programs to pay for them.

Political factors include the dramatically enhanced the ability of proprietary interests to shape the public policy agenda in ways that create change and uncertainty for the long term care industry. Home and community based care are pitted against the highly influential nursing home and managed care interests. Nonprofit community care providers are pitted against (and swallowed up by) the more powerful for-profit managed care and nursing home interests. _Economic factors_ include the rising for-profit ownership and concentration in all aspects of the medical industrial complex (Estes, Harrington & Davis, 1993) that have vastly increased the stakes in the profitability of health and long term care for private shareholders. A contradiction is that rising health costs coincide with rising profits while at the same time generating oppositional forces to the rising costs from those in the public and private sectors that pay them. Finally, _socio-cultural factors_ include the struggles and cultural shifts accompanying the pervasive and strong ideology of the market; with competition, efficiency, and rationalization as major mechanisms to achieve profits and cost containment These "means" have become goal displaced as "ends" in themselves.

❖ The Future of Long Term Care

An overarching issue concerns the effects on long term care of the growing gap between medical and social services and what Estes and colleagues (1993) have described as the capture of social services by and in service to the acute care sector. The potential new free rider problem regarding community-based LTC under managed care is a significant unanswered question.

A key question regarding the aging and LTC is whether those traditionally seen as more deserving (older persons in general and the aged, blind and disabled under SSI) are being reconstructed as less deserving with the promotion of the social construction of the "Intergenerational war" by larger political and economic interests. This, too, is an empirical question. Will the "center" hold on entitlements for groups other than the welfare population? Or will the same fate await programs for the elderly as for welfare recipients, whether on SSI, Social Security, or Medicare?

With regard to devolution, questions are whether and how states will use their policy discretion to rebalance the growing gap between social services and acute care services to assure a LTC continuum. With welfare reform, cuts were imposed in 1996 on Title XX social services block grant (SSBG). Block grants and budget cuts will decrease funding for the new needs created by shorter and shorter hospital lengths of stay (LOS), which are projected to decline another 50 percent in the next few years, the technological and managed care pressures for more home and community based care, and the sociodemographics of an aging population. There is modest decline or stability of Older Americans Act (OAA) funding in absolute dollars but a significant decline in funding for social services relative to cost of living, inflation, economic growth. Much of the social services have been shifted to Medicaid waiver programs. Their fate under managed care and increased state discretion, and Medicaid policy changes yet to come are unclear.

To summarize, with politically and economically motivated attacks on entitlement, a central question concerns the fates of the Medicare and Medicaid entitlements, for the future of LTC is inextricably entwined with them. Important considerations are:

- ❖ The existence of and extent to which a race to the bottom is occurring in LTC.
- ❖ The trade-offs that are being made between programs, population groups, and services. For example, what are the trade-offs between groups needing chronic and skilled care services? Between medical and non-medical services? Between high tech and low tech care? Between LTC institutional (nursing home), community-based, and in home services?
- ❖ The form of clinical integration brought by disease management under managed care and its incentives for, and effects on access to, LTC along

the continuum of sub-acute and post acute to chronic and supportive services.

❖ The relationships of LTC to the "rest" (currently residualized) of the nonprofit community-based LTC system (adult day care; nutrition, respite care, senior center services, personal assistance.

❖ The potential social iatrogenic effects of the U.S. health care system (e.g., managed care and technology driven medical care) on patient dependency. Will the supportive and rehabilitative services be available to promote feasible functional status improvements?

❖ On the consumer level, what are the outcomes of managed care and LTC, measuring their full economic and social consequences including: the sacrifices and transfers of costs outside of the managed care and medical care system such as informal care; the costs of empowering or dependency generating outcomes; of shifting work and increased exploitation of patients and their families?

❖ About the Author

Carroll L. Estes, Ph.D., is Director, Institute for Health & Aging and Professor of Sociology, Department of Social and Behavioral Sciences, School of Nursing, University of California, San Francisco.

Karen W. Linkins, Ph.C, is Research Associate, Institute for Health & Aging, University of California, San Francisco.

REFERENCES

Alford, 1972. The Political Economy of Health Care: Dynamics without Change. Politics and Society; 2, pp. 127-164.

Dye, T.R. 1990. Competitive Federalism: Competition Among Governments. Lexington, MA: D.C. Heath.

Eisinger, 1988. The Rise of the Entrepreneurial State: State and Local Economic Policy in the United States. Madison, WI: University of Wisconsin Press.

Estes, C.L. 1994. The Regan-Bush Legacy: Privatisation, the Welfare State, and Ageing." Community Care: New Agendas and Challenges from the UK and Overseas, (eds. David Challis, Bleddyn Davies and Karen Traske.) PSSRU Studies series in Association with the British Society of Gerontology, 1994.

Estes, C.L., J. Swan and Associates. 1993. *The Long Term Care Crisis.* Newbury Park, CA: Sage.

Estes, C.L. and Gerard, L. 1983. "Governmental Responsibility: Issues of Reform and Federalism" in Estes, C.L., Newcomer, R.J. and Associates, Fiscal Austerity and Aging: Shifting Government Responsibility for the Elderly, Sage: Beverly Hills, pp. 41-58.

Estes, C.L. and Newcomer, R.J. 1983. "The Future for Aging and Public Policy: Two Perspectives," in Estes, C.L., Newcomer, R.J. and Associates, Fiscal Austerity and Aging: Shifting Government Responsibility for the Elderly, Sage: Beverly Hills, pp. 249-270.

Estes, C.L., Swan, J.H., Wood, J., Kreger, M. and Garfield, J. 1982. Fiscal Crisis: Impact on Aging Services Final Report. San Francisco: Aging Health Policy Center.

Nathan, R. P. 1996 with assistance of E. I. Davis, M, J McGrath, W. C. O'Hearney. The 'Nonprofitization Movement' as a Form of Devolution." *Capacity for Change? The Nonprofit World in the Age of Devolution.* Eds. D.W. Burlingame, W. A. Diaz, W. F.

Peterson, P. E. and Rom, M. C. 1990. *Welfare Magnets: A New Case for A National Standard.* Washington, DC: Brookings Institution.

Peterson, P.E., Rom, M.C., and Scheve, K.F. 1995. State Welfare Policy: A Race to the Bottom? Paper presented at the National Association for Welfare Research and Statistics annual research conference, Jackson, WY.

Peterson, P.E., Rom, M.C., and Scheve, K.F. 1996. The Race Among the States: Welfare Benefits, 1976-89. Paper presented at the Annual Meeting of the American Political Science Association, San Francisco, CA.

Povlika, L., Dunlop, B.D., and Rathman, M.B. 1996. Long Term Care for the Frail Elderly in Florida: Expanding Choices, Containing Costs. Tampa, FL: Florida Policy Exchange Center in Aging, University of South Florida.

❖ Chapter 7
The Critical Role
of Nurses

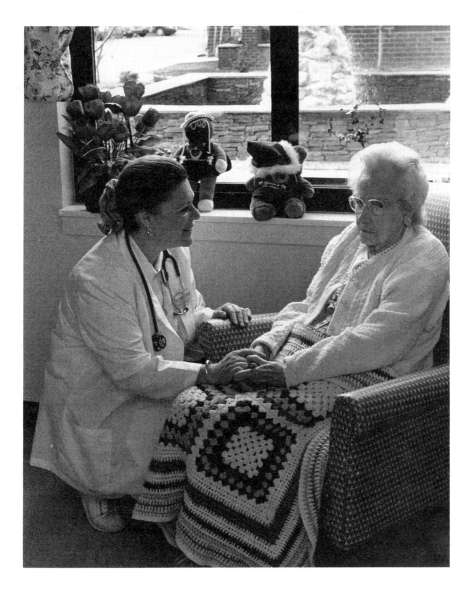

Nurses outnumber doctors, dentists, and every other group of health professionals in the United States. They are responsible for a major proportion of the coordination and delivery of health care services within institutions and are increasingly being recruited to health care settings in the community. The education, recruitment, and utilization of the over two million registered nurses (RNs) in the U.S. have serious implications for the profession itself, for every health care delivery setting in the nation, and for national health care policy. The three papers selected for inclusion in the fifth edition of *The Nation's Health* provide a broad spectrum of information about the profession, its scope and practice, and many of the challenges facing its practitioners in the 21st century.

Since the sweeping Medicare reforms of the 1980s, the profession has witnessed major changes in modes and environments for patient care that have thrust nurses into the fields of complex health care technologies and informatics. Nursing responsibilities have also been affected by federal policy changes that are rapidly transforming working conditions in acute inpatient care, acute, chronic, and long-term community care, and public health care. Nurses are employed in a wide variety of settings including public health agencies, primary care clinics, home health agencies, outpatient surgicenters, health maintenance organizations, nursing-school-operated nursing centers, insurance and managed care companies, nursing homes, elementary, secondary, and higher education settings, mental health agencies, hospices, the military, industry, nursing higher education, nursing and health care research centers, and, of course, hospitals and nursing homes (American Association of Colleges of Nursing, 1996). The major professional organizations support differentiated practice at the master's degree level which currently includes such specialty practice roles as certified nurse midwife, nurse practitioner, clinical nurse specialist, and certified registered nurse anesthetist. These specialty practitioners collectively are known as Advanced Practice Nurses (APNs) and the demand for their services is rapidly increasing.

Thousands of RNs prepared at the hospital diploma and associate degree levels are returning to colleges and universities across the nation to complete baccalaureate nursing education that focuses on health teaching, community and public health, research, leadership, and management theory and practice.

"The Registered Nurse Workforce: Infrastructure for Health Care Reform" by leading health policy analyst Linda K. Aiken, Marni E. Gwyther, and Christopher R. Friese documents characteristics of the current registered nurse workforce, identifies national trends in the nurse workforce and RN labor force participation, and assesses the adequacy of the nurse workforce to meet anticipated future health care service demands for registered nurses and Advanced Practice Nurses.

Claire M. Fagin addresses the role of nurse leaders in the nation's academic health centers in her article "Executive Leadership: Improving

Nursing Practice, Education, and Research." Professor Fagin uses the conceptual framework of the academic health center as a "learning organization" to explore the multifaceted challenges to nursing higher education leaders during this period of unprecedented change in the U.S. health care system. The evolution of strong autonomous practice in collaborative and interdependent roles necessitates the earnest commitment of executive nurse leaders in our academic health centers.

Unprecedented changes in the financing, organization, and delivery of health care services have resulted in a particularly unpredictable era for nursing personnel at all organizational levels and across nursing roles. Charlene Harrington, in her article "Nurse Staffing: Developing a Political Action Agenda for Change," discusses the implications of the Institute of Medicine's recent study of nurse staffing in hospitals and nursing homes. Professor Hanrrington encourages the profession to actively participate in long-range planning and policy formulation at the federal level by purposefully developing a coalition of nursing organizations to address public policy issues raised by the IOM report.

The relatively recent and rapid movement in the health care industry toward employment of Advanced Practice Nurses is reflected in an important article by Sister Rosemary Donley (1995) titled "Advanced Practice Nursing after Health Care Reform." Professor Donley explores a variety of areas influencing the education, employment, and practice of APNs in the future including the managed care environment, the characteristics of patient populations, and the anticipated nurse work force of the future.

❖ The Registered Nurse Workforce: Infrastructure for Health Care Reform

LINDA H. AIKEN, MARNIE E. GWYTHER, AND CHRISTOPHER R. FRIESE

The national health care reform debate brings renewed attention to the composition of the health care workforce. As America's largest group of health care professionals, registered nurses (RNs) constitute a major part of the infrastructure critical to any health care reform agenda. This article has a dual purpose—to present a statistical description of the registered nurse population, and to assess the extent to which the current nurse workforce is adequately prepared for its future role in an evolving reformed health care system.

❖ Profile of Registered Nurses

The latest survey of registered nurses estimates that, as of March 1992, there were 2,239,816 licensed RNs in the United States. Approximately 96 percent were women, 9 percent were members of racial or ethnic minorities and the average age was 43.1 years.[1] Their labor force participation rate is high, especially for a predominantly female occupation. In March 1992, 83 percent (1,853,024) were actively employed, with 69 percent working full-time. The employed RNs to total population ratio was 726 per 100,000. There were, by comparison, 255 physicians per 100,000 total population.[1,2] Most RNs practice in inpatient institutions—two-thirds in hospitals and 7 percent in nursing homes or extended care facilities.

Educationally, RNs are a heterogeneous group. Three educational pathways qualify graduates to take the national registered nurse licensing exam: 3-year hospital-based diploma programs, 2-year associate degree programs in community colleges, and 4-year baccalaureate programs in colleges and universities. Of employed nurses in 1992, 30 percent held diplomas from hospital training schools, 31 percent had associate degrees in nursing, 31 percent earned baccalaureate degrees in nursing or a related field, and about 8 percent had a master's or a doctoral degree in nursing or a related field.[1]

The average income of a full-time RN in March 1992 was $37,738[1] with full-time hospital-employed staff RN annual salaries ranging from $27,625 to $41,559.[1,3] Starting incomes for registered nurses have increased steadily in recent years, making the short-term financial return of an associate degree favorable, resulting in oversubscribed community college programs. Nursing, however, has historically faced wage compression. Moreover, while starting wages are currently high compared to other occupations, the career wage progression continues to be low, producing an overall modest average income for RNs.

❖ Trends

The national RN population has grown consistently over past decades, as has RN labor force participation. Since 1977 the RN supply has increased, on average, by more than 50,000 annually. Employment rates have increased in parallel with those of American women in general, but at a higher overall rate. To illustrate, 55 percent of RNs and 38 percent of all American women were employed in 1960. By 1992 these proportions had increased to 83 and approximately 58 percent, respectively.[1,4]

Over the past three decades, the locale of nursing education has moved from hospital-based apprentice-type education into the mainstream of higher education. In 1960, 80 percent of RNs received their education in hospital diploma schools versus less than 10 percent in 1992. Hospital-based diploma training has been largely replaced by associate degree training from community colleges; the proportion of RNs graduating with associate degrees increased from 3 to 51 percent between 1960 and 1992. Currently, 1,484 programs prepare students to practice as RNs, including 501 baccalaureate programs, 848 associate degree programs, and 135 diploma schools. Increasing numbers of RNs are pursuing advanced practice careers (e.g., nurse practitioners, nurse-midwives) that require graduate study.

The most noticeable demographic change in the RN workforce is its aging. Between 1980 and 1992, the proportion of RNs under age 30 declined from 25 to 11 percent while the proportion over 40 increased significantly. By 2000, two-thirds of all RNs are expected to be over age 40. The two primary reasons for this trend are: an overall greater labor force participation of RNs at all age levels and an increasing average age at graduation from basic nursing education. In 1992 the average age at graduation from associate degree programs (the largest producers of RNs) was 29.2 years; from baccalaureate programs, 24.2; and from hospital, diploma programs, 22.3 years.[1]

The practice settings of RNs are becoming more varied. Although hospital inpatient facilities continue to employ the majority of RNs, the most rapid job growth has occurred in the outpatient sector. Even within hospital settings, RN employment in outpatient departments grew by 68 percent between 1988 and 1992, while growth in inpatient bed units remained at 5.5 percent. Over this period the number of nurses working in community/public health positions increased 38 percent, due in large part to the rapid expansion of home health care services.[1]

❖ Adequacy of the Nurse Workforce to Meet Future Needs

Registered Nurses

The national supply of RNs is large by international standards, and continues to grow at a faster rate than the U.S. population. However, the distribution of RNs is not uniform. Cyclical national nursing shortages, as measured by the number of budgeted full-time-equivalent hospital RN vacancies, have occurred since World War II. These shortages are more attributable to increases in employer *demand* than the result of supply factors.[6] Rising complexity of care and relative wages are two components of that demand. The number of intensive care beds has more than doubled since 1973, increasing to over 90,000 today.[7,8] The increasing severity of illness of hospital inpatients creates an elevated demand for the clinical expertise of RNs. Second, hospital cost pressures have often resulted in lower wage growth for nurses than for other workers. Because RNs are so versatile in a hospital context, when their wages decline relative to alternative workers, hospitals tend to substitute RNs for less skilled personnel, creating cyclical RN shortages.

At present, RN incomes are relatively high and the job market is tighter than usual. However, if the past is a good predictor, salaries will begin to erode again with increased pressures for hospital cost containment under health care reform, creating the possibility of another national nursing shortage. The number of RN positions is projected to increase by 42 percent between 1992 and 2005, placing nursing at the top of the list of 25 better-paying occupations that are expected to grow.[9] One factor that makes predicting nursing job growth difficult is the diminishing size of the hospital inpatient sector. Inpatient hospital days decreased by 23 percent between 1982 and 1992.[8] While hospitals continued to employ more RNs over this period, it is unclear whether this trend will continue if hospitals experience greater future budget pressures. The large growth in jobs predicted by the Department of Labor assumes continued job growth for nurses in hospitals.[9]

A national nursing shortage does not currently exist, but there is growing concern in nursing, as in medicine, that the workforce is not optimally trained for the present or future needs of the population. It is predicted that by the year 2000 there will be 848,000 associate degree nurses to fill 692,000 positions, while there will be only 591,000 baccalaureate RNs to fill a need for 1,019,000 of these graduates.[10]

The need for baccalaureate graduates across practice settings is particularly apparent in statistics showing the proportion of RNs pursuing formal educational programs leading to nursing or nursing related degrees. In 1992, 61 percent of these RNs were in educational programs leading to a BSN (bachelor of science in nursing) degree.[1] Rising complexity of care and anticipated reductions in the number of medical residents in hospitals (a proposal included in some federal health reform legislation) are factors that will increase the demand for the clinical expertise and autonomous decision making of baccalaureate nurses. With the likely continued downscaling of the inpatient sector, job growth is and will continue to be most rapid in community-based, outpatient settings. While associate degree programs typically train students for structured inpatient settings, baccalaureate graduates are more suitably educated to provide clinical care and case management in ambulatory and home care settings, as well as in managed care organizations which are expected to enroll much larger shares of the population.

❖ Advanced Practice Nurses (APNs)

Nurse practitioners, nurse midwives, nurse anesthetists, and clinical nurse specialists are advanced practice nurses (APNs) with post-RN graduate clinical training. Thus, APNs are qualified to conduct health assessments, diagnose and treat a range of common acute and chronic illnesses and manage normal maternity care; they play critical roles in expanding access to high-quality, cost-effective health care services.[11-13] Nurse-midwives now attend about 4 percent of births, nationally;[14] nurse anesthetists are involved in providing an estimated 65 percent of all anesthesia services;[15] and nurse practitioners are now utilized extensively in managed care settings such as health maintenance organizations (HMOs).[16] The Division of Nursing projects about 392,000 masters- and doctoral-prepared full-time-equivalent RNs will be required by the year 2000, while the supply for that year is estimated at 185,000.[10]

Practice barriers currently prevent the increasing numbers of APNs from being fully utilized, i.e., only 21,000 of an estimated 43,000 trained nurse practitioners now practice with that job title.[1] These barriers have been grouped into three categories: 1) *legal barriers*, state-by-state practice laws which prevent APNs from practicing fully within their scope of training; 2) *financial barriers* that prevent public and private third-party payers from reimbursing APNs for the services they perform; and 3) *professional barriers* that exclude APNs from working in certain settings or prevent them from purchasing malpractice insurance.[17] A Bureau of Health Professions analysis shows that states with favorable legal, financial, and professional environments for nonphysician providers are generally successful in attracting nurse practitioners, regardless of whether an adequate level of primary care physicians is achieved.[18] Moreover, APNs are considered critical primary care providers in chronically medically underserved inner-city and rural areas.

Demand for APNs is likely to increase during discussions of health care reform as a greater portion of the population is expected to gain access to health care services, and as more of the population is enrolled in managed care arrangements. The Council of Graduate Medical Education (COGME) predicts a shortage of 80,000 primary care physicians by the year 2020 if there is no change in medical education in the interim.[19] Even if COGME reform recommendations were achieved, it would take until at least the year 2020 to produce an appropriately balanced physician workforce.[19] Therefore, APNs will continue to play a critical gap-filling role in both inpatient and outpatient settings. Furthermore, their cost-effective practice and lower salaries will make them competitive with physicians over the long term, especially in cost-conscious managed care settings. Therefore, working for the removal of existing impediments to APN practice should be one of nursing leadership's highest health care reform priorities.

❖ Conclusion

In general, the incentives put forth in the health care reform debate—expanded health insurance coverage, integrated health care delivery systems, and cost-effective practice—are favorable to nursing, as nurses provide a large volume of inpatient and outpatient services to a broad portion of the population, including the underserved. The nursing profession has had a dynamic nature over recent decades. Its responsiveness to change will be a critical variable in the future course of the profession, as it confronts the many challenges and opportunities of health care reform.

❖ About the Authors

Linda H. Aiken, Ph.D., R.N., is Trustee Professor of Nursing and Sociology and Director, Center for Health Services and Policy Research, School of Nursing, University of Pennsylvania, Philadelphia.

Marni E. Gwyther, B.A., and Christopher R. Friese are with the Center for Health Services and Policy Research, School of Nursing, University of Pennsylvania, Philadelphia.

REFERENCES

1. Moses, E.B. *The Registered Nurse Population: Findings from the National Sample Survey of Registered Nurses, March 1992.* U.S. Dept. of Health & Human Services, Public Health Service, Health Resources and Services Administration, Division of Nursing. Washington, DC: U.S. Gov. Print. Off., 1994.

2. Roback, G., Randolph, L., Seidman, B. *Physician Characteristics and Distribution in the U.S.: 1993 Edition.* Chicago, IL: American Medical Association, 1993.

3. University of Texas Medical Branch at Galveston. *1992 National Survey of Hospital and Medical School Salaries.* Galveston, TX: University of Texas Medical Branch, October 1992.

4. U.S. Bureau of the Census. *Statistical Abstract of the United States:*

1993 (113th edition). Washington, DC: U.S. Gov. Print. Off., 1993.

5. National League for Nursing, Division of Research. *Nursing Data Review: 1994*. New York, NY: National League for Nursing Press, 1994.

6. Aiken, L.H., Mullinix, C.F. "The nurse shortage: Myth or reality?" *New Engl. J. Med.* 317(10):641-646, 1987.

7. Aiken, L.H. "The hospital nursing shortage: A paradox of increasing supply and increasing vacancy rates." *West. J. Med.* 151(1):87-92, 1989.

8. American Hospital Association. AHA. *Hospital Statistics: 1993-1994 Edition*. Chicago, IL: American Hospital Association, 1992.

9. Knight-Ridder analysis of data from Bureau of Labor Statistics and U.S. Commerce Dept. "The workforce in 2005." *The Philadelphia Inquirer*. Business Section, September 4, 1994.

10. U.S. Dept. of Health & Human Services, Public Health Service, Health Resources and Services Administration, Bureau of Health Professions. *Seventh Report to the President and Congress on the Status of Health Personnel in the United States*. Washington, DC: U.S. Gov. Print. Off., March 1990; and *Eighth Report to Congress on Health Personnel in the United States, 1991*. Washington, DC: U.S. Gov. Print. Off., September 1992.

11. U.S. Congress, Office of Technology Assessment, *Nurse Practitioners, Physician Assistants, and Certified Nurse-Midwives: A Policy Analysis*. (Health Technology Case Study 37), OTA-HCS-37, Washington, DC: U.S. Gov. Print. Off., December 1986.

12. Safriet, B.J. "Health care dollars and regulatory sense: The role of advanced practice nursing." *Yale Journal of Regulation*. 9(2):417-188, 1992.

13. Brown, S.A., Grimes, D.E. *A Meta-Analysis of Process of Care, Clinical Outcomes, and Cost-Effectiveness of Nurses in Primary Care Roles: Nurse Practitioners and Certified Nurse-Midwives*. Report prepared for the American Nurses' Association Division of Health Policy, Washington, DC. Revised, 1993.

14. National Commission on Nurse-Midwifery Education, 1993. *Educating Nurse-Midwives: A Strategy for Achieving Affordable, High-Quality Maternity Care*. Washington, DC: American College of Nurse Midwives, 1993.

15. National Commission on Nurse Anesthesia Education. "Chapter 1: The report of the commission on nurse anesthesia education." *National Commission on Nurse Anesthesia Education*. Washington, DC: American Association of Nurse Anesthetists, 1990.

16. Weiner, J.P. "Forecasting the effects of health reform on US physician workforce requirement: Evidence from HMO staffing patterns." *JAMA*. 272(3):222-230, 1994.

17. Aiken, L.H., Sage, W.M. "Staffing national health care reform: A role for advanced practice nurses" *Akron Law Review*. 26(2):187–211, Fall 1993.

18. Sekscenski, E.S., Sansom, S., Bazell, C., Salmon, M.E., Mullan, F. "State practice environments and the supply of physician assistants, nurse practitioners, and certified nurse-midwives." *New Engl. J. Med.* 33(19):1266-1271, 1994.

19. Council on Graduate Medical Education. "Recommendations to improve access to health care through physician workforce reform." *Fourth Report to Congress and the Department of Health & Human Services Secretary*. Washington, DC: U.S. Dept. of Health & Human Services, 1994.

❖ Executive Leadership
Improving Nursing Practice, Education, and Research

CLAIRE M. FAGIN

Nurse executive leadership in academic health centers is essential to the improvement of nursing education, practice, and research. The author raises questions to highlight the dilemmas in which nursing finds itself at this time of dramatic transformation of health systems. The framework of the "learning organization" is used to examine the way in which leaders are defined in nursing and the way in which they perceive their roles. Comparisons are drawn between educational and practice administrators, and similarities and differences between these two groups are discussed. Integrative faculty practice roles are summarized, and innovations in advanced nursing practice are described briefly. Specific aspects of the research enterprise discussed are collaboration among members of the nursing discipline and examination and evaluation of quality-of-care issues. For improvement to occur, the author advocates involved, participatory problem solving by nurse colleagues in education and practice.

To find the right answers to how executive leadership can improve nursing education, practice, and research, some new questions must be raised that will better define the dilemmas in which nursing finds itself. First, some of assumptions underlying this article are examined.

The first assumption is that nursing practice, education, and research need to be improved. The second assumption is that professional advances in nursing have become far too complex for one person to deal with them comprehensively. The third assumption, perhaps more covert than overt, is that the question of how to improve nursing education, practice, and research, which has been asked and answered hundreds of times in the past, must be looked at anew, from a different perspective, from a different context, and with a new paradigm. Thus, the answers to the question must be different from those given previously. The fourth assumption is that current changes will take us into the 21st century; however, I would *not* assume that we should shape our thinking on the current situation. We have seen dramatic changes in the healthcare field over its history and very rapid changes in the past decade. I expect that the current turmoil may be an in-between step to new solutions that will occur in a 5- to 10-year period as managed care is evaluated and other contemporary developments surface. The fifth and final assumption is that we are experiencing a crisis of national leadership in healthcare. Our institutions can boast of superb leaders in nursing and medicine responding to current political and managerial challenges. However, there seems to be an absence of the visionary, transforming nursing and medical leaders who not only respond to their institutional challenges but also speak for their professions and for the public they serve. Such leaders help to set the national healthcare agenda rather than react to it.

Given these five assumptions, and particularly because of the fifth, I discuss education, practice, and research by focussing first on executive leadership in nursing. Questions are raised and recommendations are made for the present and the future.

❖ Leadership

A useful framework for linking the worlds of the nursing educator and practitioner is Peter Senge's learning organization.[1]

A learning organization . . . is continually expanding its capacity to create its future. For such an organization, it is not enough merely to survive. "Survival learning" . . . is important . . . But for a learning organization . . . [it] must be joined by "generative learning," learning that enhances our capacity to create.[(p14)]

This definition is very appropriate as we examine the organizations that nurse lead. Looking at academic health centers as learning organizations suggests several questions:

1. How do we define leaders?
2. Why are we leading?
3. How do we prepare leaders?
4. Do leaders of practice disciplines such as nursing and medicine have a responsibility for building their disciplines?
5. Does nursing leadership differ from medical leadership in academic health centers?

Answers to the last question provide a distinctive picture to the nurse executive. The professions of medicine and nursing are vastly different in many aspects including their cultures, hours and patterns of work, and income expectations. Friedson defines critical aspects of a profession as its power to control the terms, conditions, and content of its work.[2] It is this power that has been the principal differentiation between the ways in which medicine and nursing have progressed, organized their systems, and maintained their hegemony—at least until very recently. It probably is this characteristic that influences the sharp differences in executive leadership among nursing professionals, and particularly between nursing administrators in education and practice.

❖ Educational Administrators

There are few ambiguities in the answers to my questions about leadership among nursing education administrators in major academic health centers. Although particular administrative styles may differ greatly, there is clarity in the who, what, and what-for of leadership.

How Do We Define Leaders?

When any of our institutions is searching, the desired candidate usually is described as a scholar with a track record of achievement in the discipline. That record should include some demonstrated skill in managing in a similar organization, examples of influencing others in the advancement of the profession, interpersonal skills within and outside the discipline, impressive publications, and in the major academic health center world about which we are concerned here, an imposing reputation. We seek such people because we believe that the organization is in need of leadership to move the discipline forward and to represent the institution in the best way possible. From the standpoint of the faculty, they want their leader to represent them to the administration, to help them achieve their full rights and respect, to present the discipline in the most reputable way, and to be able to engage in the broad campus and alumni arenas in a way that brings nursing positive attention. These administrators know why they are leading. During their extensive pre-employment interviews, they give the search committee and the administration confidence that they share a creative view of leadership related to the needs of the school and discipline, as well as their fit in the university.

Do we prepare academic leaders for these roles? Certainly not in any educational program of which I am aware. One of the reasons for seeking a tested person is that learning how to use one's leadership skills comes from testing various modes of behavior in small and large venues, finding what works, seeking to develop a new and wide repertoire of responses, and evolving a persona that has enough constancy to be recognizable as one's own individual leadership style while maintaining the flexibility to continue to develop. These administrators generally are awarded tenure in an academic title (not in the administrative title) on appointment, thus meeting the professional characteristics of control and autonomy.

❖ Administrators of Nursing Practice

I will briefly address the same questions for practice leaders. Although searches in academia are influenced by the higher administration or the trustees, faculty members have a major or dominant role in the choices. This differs from the practice situation, in which nurses in the institution play some part in the recruitment and selection; however, in most institutions, this is a less powerful and decisive role than faculty members play in universities. The expression "team players" appears in many current advertisements, but even when this characteristic is not in print, the degree to which a candidate is a good team player is always asked when calling for references and when describing incumbents. Rarely does a chief executive officer or chief operating officer of an academic health center view the applicant first as a practice leader and second as a member of his/her hierarchy. Further, when the chief nursing officer is a member of the school of nursing faculty, to what degree is that role stressed in the health system search process? That answer varies with the institution, but whatever the answer, it will suggest the definition of nursing leader in the specific institution.

The cultures of academia and practice differ substantially in such dimensions as control of the terms of work, autonomy, and independence. For the nurse executive in educational institutions, there generally is parity with other professionals. For the nurse executive in service institutions, the potency of professional characteristics is more cloudy, and rewards in the current environment more often stress abilities to manage within a cost-constrained organization over discipline-building goals. There are inevitable conflicts for the nurse executive trying to maintain and strengthen a care-giving cadre of professionals in situations in which the reward system is valuing that goal less than in former years.

Why Are We Leading?

Many of our institutions are changing the role of the nursing executive. Many are adding responsibility for patient care related departments in addition to nursing; more often than not, the nurse executive is the vice president of patient care services, not of nursing alone. This suggests that new answers must be given to the definition of leader and to the questions of why and who we are leading. Is the leader of nursing practice the generative and regenerative leader of nurses? Do nurse executives see themselves as increasing their scope and prestige by minimizing or, even in some cases, obliterating their nursing identification? Are nurse administrators and other nurses taking an active role in creating nursing's future? Are nurse executives reacting to the administrative and managerial hierarchies with plans for survival or with active and inspiring participation in the planning process for change? Are the responses we hear from nurses all over the country reacting to threat, rather than acting to regenerate our systems to reflect both cost and quality from the nursing frame of reference? Answers to these questions can lead to strategic actions.

Some healthcare institutions are substituting minimally prepared workers for nursing personnel. Others are describing new models of care using cost-effective health service teams, but with incomplete information about the preparation of the various team members. In examining some written descriptions of these models, one notes that discipline-specific requirements exist only for physicians. Surely nurses exist and participate in some of the leadership roles, but the credentials do not appear. This dangerous situation appears to be part of a growing trend that has implications for the profession and for the public. For the profession, by deliberately leaving out the credential of the nursing license, nursing's power, ethic, roles, and future are made as invisible as the most stereotypic view of nursing we all decry. For the public, the potential absence of professional nurses could lead to lower quality care and in some cases to life-threatening events.

These trends are of great concern. The problems that nursing practice and education executives have had previously in seeking unity will only be exacerbated by the immediate threats to the practicing nurses in these settings and the delayed, but already clear, dilemmas these changes imply for the students currently in our educational programs.

To whom must practice leaders prove themselves? As I said earlier, practice leaders do not have benefits of autonomy and control compared with education leaders. When forced into a survival mode, can practice leaders focus on building the discipline and on the visionary, regenerative aspects of leadership? Yet this is exactly what must be done despite the difficulty of moving our mission of care forward while we respond to current crises.

Our focus must be how we move forward in a new paradigm of delivery of health services. Recognizing that our leadership role is often a position in the middle—between our staff and the administrators we also serve—our methods must include developing strategies for involving all of our nursing staff in problem solution, taking account of the present and future, and most important, recognizing that our special mission of quality nursing care must be our primary concern within the broader context. Peter Senge says that "Most of the leaders with whom . . . [he has] worked agree that the first leadership design task concerns developing vision, values, and purpose or mission."[1(p343)] Stewardship of the vision and mission is a vital function of the leader, and improvement in the three arenas of nursing education, practice, and research requires recognition of our mutual stake in managing this leadership design task. There is no way that leaders in nursing education and practice can move ahead in parallel play at this time. How we work together in the strategies we design will probably tell the tale for our profession in decades ahead.

❖ Improving Nursing Education, Practice, and Research

For some years, I have advocated a model of integrative nursing that includes faculty status for all appropriately credentialed practitioners in academic health centers.[3] I also believe that those faculty members whose work is predominantly in research and teaching need to be part of the health delivery arena but, perhaps, in somewhat different ways. The development of the discipline, the quality of nursing education, and the quality of nursing practice is enhanced by models that permit the pronouns "my" and "our" to be used to describe the school and health system by all nurses in the setting.

Such models require a high degree of job security so that a sense of continuity pervades the care and teaching components of the institution. For example, at the University of Pennsylvania there is a commitment to the clinician/educator/faculty member for a period of time from the University School of Nursing. In fact, although the initial appointment may be with the university hospital, there is no requirement that this be a permanent arrangement, provided that the faculty member and the school agree on a new role. Since the program started, several faculty members have changed their clinical employment, most from a hospital setting to some form of community healthcare.

The University of Pennsylvania's system, which grants faculty status to fully credentialed clinicians, is unusual in its flexibility and fits a variety of circumstances. It guarantees academic freedom and unites people rather than organizations.[3] At the time the system was designed, down-sizing of nursing personnel was not an issue. In fact, the issue at the time was how to make the hospital more attractive to nurses at all levels. Building nursing leadership through integrating practice and education was one attractive and successful strategy. Currently, down-sizing nursing organizations presents questions about the potential security of hospital-based faculty positions. These questions do not lead necessarily to negative answers because the program is being maintained and enlarged.

The irony about down-sizing is that its inevitability had not been planned for by the nursing community (back to the leadership issues of survival versus generative leadership). A striking example of lack of foresight is that few of us took seriously the predictable outcome of the large increases in nurses' pay. Some of us warned that higher salaries would end the nursing shortage, not by recruiting new nurses but by presenting a more costly solution to hospital care than managers were willing to pay. Although it is not necessarily a bad thing to have fewer and better paid professional nurses than we were accustomed to, the nursing community did little to prepare in advance for this eventuality.

For at least four decades, goals of quality improvement have been confounded by a contradictory strategy of preparing large numbers of registered nurses at the lowest level, the 2-year program, to meet the nursing needs of the public. This strategy, to produce nurses quickly to meet the needs of hospitals and nursing homes, was assumed to be sufficient to the needs of the times, attractive to a racially and ethnically diverse population, and inexpensive. The programs are supported financially by a wide variety of local, state, and federal funds, which are not easily calculated to show cost, and, contrary to myth, the programs graduate a population less racially diverse than baccalaureate programs. Further, nursing administrators and many educators have never urged differentiation of nurses' salaries by education so that the fast track to the registered nurse license has led to an irrationally expensive work force based on the outworn philosophy of "a nurse is a nurse is a nurse."

Although the nursing profession (among others) did not forecast the chaotic changes in healthcare of the mid 1990s and plan its work force requirements of entry-level nurses for these changes, forward-looking developments were occurring at the higher end of nursing education and practice. Practice and education leaders have collaborated in building programs of innovative nursing practice in a wide variety of settings. Advanced practice nurses (APNs) are at the heart of these innovations. The American Association of Colleges of Nursing[4] has agreed that APNs should hold a graduate degree in nursing and be certified.

The innovations in advanced nursing practice offer us the direction in which our improvements in nursing practice and education must continue. These roles fit well with the assumptions stated earlier and with integrated roles in schools of nursing.

Until recently, roles for APNs have been quasi-independent roles, and two of them, the nurse practitioner and the certified nurse midwife, were community roles. The newest model of the APN is a hospital-based tertiary care practitioner who blends the nurse practitioner role with the clinical nurse specialist role.[5]

The Columbia-Presbyterian Medical Center in Manhattan offers two interesting examples of improved practice by implementing both the community and hospital APN roles. On selected units of the hospital, APNs do initial assessments, write admission orders, work with attending physicians to review plans of care and with the nursing staff to interpret clinical information, and explain the rationale for treatment plans. Further, APNs managing clinics in the Columbia system have admitting privileges for all of Presbyterian's hospitals. In New York, APNs have prescriptive privileges for their patients.

Henry Silver, Loretta Ford's co-pioneer in the nurse practitioner movement, predicted and recommended the development of a hospital-based nurse practitioner role in an article published in 1988.[6] Describing the role, he and McAtee stated, ". . . they would perform many functions and provide many services given by first-year residents in teaching hospitals.[6(p1671)] They estimated that these nurses could reduce physician needs by 5% to 10% and reduce healthcare costs significantly.

❖ Nurse Specialist Transitional Care

It is no secret that the current payment structure for hospitals is increasingly reliant on managed-care organizations. In efforts to compete for business, hospitals aim to shorten hospital stays or eliminate hospitalization completely for many surgical procedures. Nurse specialist transitional care helps counter the fragmentation of care that many consumers experience as they navigate among different providers, treatments, and settings. Nurse-managed, hospital-based programs to provide transitional care for patients diagnosed with cancer, for perinatal care of mother and infant, for the frail elderly, for patients with acquired immune deficiency syndrome, and for many other populations have been shown to be extremely effective.

Many of these innovations were stimulated by the research of Dorothy Brooten,[7] whose first study on early discharge of low birth weight infants demonstrated important quality and cost results. The Brooten model has since been studied for patients with a variety of conditions who are discharged earlier from the hospital by substituting a portion of hospital care with a comprehensive program of home follow-up by APNs. Highly successful interventions have been documented for low birth weight infants, mothers undergoing Cesarean births, high-risk mothers (i.e., pregnant women at high risk for complicated pregnancies and deliveries), women undergoing hysterectomies, and the hospitalized elderly.

Nursing has demonstrated that it can improve care for a wide variety of patients currently considered chronic or not amenable to care. For example, treatment options for patients with pain, incontinent clients, patients with asthma, patients with diabetes, and others have been initiated or assumed by nurses, and are being documented increasingly. Preparation and use of nurses in these roles are fundamental to improvement of nursing practice and nursing education.

❖ Managed Care and Nurse-Managed Clinics

We are seeing increasing interest in nurse practitioners in managed-care organizations and other innovative practice settings that are community based. Day hospitals for the elderly are natural nurse-managed facilities, and working in tandem with hospitals and health maintenance organizations can offer appropriate care for less cost than more traditional 24-hour care or home care. We are learning that health maintenance organizations and other managed-care settings are relying heavily on the cost-effective APN. Further, health maintenance organizations have the highest percentage of baccalaureate and higher degree nurses among employers in the United States.[8]

Some of these nurses are in direct primary care roles. Others are in case manager roles. Under the best of circumstances, these roles can be exciting and satisfying; however, if efforts to cut costs become the paramount aim of the organization, the roles, innovative as they may be, are dissatisfying and frustrating. Further, they may conflict sharply with the values of the nursing professional. Managed care has great promise, provided that it maintains a focus on the client and family and offers a strong array of services from prevention to specialty treatment.

In many parts of the United States, nurses are involved in value-added roles in managed care, including those offered in the 300 or so nurse-managed centers throughout the nation.[9,10] Most of these centers offer a range of primary care, case management, and wellness care. They compete with other primary care providers for clients and contracts.

School and community center clinics, expanded home health visits, and work site health programs have mushroomed in recent years and use nurse practitioners almost exclusively. The settings may differ one from the other in the type of services and the background of the nurse provider. All stress prevention and maintenance of health. Many of them involve the community in planning and monitoring services. The notion of marketing prevention and risk reduction with vulnerable populations is implicitly or explicitly part of many nursing centers.

All of the changes we are seeing have relevance for improvement in both nursing practice and nursing education. They suggest issues and questions. Just as hospitals are changing rapidly, many of our schools are moving rapidly to prepare for the newer models of practice. Our leading centers of nursing education must focus on the kind of generative leadership necessary for their students to be able to take their places in contemporary healthcare with clarity about their current and changing roles and the awareness of the heavy responsibility that the nursing roles entail. To ensure improvement in nursing practice and nursing education, we need to have shared answers to some vital questions. These shared answers require commitment and planning so that fragmentation and fracturing do not continue.

1. Do our academic health center schools have the faculty and clinical settings to provide a quality education for the innovative practice models developing?
2. Is there stress on nursing roles vis a vis prevention and maintenance of health?
3. Do our students understand the differences between case management and care management?
4. Are we preparing for the hospital environment as well as for community health settings?
5. Are we in one of our historic pendulum swings as we see the hospital market shrinking and changing in threatening ways? Are we allowing the pendulum to take precedence over long-term strategies and considerations?
6. To what extent are practice and education leaders collaborating to forge a new paradigm for practice and education?
7. To what extent are practice and education leaders collaborating to sell this new paradigm to managers and administrators?
8. How are nurses uniting to examine the risks of a down-sized nursing population in hospitals?
9. How are nursing practice and education leaders teaching and supporting continuity of care and accountability of nurse providers?

10. What are education and practice leaders doing in recognition of the extreme burden young nurses have in accountability and advocacy?
11. To what extent are our students and young nurses cognizant of their responsibility to protect the patient?

Whether in hospital or community care, if we lose our accountability, we lose our discipline. In recent months, we have read about tragic outcomes for patients in hospitals around the country. We do not know the extent of nursing involvement in these incidents. Are we seeing a denigration of the nursing ethic of advocacy and accountability as our nursing staffs are being down-sized, as our health systems' administrators downgrade the nursing role in development of generic teams, and as our chiefs of nursing services leave out the nursing role in development of generic teams, and as our chiefs of nursing services leave out the nursing word in their assumption of broader portfolios? Implicitly and explicitly, the statement of the senior nursing officer about the mission of the hospital and the principal caring profession has never been more important.

The research, education, and managerial missions are key to all of us in the healthcare field, but it is the nursing service mission that forms our center, gives meaning to our lives, puts us all in this frustrating and fascinating field, and must be dealt with now and not later as we move to new problems and solutions for the decades ahead. Although I endorse completely the broader portfolio that is part of the trend for nurse executives, I urge maintaining clarity about the nursing discipline, its continued development, and its centrality to the hospital mission. The discipline and the patient will both be better served by our own clarity.

❖ Nursing Research

The aspect of the research enterprise most germane to my central themes is collaboration among members of our own discipline in the examination and evaluation of quality-of-care issues.

I will highlight a few questions nurses and others need to be investigating under the rubric of what I will call the bandwagon phenomenon. Whether we are talking about restructuring our hospitals, reengineering our universities, moving rapidly into a managed-care world, virtual integration, or the like, the bandwagon phenomenon seems more prevalent currently in the healthcare industry than at any time in the past few decades. An example of questions which might be explored are:

What evaluations are occurring with regard to rapid changes of restructuring and shifting of modalities for healthcare delivery?

What are the posthospital experiences of patients discharged earlier than formerly who do not have the expert care described by nursing researchers?

What steps are being taken to change the culture of most managed-care organizations from the healthy, young employed family to the older, often less healthy populations they currently are seeking and for whom they are being mandated to care?

What additional costs, if any, are being incurred as a result of a reduced Medicaid budget—e.g., are there changes in emergency room use with Medicaid and Medicare managed-care organizations?

Recent reports on the last question give us cause for concern. Evaluations of the changes being made by the industry and by government are vital and are at least as much nursing's business as that of any other discipline. We must keep our eye on the mission—quality patient care. What are we doing to assess change in relation to the core values of all healthcare providers? Some hospitals have used dedicated small grant funds to help clinicians test efficacy of particular patient care interventions.[11] It would seem that the bandwagon phenomenon changes should be accompanied by funding for evaluative programs that focus on cost and qualitative and quantitative results of the change. These studies will benefit from collaboration within nursing as well as between nursing and medicine.

Collaboration in the research enterprise also implies a collaborative approach to implementation of innovations into practice. What should be included among the saddest examples of dysfunctionality among nursing leaders is the poor record of implementing research-based innovations into practice. According to Bostrom and Wise,[12] a 10- to 15-year gap exists between discovery of potential innovations and implementation of these innovations into nursing practice. This gap is particularly troubling when it exists in one's own academic/clinical environment. Closing this gap must move to the near top of our collective priorities.

What is crucial is that we approach our research initiatives of the future recognizing that nursing education and nursing practice have a common agenda. Partly because of health system changes, this agenda will be shared, more often than not, with clinician/physician colleagues. Thus, I would suggest that a collaborative approach with each other and with physicians is an important component for improvement of nursing research.

❖ Conclusion

Improvement of nursing practice, education, and research must remain a major focus of executive nurse leaders in academic health centers. Any restructuring must include the maintenance or improvement in autonomy in the nursing roles with collaboration and interdependence in broader healthcare roles. Any restructuring should engage practicing nursing in job improvement and patient care improvement, not job protection. Any restructuring should address the challenge of how nursing can be positioned in academic health centers so that patient care services that are non-nursing can serve patients and facilitate nurses' work in their service. Executive nurse leaders must address together the nursing work force issues of reducing the production engine of the associate degree programs, recognizing the importance of nursing knowledge and skills; building and using them; and restructuring their nursing table of organization with an eye on both the short-term and long-term maintenance and building of the discipline. Improvement is not possible without extremely involved, participatory membership in problem solving of nursing colleagues representing the education and practice arenas.

So our work is cut out for us in the practice, education, and research arenas:

* Take control of our current and future destiny.
* Unite to whatever extent is possible in particular settings.
* Do not sacrifice the long term for the short term.
* Keep your eye on your mission.
* Identify where the nursing strength is in your institution and gather round that strength for forward movement. If that means giving up your own hegemony, so be it.

❖ About the Author

Claire M. Fagin, PhD, RN, FAAN, is Leadership Professor, at the School of Nursing, University of Pennsylvania, Philadelphia.

Based on paper presented at Invitational Conference on Executive Leadership in Major Teaching Hospitals and Academic Health Centers; June 22, 1995; Cambridge, Massachusetts.

REFERENCES

1. Senge PM. *The Fifth Discipline.* New York: Doubleday; 1990.
2. Friedson E. The future of professionalization. In: Stacey M, ed. *Health and the Division of Labor.* New York: Prodist; 1977:14–38.
3. Fagin C. Institutionalizing practice: historical and future perspectives. In: Barnard KE, Smith GR, eds. *Faculty Practice in Action.* Washington, DC: American Academy of nursing; 1985:1–17.
4. American Association of Colleges of Nursing. *Certification and Regulation of Advanced Practice Nurses.* Washington, DC: AACN; 1994.
5. Keane A, Richmond T. Tertiary nurse practitioners. *Image.* 1993;

25(4):281–284.
6. Silver H, McAtee P. Should nurses substitute for house staff? *Am J Nurs.* 1988; 12:1671–1673.
7. Brooten D, Kumar S, Brown L, et al. A randomized clinical trial of early hospital discharge and home followup of very low birthweight infants. *N Engl J Med.* 1986; 315: 934–939.
8. Public Health Service, Health Resources and Services Administration, Bureau of Health Professions. *The Registered Nurse Population: Findings From the National Sample Survey of Registered Nurses, March 1992.* Washington, DC: U.S. Department of Health and Human

Services, Division of Nursing; 1994.

9. Barger S, Rosenfeld P. Models in community health care: findings from a national study of community nursing centers. *Nurs Health Care.* 1993; 14(8):426–431.

10. Holthaus R. Nurse-managed health care: an ongoing tradition. *Nurse Pract Forum.* 1993; 4(3):128–132.

11. Franklin PD, Panzer RJ, Brideau LP, Griner PF. Innovations in clinical practice through hospital-funded grants. *Academic Med.* 1990; 65(6):355–360.

12. Bostrom J, Wise L. Closing the gap between research and practice. *J Nurs Adm.* 1994; 24(5):22–27.

❖ Nurse Staffing:
Developing a Political Action Agenda for Change

CHARLENE HARRINGTON

Critical provider concerns, such as downsizing and staffing levels—as well as quality of care and staffing standards—were recently identified in the Institute of Medicine's (IOM) report. *Nursing Staff in Hospitals and Nursing Homes: Is it Adequate?* Released to Congress in January 1996, this landmark document represents the culmination of 22 months of study by the Committee on the Adequacy of Nurse Staffing in Hospitals and Nursing Homes.

Appointed by IOM in 1994, the 16-member expert committee included nurses, physicians, lawyers, academics, consultants, and administrators. This committee was charged by Congress with determining "whether and to what extent there is need for an increase in the number of nurses in hospitals and nursing homes to promote the quality of patient care and to reduce the incidence among nurses of work-related injuries and stress" (P.L. 103–43) (Institute of Medicine [IOM], 1996, p. 3). For the purposes of the study, Congress defined "nurse" to include registered nurses (RNs), licensed practical or licensed vocation nurses (LPNs/LVNs), and nurse assistants (NAs).

As part of its directive, the committee analyzed available data and literature, commissioned papers, heard expert testimony, held public hearings, and conducted onsite visits. After assembling this information, members deliberated, approaching the question of nurse staffing in terms of an evolving delivery system and how increasingly aging and minority populations will impact health care in the next century.

While the committee found that current staffing concerns in hospitals and nursing homes are intense, the future of nursing services is equally critical, both to long-range planning and policy formulation. As managed care grows, and more hospitals move toward patient-centered services, nurses will provide increased care across the continuum—and documentation of quality outcomes will become even more essential.

By building a consensus on outcome measures and staffing, documenting quality indicators and collecting data, and educating the public and Congress on the value of nursing care, the profession can promote greater regulation of, and compliance by, all health facilities. Nursing organizations have the opportunity—indeed, the responsibility—to develop a broad political action strategy that will ensure quality health care for consumers and communities alike.

❖ Supply Vs. Demand

In order to determine the adequacy of nursing personnel, the IOM committee reviewed current employment data and considered potential ramifications of shifting demand for services. Today, the nursing labor force consists of over two million RNs, 700,000 LPNs/LVNs, and 1.3 million NAs (IOM, 1996). Hospitals remain the major employers of RNs, while many LPNs/LVNs and NAs work in nursing homes. As hospitals downsize and nursing homes experience increased demand for rehabilitative services, however, some professional positions are being eliminated or transferred to ambulatory and community settings. In fact, nursing is increasingly moving away from the hospital bedside and into the community, providing a continuum of patient care.

With such instability in the health system and the labor market, the committee was uncertain whether there was an excess supply of 300,000 nurses—as noted in a recent Pew Commission (1995) report. Members concluded that the current supply of nurses was adequate to meet national needs, but that "the educational mix may not be adequate to meet either current or future demands in a rapidly changing health care system" (IOM, 1996, p. 88).

This led to the view that health care professionals require a broad education to acquire the necessary knowledge and skills for future practice environments. The committee particularly emphasized the need for training nurses in advanced practice, urging that state barriers to expanding the roles of these nurses be eliminated. Moreover, members stated that there is a need for "a thorough evaluation of the current funding of training" (IOM, 1996, p. 88) and a possible redirection of efforts.

❖ Staffing Levels

As cost containment efforts increase throughout the health care industry and new delivery systems emerge, demand for nursing care changes. In turn, staff mix and roles of nursing personnel—both professional and ancillary—are affected.

Hospitals

One of the major challenges facing the IOM committee was the lack of data on nurse staffing in hospitals. The Health Care Financing Administration (HCFA), the Joint Commission on Accreditation of Health Care Organizations (JCAHO), and the American Hospital Association (AHA) do not publish data on staffing levels or on type of nurse for individual hospitals or for units within hospitals.

Still, AHA did report that total RN full-time equivalents (FTEs) were increasing slightly while LPN/LVN FTEs had declined a bit (see p. 45 and

p. 78 of the IOM report). However, this growth in total number of RNs in hospitals masks the changes in nurse staffing levels and the changes in nursing roles. Although some suspect that there are substantial reductions in the number of RNs providing direct care to patients, the IOM committee could only urge that data be collected and made public in the future.

Nursing Homes

Information on nursing home staff is available from the federal online survey and certification reporting system (OSCAR) maintained by HCFA. Although the data are crude and unaudited, they show some minor improvements over the past few years in RN staffing ratios, primarily in hospital-based units. More importantly, they illustrate inadequate levels of care for the average facility. For example, data show that for all 16,000 nursing homes in the U.S., residents received only 24 minutes of RN care, 36 minutes of LPN/LVN care, and two hours of NA care, on average, over a 24-hour period.

❖ Lack of Staffing Standards

In the author's opinion, part of the explanation for inadequate staffing in some facilities may be the lack of standards. While nursing organizations have developed professional standards for individual nursing specialists, none have been recommended for hospitals or nursing homes. Moreover, very little nursing research has been conducted on minimum or ideal staffing standards for either of these types of facilities. In fact, at the present time, health care organizations develop their own patterns, without professional guidelines. Private health care consultants provide guidance to organizations using commercial staffing systems, but clear regulations are only available for nursing homes.

In the absence of standards, the IOM committee was unable to address the question of minimum or ideal patterns. Additionally, it could not consider how adjustments should be made to take into account patient acuity levels and/or characteristics.

❖ Quality of Care

Defining quality of care in hospitals and nursing homes is a complex process. While recent advances have been made in measuring outcomes for individual patients and specific populations, methods have not focused on nursing's contribution to quality. Despite these challenges, the committee attempted to determine how the level of nursing care in these facilities could be evaluated and whether the quality of care was changing or declining.

Defining and Measuring Quality

In the past, the general focus on quality of care has been on *process measures:* diagnosis, assessment, planning, care delivery, monitoring, and evaluation (IOM, 1996). While these elements are important, the committee supported the recent national focus to develop outcome measures of quality.

Hospitals

Historically, hospital measures have been limited to mortality rates and medically related outcomes. Some hospital outcomes such as staff courtesy and satisfaction with meals, are designed more for marketing services than for measuring quality. Others, including the report card measures for managed care organizations, emphasize preventive screening services. Many of the hospital outcome measures under development are not *sensitive* to nursing care.

The IOM committee considered that negative outcomes for hospitals related to nursing care would include adverse events, such as falls or injuries; reductions in physiological characteristics, functional status, mental and emotional status; poor patient and family satisfaction: and negative post discharge events, like unexpected death and readmission (IOM, 1996).

Nurse-sensitive outcomes are those where nursing care can make a difference in the prevention, mitigation, or treatment of patient problems. For example, the American Nurses Association (ANA) has identified outcome measures as decubitus ulcers, nosocomial infections, and accidents in hospitals. While nursing has not generally agreed upon a list of nurse-sensitive outcome measures for hospitals, ANA has recently developed a set of recommended quality indicators.

Nursing Homes

For these facilities, outcome measures have been examined in a number of studies. They include: hospitalization: pressure sores: and reductions in functional, mental, or psychological status. Weight loss, infections, injuries, incontinence, depression, and poor satisfaction are additional criteria (IOM, 1996; Zimmerman et al., 1995).

Evaluating and Reporting

Another challenge facing the IOM committee was reviewing research on quality of care in these two types of facilities. While information on quality of nursing home care has been available to some extent since the enactment of the Nursing Home Reform Act of 1987, few studies on hospital quality currently exist.

Hospitals

In fact, when searching for answers, members were "shocked by the lack of current data relating to the status of hospital quality of care on a national basis, apart from information on indicators such as hospital-specific mortality rates (which HCFA no longer makes easily accessible)" (IOM, 1996, p. 116). JCAHO, which surveys hospital quality every three years on a voluntary basis, has not made its data publicly available on individual hospitals. Meanwhile, AHA, which has the most extensive data on hospitals, does not collect or report on outcomes.

Additionally, while the 1986 Rand Study, one of the most definitive surveys supported by HCFA, examined nursing as a part of hospital services, no research has been published on nursing issues. However, study findings showed that quality of hospital care had generally been improving but that there were some problems, particularly when patients were discharged in medically unstable conditions (Keeler et al., 1992).

In an effort to describe current quality of care problems in hospitals, a number of nursing organizations presented extensive testimony before the IOM committee. Most of the data were anecdotal reports, such as examples of decreased quality for individual patients or hospitals.

Without concrete statistics to show a pattern of poor quality in many hospitals, nurses were not able to make a strong case that hospital quality is declining in general. However, the nurses' presentations did indicate the *potential* for this occurrence. Because the reported anecdotal data did concern the IOM committee, it concluded that the "investigation of hospital quality of care warrants increasing and immediate attention" (IOM, 1996, p. 9).

Members also reaffirmed the importance of the regulation of hospitals to ensure quality. Under federal certification, hospitals can participate in the Medicare and Medicaid programs if the facilities meet the accreditation standards set by JCAHO. Thus, the committee supported JCAHO's general requirements for nursing care, especially the matching of nursing resources with patient needs. In other words, hospitals need to ensure that staffing patterns are sufficient to meet the needs of patients. Staffing levels would be expected to vary based upon patient acuity of illnesses, where higher staffing levels are provided for patients with greater acuity.

Nursing Homes

In contrast to hospitals, federal reporting is required for all 16,000 nursing homes in the U.S. to be certified for participation in Medicare and Medicaid programs. Under the Nursing Home Reform Act of 1987—which enacted greater enforcement and even higher nurse staffing requirements—facilities were mandated to conduct comprehensive assessments for all residents on a periodic basis. Moreover, nursing homes must complete a minimum data set for each resident. Data from this reporting system are being used to develop quality indicators that can identify problem care (Zimmerman, 1995).

Data on quality of care for nursing homes are available from the federal certification surveys conducted by states. The data include staffing information, facility characteristics, and residents' demographics and process and outcome measures. State surveyors evaluate quality and document problems which are then made available to the public. As shown in the IOM report (see p. 137), 30 percent of all nursing homes were cited for unsanitary food, 25 percent for inadequate care plans, 18 percent for improper restraints, and 15 percent for inadequate infection control in 1993. In terms of outcome measures, 19 percent of facilities failed to maintain the dignity of residents, 12 percent had inadequate treatment for incontinence, 9 percent did not prevent pressure sores, and 9 percent provided poor nutrition.

Other anecdotal reports and testimony confirmed the problems that have long been endemic to the nursing home industry. The IOM committee, concerned about poor quality of care delivered by some nursing homes, reaffirmed the importance of the regulatory process, including the use of the comprehensive resident assessment and care planning system.

❖ Linking Nurse Staffing and Outcomes

After assessing data on supply and demand, staffing levels, and quality for hospitals and nursing homes, the committee was asked to examine the link between nurse staffing and outcomes.

Hospitals

Although little research currently illustrates declining quality of care and how low staffing ratios can affect outcomes, the committee was able to identify a few studies of hospital staffing that suggested RN presence was sometimes associated with improved outcomes. Members pointed out the difficulty of isolating the factors influencing outcomes and, particularly, the role of nursing in relation to other factors, such as patient acuity.

In general, the conclusion was that "a high priority should be given to obtaining empirical evidence that permits one to draw conclusions about the relationships of quality of inpatient care and staffing levels and mix" (IOM, 1996, p. 121). Because policymakers cannot solely rely on anecdotal data about poor quality, the committee urged the National Institute of Nursing Research (NINR) and other federal agencies to fund more studies on the relationship between quality and staffing and to develop a research agenda on staffing and quality. In the absence of this type of data, the downsizing of professional and total nursing staff levels in hospitals may continue to be a common practice.

Nursing Homes

For nursing homes, members concluded that "the preponderance of evidence from a number of studies using different types of quality measures has shown a positive relationship between nursing staff levels and quality of nursing home care, indicating a strong need to increase the overall level of nursing staff in nursing homes" (IOM, 1996, p. 153).

Based on these findings, the IOM committee recommended 24-hour RN care for nursing homes as a starting point for improving staffing. "The committee, therefore, supports the need to increase professional nurses in nursing homes on all shifts" (IOM, 1996, p. 153). Because 75 percent of nursing homes are for-profit, and many are investor-owned chains, these organizations would be unlikely to improve staffing on a voluntary basis (Harrington, 1996). Therefore, legislation and funding are needed to mandate increased staffing and to pay for the expense of implementing such standards in the Medicare and Medicaid programs (IOM, 1996).

Interestingly, only a few of the studies reviewed were conducted by nurses. Most nursing research funded by NINR does not examine organizations and staffing issues. Focusing primarily on the clinical care of individual patients, such studies limit the ability of nurses to make policy recommendations about staffing. Clearly, changes in the priorities for nursing research are necessary if the problems of hospital and nursing home quality are going to be addressed.

❖ Developing A Political Action Agenda

Hospital restructuring and the shifting of registered nursing roles to less skilled staff is a serious concern that affects nurses' professional and economic survival. Nursing organizations must unite, forming coalitions of consumer and provider groups to address these and other problems identified by the committee.

History has shown that such an action agenda can have great impact, regardless of economic or political climate. For example, in 1986, the IOM Study of Nursing Home Regulation recommended stronger regulation when there were severe economic pressures on government and an anti-regulatory mood in Congress (IOM, 1986). Efforts by the National Citizens' Coalition for Nursing Home Reform—which organized representatives from the ombudsman, nursing home associations, nursing groups, and senior organizations in Washington to advocate for adoption of the report—resulted in passage of the Nursing Home Reform Act of 1987.

Today, a similar process needs to be undertaken to strengthen the existing staffing standards for nursing homes and to develop standards for hospitals. The major concern should be to protect the quality of health care for the public and to respond to consumer needs for high quality of care.

When developing short- and long-term political agendas for change, nursing must address a variety of issues. Some key areas, from the author's perspective, include:

Building a Consensus on Outcome Measures and Staffing Standards

Nursing groups need to agree on the most important quality indicators—that are sensitive to nursing care—for different types of health care organizations. Since there are few research studies on hospital outcomes, nurses will have to make *their* best judgment about what key outcomes should be examined. First, nurses should review ANA's proposed outcomes, then work toward adopting these measures, and consider expanding this list to include new outcomes.

If a broad spectrum of nursing organizations—along with quality experts and researchers—could build a consensus, these measures would likely be more easily recognized by health care organizations that are creating new reporting systems. Consequently, nurses could ensure that nursing outcome measures would be included in any system under development. Nurses also need to collaborate on determining the minimum staffing levels for hospitals and nursing homes, as well as for different types of settings, such as ambulatory and home care. For optimal success, providers must take into account the acuity and characteristics of patients in each instance.

All of these actions are best undertaken by consensus conference(s), comprised of representatives of major nursing organizations who are knowledgeable about clinical practices in different settings. For a relatively low cost, nursing groups could sponsor separate consensus panels to develop staffing standards, relying on clinicians who are experienced in bedside care and best practices to make these judgments. If standards are developed based on these criteria, then they can be tested by researchers and could be monitored during the licensing and certification process, just as the standards for nursing homes are reviewed on a regular basis by the federal and state governments.

Nurses from different local organizations should encourage their leadership at the state and national levels to make this activity a high priority. The broader the agreement on quality outcomes and staffing standards, the more quickly nurses can begin to collect statistical data on staffing patterns and outcomes within their own organizational settings.

Advocating for Full Disclosure of Data

Once general standards for reporting outcomes and staffing have been developed, data on staffing ratios and nurse-sensitive outcomes by individual health organizations and special units should be disseminated. Disclosure—a top legislative priority of nurses in Washington and, to a greater extent, in California—should be mandatory, reported on a regular basis, such as quarterly, and audited by government agencies or their designees to ensure accuracy.

If a few large states were to adopt such reporting requirements, then greater pressure could be placed on Congress for national data on staffing. In fact, such reporting requirements could be made a part of federal legislation for Medicare and Medicaid certification by working with organizational lobbyists at the national level.

Documenting Quality Indicators and Collecting Data

Nursing also needs to document quality indicators and to collect statistical data for health organizations in a systematic way that can make organizations more accountable. Individual nurses can collect and analyze data from their own employers on quality and outcomes.

If formal complaints need to be filed, nurses could contact state regulators, including the Department of Health and/or the state Medicaid program, or federal agencies, such as HCFA's Bureau of Health Quality and Standards. As complaints accumulate, state and federal agencies investigate, building a record on those health facilities that maintain lower standards or jeopardize patient care.

This is happening for nursing homes but generally not for hospitals. Nurses have been reluctant to report complaints about these facilities. Where staffing problems negatively affect quality, such complaints should be filed to appropriate agencies in order to protect the public.

Supporting Increased Regulation of Quality and Higher Staffing Standards

It is imperative that nursing groups advocate for more regulation of quality of care and higher standards for nurses in all practice settings with mandated minimum staffing levels. In hospitals, the major emphasis should be on advocating for an appropriate mix as a means of ensuring high quality of care.

Nursing home outcome and staffing standards, as noted in the IOM report are not established at a high enough level to be effective. Nurses need to urge their state and national organizations to make this a legislative priority. In addition, funding should be requested from Congress and the

Department of Health and Human Services (DHHS) for developing staffing standards and guidelines for hospitals and nursing homes.

Educating the Public and Congress on the Value of Nursing Care

Many reports have noted that the public generally does not understand the crucial role that nursing care plays in health service outcomes. After measures are developed, nursing organizations need to educate consumers, and Congress, about the importance of these elements and the need for regular reporting by facilities.

Nurses can accomplish this goal through a number of methods. Letters to the editor, newspaper editorials, and radio commentaries are but a few. Holding public forums and conducting campaigns for ballot initiatives that will ensure high quality of care are other ways to increase public awareness. In addition, nurses can write letters to elected officials, attend congressional town hall meetings, or personally visit state and / or federal representatives.

Involving consumer groups with nursing organizations will expedite the educational process and build political coalitions. Remember, to achieve nursing's goals, political action is needed at all levels—local, state, and federal.

Advocating for Research that Links Staffing and Outcomes

To follow-up the IOM recommendation for more study of hospital quality, nursing organizations should support the funding of research that collects and analyzes data on both the process and the outcomes of hospital quality of care. Such a survey should be on the scale of the 1986 HCFA-funded study of hospital quality.

Nurses also should advocate the funding of new research on health care organizations that examines the link between staffing and outcomes. One aspect that is of particular importance to policymakers would be scientific pre- and post-studies of the impact of restructuring of nurses' roles on hospital outcomes.

Again, letter-writing campaigns and personal visits to legislators are important ways to lobby for these goals. Encouraging national organizations to direct pressure on Congress, DHHS, and NINR is another effective approach.

❖ A Clear Message

The findings of the latest IOM report leave little room for doubt: All nurses, regardless of specialty area or educational background, must raise each other's consciousness about these crucial issues.

Indeed, nursing organizations need to unite together with a coalition of consumer and provider groups to address the serious problems identified by committee members. Without the backing of consumer organizations to protect the health of the public, such initiatives are unlikely to be successful with state and federal representatives. In fact, nursing will need to exert political leadership for congressional legislation if the committee's recommendations are to be implemented during the current conservative political and fiscal climate. With the nation's competitive market, if nursing advocates and professionals do not make the most of this opportunity and design a specific action agenda for change, quality of patient care—perhaps even nursing itself—may become compromised.

❖ About the Author

Charlene Harrington, Ph.D., RN, F.A.A.N., is Professor of Social and Behavioral Sciences, Department of Social and Behavioral Sciences, School of Nursing, University of California, San Francisco.

REFERENCES

Harrington, C. (1996). Nursing facility quality, staffing and economic issues. In G.S. Wunderlich, F.A. Sloan, & C.K. Davis (Eds.). *Nursing staff in hospitals and nursing homes: Is it adequate?* (Volume II. pp. 453-502). Washington, DC: National Academy Press.

Institute of Medicine (1986). *Improving the quality of care in nursing homes.* Washington, DC: National Academy Press.

Institute of Medicine, (1996). *Nursing staff in hospitals and nursing homes: Is it adequate?* Washington, DC: National Academy Press.

Keeler, E.B., Rubenstein, L.V., Kahn, K.L., Draper, D., Harrison, E.R., McGinty, M.J., Rogers, W.H., Brook, R.H. (1992). Hospital characteristics and quality of care. *Journal of the American Medical Association, 268.* 1709-1714.

Pew Health Professions Commission. (1995). *Critical challenges: Revitalizing the health care professions for the twenty-first century.* San Francisco. CA: UCSF Center for the Health Professions.

Service Employees International Union. (1993). *The national nurse survey: 10,000 dedicated healthcare professionals report on staffing, stress and patient care in U.S. hospitals and nursing homes.* Washington, DC: SEIU AFL-CIO.

Zimmerman, D.R., Karon, S.L., Arling, G., Clark, B.R., Collins, T., Ross, R., Sainfort, F. (1995, Summer). Development and testing of nursing home quality indicators. *Health Care Financing Review, 16*(4). 107-127.

BIBLIOGRAPHY

American Nurses Association. (1995). *Summary of the Lewin-1 HI. Inc. report: Nursing report card for acute care settings.* Washington, DC: American Nurses' Association.

Harrington, C., Thollaug, S.C., & Summers, P.R. (1995). *Nursing facilities, staffing, residents and facility deficiencies, 1991-1993. Report prepared for the Health Care Financing Administration.* San Francisco. CA: University of California.

PART IV

Health Care System Issues

❖ Chapter 8
Health Care and
Health Care Reform

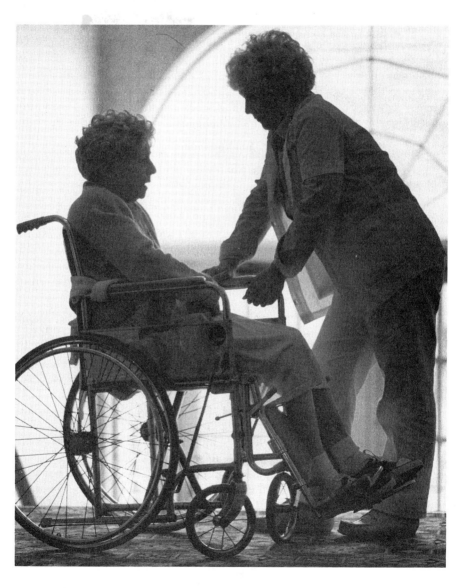

The health care revolution of the 1990s has its roots in a number of developments during the past 30 years, particularly the continuing impact of technology on the quality and costs of health care. Both the volume and the intensity of services, which are the major factors affecting health care costs, are driven by technologies—old and new.

The initial response to the rapidly rising costs in the 1970s was eliminating federal subsidies for hospital construction and other health facilities construction, termination of direct subsidies for support of medicine, nursing, pharmacy and dental education, scholarships for students were shifted to loans, then loan guarantees. Three subsidy programs continue: the support of biomedical research through the National Institutes of Health (NIH), the support of graduate medical education (GME) and, to a lesser extent, nursing education, through Medicare. Medicare and Medicaid subsidies continued, but the expansion of these programs was halted after the mid-1970s.

Attempts were made to slow the increasing costs of health care, through industry-wide wage and price controls initiated in 1971 by Present Nixon and continued in the health sector through 1974. This broad-based regulatory effort to control prices was followed by Medicare policies to slow price increases by physicians and hospitals and deter unnecessary utilization, particularly of hospital services, through the establishment of professional standards review organizations by Congress in 1972. In addition, steps were taken in the 1970s to strengthen health planning and make it a more effective policy tool to slow the rate of increase in health care costs. These efforts were not particularly successful.

An attempt was also made to control costs through the stimulation of greater competition. Legislation was enacted in the early 1970s to stimulate the development of group practice, prepayment plans—particularly health maintenance organizations (HMOs). Although the initial impact was slight, the growth of HMOs and other managed care arrangements was to dominate the 1990s.

In the late 1970s, President Carter attempted to convince Congress of the necessity to directly regulate hospital expenditures. While this effort failed because of effective lobbying by the hospitals, it set the stage of the Medicare hospital cost containment policies of the 1980s.

Congressional actions to control the rising costs of Medicare began in 1972 when Congress called for the establishment of the Medicare Economic Index (MEI) to adjust the prevailing charges by physicians. The MEI broke the link between physician charges and actual Medicare payments. The MEI went into effect in 1975 and remained a major tool to control physician payment for over 15 years.

The big change occurred in 1983 when Congress mandated the establishment of a system of prospective payment for hospitals. This system dramatically restructured the financial incentives for hospitals by defining specific diagnosis related groups (DRGs) to represent conditions for which

Medicare patients were hospitalized and setting specific payment amounts for each diagnosis related group. This policy turned on its head the previous policy of paying hospitals on the basis of costs incurred in treating patients (cost–based reimbursement).

Beginning in 1984, Congress began to regulate direct Medicare payments to physicians and the charges by physicians to patients that were above the permissible Medicare payments (balance billing). The following year, Congress directed the Secretary of Health and Human Services to develop a a resource-based relative value scale for physician payment and established the Physician Payment Review Commission to advise it on physician payment policies. In 1988, the Commission endorsed the concept of replacing the customary, prevailing, and reasonable (CPR) system of payment with a fee schedule. In 1989, a resource-based fee schedule with limits on balance billing and an annual expenditure target to restrain rising costs were recommended by the Commission. These recommendations were basically adopted by Congress in 1989, with the fee schedule implemented in 1992 (Culbertson and Lee, HCFA Review, 1997).

While Medicare was adopting a regulatory approach to both hospital and physician payments, the private sector, driven by employer's desires to slow the rising costs of health care, turned to managed competition. The most significant changes have been the shifts from indemnity insurance, with fee-for-service payments to physicians and charge based on cost based payments to hospitals, to capitated payments for both and the integration of the financing and the delivery of medical care. In addition, employer health benefits have been reduced, particularly the coverage of dependents, and restrictions have been placed on individuals with preexisting conditions. Until the recently enacted Kennedy-Kassenbaum law by Congress, there was great uncertainty about an employee keeping his/her health insurance when moving from one job to another.

While managed care had its roots in the development of group practice pre-payment plans after World War II (e.g., Kaiser Permanente), it was not until the early 1970s that federal policy began to explicitly encourage the development of health maintenance organizations (HMOs). The growth of HMOs was slow in the 1970s, in part because Medicare and Medicaid policies gave little support for HMOs until the 1980s.

Between 1980 and 1988, enrollment in health maintenance organizations and other managed care plans more than quintupled, from 9 million to 51.5 million people. One in five Americans now receives health care from among the 574 HMOs available. While HMOs were initially primarily staff and group model plans, the most rapid growth has been among individual practice associations and preferred provider organizations. In many of these managed care plans (e.g., IPAs), cost controls are achieved through price reductions, by fee-for-service practitioners, and by stringent utilization review. The growing limitations on consumer choice of health plans and practitioners is causing a rising tide of consumer complaints. Congress recently mandated that health insurance plans, including managed care plans, pay for at least two days of hospital care after a normal delivery. Many states are considering legislation to curb the growth of HMOs, much of it stimulated by physicians and nurses who find their incomes and job options limited in the managed care environment.

While the pace of change in the private sector has been dramatic, it is beginning to affect state Medicaid programs, with most states requesting federal waivers in order to implement managed care plans, at least for AFDC (Aid to Families with Dependent Children) beneficiaries. Medicare is also gradually expanding its Medicare Managed Care options. At the beginning of the program, Medicare allowed certain prepaid organizations to receive a cost reimbursement, instead of a fee–for–service payment, for Medicare enrollees. A risk sharing contract option for HMOs was instituted in 1972, one year before the federal HMO Act was passed. This program did not begin until 1978, as a five state demonstration program. It required five years, from 1982 to 1987, to enroll the first one million Medicare beneficiaries under risk contracts. In 1982, Congress authorized managed care payments based on a prospective payment methodology.

Medicare HMO enrollment has increased steadily since risk contracting began in 1985. One million new beneficiaries enrolled in HMOs from 1987 to 1991 and by 1993, a third million beneficiaries enrolled. While the Medicare beneficiaries in risk contracting plans continues to grow, the number of beneficiaries in cost reimbursement plans has been relatively steady for the past decade.

In 1996, nearly nine percent of Medicare beneficiaries were enrolled in risk contracting HMOs. In recent years, Medicare risk contracting has grown rapidly, particularly in California, Oregon, Arizona, and Hawaii.

Recently, Professor Victor R. Fuchs (1996) provided an excellent overview of the basic issues in health care economics and a road map for future policy choices. Unlike many economists, he is not a blind advocate of the market, but provides a strong rationale for an essential role for the government. We highly recommend reading this important paper in its entirety but are unable to include it due to space limitations.

We have also included the poignant paper "Whatever Happened to the Health Insurance Crisis in the United States?" by Karen Donelan and associates. National data indicate that the ranks of the uninsured continue to swell, yet there is a conspicuous absence of public debate or political attention to this now apparently invisible problem. The authors explore results of nearly 4000 focused interviews to answer questions about the uninsured and why they do not have insurance and the insured and what difficulty they face in obtaining care. Their results clearly indicate that there are millions in precarious situations regarding their basic health care. Whether or not this crisis situation for a segment of our society indicates that there is a crisis in the U.S. health care system at-large is a question that cannot be answered by quantitative data.

In the Winter 1995 issue of *Health Affairs*, there was a comprehensive review of Medicare and its future from a variety of perspectives. We have chosen to include the article by Marilyn Moon and Karen Davis, "Preserving and Strengthening Medicare," because it argues first and foremost for preserving the integrity of the program. In their article, Moon and Davis describe the strengths of Medicare (universal for all those age 65 years and older, risk is shared across a large population group, strong cost containment policies) and its problems (the high cost of health care and the continuing of growth of Medicare outlays). They analyze the Medicare managed care option, and believe this could be expanded incrementally, while still protecting beneficiaries. They squarely address the issue of future cost increases and the need to meet them through social security and general tax increases or greater beneficiary cost sharing.

Other leading students of the Medicare program propose different solutions. Henry Aaron and Robert Reischauer (see Recommended Reading) propose a major shift in Medicare from a "service reimbursement" system to a "premium support" system. In this approach, they include both the basic Medicare program and supplemental plans (Medigap) that most beneficiaries purchase. In their article, they detail the steps necessary to move to this new system. They also note, as did Moon and Davis, that the program cannot be sustained without new taxes in the future. Another approach similar to the Federal Employees Health Benefits Program (a defined contribution rather than a defined benefit) is proposed by Butler and Moffit in the third major paper in this issue of *Health Affairs*. There are a variety of other perspectives included in this issue that make it very interesting and provocative reading.

Medicaid has been the principle source of payment for medical care for those eligible on public assistance (AFDC, SSI) for the past 30 years. Because of expanded enrollments in recent years which were mandated by Congress in the late 1980s, rising costs have contributed to putting more and more pressure on states' discretionary budgets. In recent years, the Henry J. Kaiser Family Foundation Commission has provided a wealth of information about the programs. We include one of the Commission Policy Briefs to illustrate the type of material produced.

The pressures to curtail costs in the Medicaid program have lead states to turn increasingly to managed care. Several states, including Oregon and Tennessee, used Section 1115 waivers to both broaden access for low income populations and slow the increase in costs. In Tennessee, the emphasis was on managed care. In Oregon, limits were placed on benefits, particularly those that were not considered cost effective. In this article, included in this chapter, Bruce Vladeck reviews the developments in the 1115 Waiver Program in 1995. The pace of state applications continues despite the plea for caution by Andrulis et al. who note: "The lack of critical information, however, suggests the need for caution before accelerating this process. Today, there has been little or no assessment of state Medicaid initiatives in either waivered or unwaivered states" (p. 163).

There have been a number of potential problems with the rapid shift to managed care. Many of the traditional safety net providers, particularly urban public hospitals, may lose the disproportionate share funding to cover their costs of the uninsured population that they serve. There have been concerns expressed about access to care for the chronically mentally ill, those with substance abuse, the homeless, and those with chronic illness. If public hospital systems lose Medicaid patients to competing private health plans, their capacity to meet community-wide needs for emergency care, trauma and neonatal intensive care services may be compromised as noted by Andrulis et al. in the article included in this chapter.

The jury is still out on Medicaid managed care. Although there are opportunities to improve the quality of care and contain rising costs, the access and other issues must be addressed.

At one time Americans believed that theirs was the best health care system in the world. However, a 1989 Louis Harris and Associates survey reported that Americans are most dissatisfied with their health system than either Canadians or Britons, despite the higher levels of health care spending by Americans. The poll reported that 89 percent of U.S. residents called for fundamental changes in the delivery of health services, and 61 percent would be pleased to trade the U.S. system for a model like that in Canada.

More recent polls indicate continuing discontent with the present system. A 1991 Time and Cable News Network poll found that the number of those who called for fundamental reform in the health care system was as high as 91 percent. A *Wall Street Journal* poll in March 1993 also found that a significant majority of Americans believe the U.S. health care system needs major change. In a November 1991 poll, Pennsylvanians were asked what they thought was the biggest problem with health care, and 77 percent responded that the biggest problem for themselves and their families was cost. A Roper survey estimated support for extending Medicare coverage to everyone to be as high as 69 percent. An analysis of U.S. polls taken between 1989 and 1991 by Blendon and Donehue concluded that support for a national health plan was indicated by well over half of the nation. This reflected a dissatisfaction with a number of aspects of the current system, including limitations on access to services, high costs, complex technologies, fragmentation of services, and uneven quality. These attitudes did not translate into support for the health care reforms proposed by President Clinton in 1993.

Some say this is but another expression of the basic American wish to "have our cake and eat it too." We want miracle cures, but we do not want prices to go up. Although the system is meeting the personal needs of many people, collectively there are failures. These failures reflect the tradeoffs that are necessary under the current payment system. For example, over 41 million low-income people have no insurance coverage and thus no direct means of payment for health care, and these are often the people who most desperately need care. Those who have health insurance do not want their choices restricted, but they do want costs, particularly costs that they bear directly, controlled. There seems to be less willingness than in the past to support universal health insurance.

The great expense of many advanced technologies forces health care providers to weigh individual circumstances of patients against economic constraints in making therapeutic decisions. Thus, providers find they must limit resources and withhold treatment from patients who could benefit from the care. A recent report that infant mortality was higher in the United States than in Singapore and that the United States ranked twenty-second in infant mortality worldwide raised many questions about the lack of availability of prenatal care to certain groups in this country, which experts say could prevent needless deaths. African-American infants are more than twice as likely to die in their first year as are white infants. Although infant mortality has declined, the ratio of African-American to white infant mortality has increased in recent years, from 1.8 in the early 1970s to 2.2 in 1990. Life expectancy in the U.S. at birth ranks twentieth for men and fifteenth for women worldwide. A 1991 study found the in-hospital death rate of uninsured patients to be 1.2 to 3.2 times higher than the rate for insured patients. African-American women have been found to show higher rates of invasive cervical cancer, and this has been connected to their lower access to Pap tests. There is no disputing that under the current system one's health status and access to services are statistically tied to one's income, race, education, and health insurance status.

Though the problems are apparent to everyone, there is by no means a consensus about how to reform the system. In the 1980s, the trend toward for-profit medicine emerged in the form of privately owned proprietary hospital chains or systems and a shift in many other nonprofit organizations to for-profit status. This was coupled with an increase in centralized ownership and investor-owned national chains, which tend to seek out affluent, well-insured markets. The policies under Presidents Reagan and Bush favored employment of market principles in allocating health resources, thus progressing toward greater competition in health care and away from strict regulation of the industry and universal coverage. President Clinton's proposals for health care reform in 1993 included elements of both competition and regulation in an attempt to assure universal coverage and curtail costs. These conflicting goals, the complexity of his proposals, the lack of benefits for the already insured middle class, and the attack by special interests (e.g., health insurance industry, small business) killed the plan in Congress in 1994.

The problems addressed in President Clinton's plan—rising costs, the growing number of uninsured, inequitable access to care, variations in quality—remain, and, in many cases have grown worse since the failure of Congress to act in 1994 (e.g., the growing number of uninsured). Many of the ideas that were incorporated in the Clinton Health Plan, albeit modified from the original, remain the basis for the current debate about how much to control costs and assure universal access to care.

Professor Alain Enthoven, a Stanford University economist, has long been one of the advocates of competition in health care as a means to address the underlying causes of uncontrolled cost increases and to result in the survival of health plans that offer good value to their customers. Out of this grew an approach he labeled "managed competition," the goal of which is "to divide the providers in each community into competing economic units and to use market forces to motivate them to develop efficient delivery systems" (1993, p. 24). This policy was adopted in a modified form by President Clinton and woven into his plan presented to Congress in 1993. In describing his plan, the President said it would "give groups of consumers and small businesses the same market bargaining power that large corporations and large groups of public employees have now" (1992, p. 79). He said it would allow plans to compete on the basis of price and quality rather than by excluding sick people. Part of the strategy is to make both providers and consumers more cost conscious by offering everyone a choice of plans. This would foster competition among the provider networks, all of whom would have to offer a guaranteed benefit package.

Other proposals introduced in Congress deviated in various ways from the President's plan, including universal, single-payer plans and private vouchers, but none attracted sufficient support to move forward. Republicans in Congress introduced a number of proposed health plans, all of which favor less government intervention than the President. Although some of the more conservative plans have similarities to the one proposed by President Clinton, in general they would not include an employer mandate; they call for gradually achieving universal coverage, and they do not favor sweeping restructuring of the nation's health care system. Many policymakers who hesitate to embark on uncharted waters support the concept of providing tax credits or other means to make insurance more affordable for the unemployed and others who are uninsured in order to provide easier access to benefits, but many of them consider universal coverage to be an unrealistic first step. Much of the debate centers on how much reform will cost and how to pay for it. No one expects it to come cheaply.

One prominent theme that has taken a variety of forms during the past 25 years is the call for a national health plan, often referred to as the single-payer option. The model favored by many is the one adopted by Canada, where the provincial government is the single payer, everyone is covered, and people freely select their providers. Considerable administrative savings would be realized through elimination of private health insurance. Proponents predict that such a government-run program could be financed by money that is already in the system.

An overview of health care reform by policy analysts Philip R. Lee, Denise Soffel, and Harold S. Luft, included in the fourth edition of *The Nation's Health* (1994), provides an insight into the root causes of the current crisis: rising costs and the growing ranks of uninsured. Factors contributing to rising health care costs include market failure, high technology, administrative costs, unnecessary care and defensive medicine, patient complexity, excess capacity, and low productivity. Lee and associates also assess attempts to control costs by the federal government and the private sector, which have been largely unsuccessful.

Veteran health policy analyst, Eli Ginzberg, provides us with a capsule summary, also in the fourth edition of *The Nation's Health* (1994), of the positions the various interest groups have carved out for themselves on the subject of reform. Despite the intransigence of most of these groups, Ginsberg predicted that some reform would be undertaken because of the simple fact that the nation cannot possibly afford to continue on its present path through the rest of the 1990s. He followed with a discussion of the urgent need for global budgeting, which would place a cap on annual expenditures in order to limit health care spending. Global budgeting, proposed by President Clinton in his health care reform plan, would have placed a cap on annual expenditures in order to limit growth in health care spending.

While he echoes many of Dr. Ginzberg's concerns about the urgent need for reform, David Blumenthal, in his article included in this chapter, was less optimistic about the prospect for policymakers to "brave the adverse consequences" endemic in any attempt at sweeping reform. In "The Timing and Course of Health Care Reform," Blumenthal predicts that any package implemented in the near future "will perpetuate at least some of the current system's inequities and inefficiencies" (Blumenthal, 1991, p. 198). Thus the crisis atmosphere surrounding health care will continue to build until its catastrophic effects are experienced first hand by a greater proportion of the electorate and the national economy is threatened.

An important element in the Clinton Plan, managed competition, was embraced, at least in part, by a number of health care reform plans that have been considered by Congress in recent years. The second concept, managed care, is already a reality for many Americans, and we can expect that more and more of us will come to experience it in the coming years. Managed care plans integrate the delivery and financing of care, usually placing constraints on both patients and providers.

Others have dealt with key issues that must be addressed in any proposed health care reform. Public hospitals, as Andrulis, Acuff, Weiss, and Anderson (1996) point out, are a key element in the safety net for the poor. Not only do they provide essential inpatient, emergency room, and outpatient services for the poor, they are also one of the major centers for graduate medical education in the country. To date, no solution has been found to the issues related to safety net providers.

The academic medical center is another challenged institution. In his *New England Journal of Medicine* editorial, Kassirer raises a number of the key issues that these institutions will confront. The loss of faculty practice revenue attributable to managed care is a key issue facing academic medical centers. Many feel that the support of clinical research is threatened. Others are alarmed by the trend toward primary care. In the fact of multiple challenges, many of the nation's academic medical centers are responding with a wide range of organizational changes, particularly mergers and downsizing of their hospital systems.

❖ Whatever Happened to the Health Insurance Crisis in the United States?

Voices From a National Survey

KAREN DONELAN, ROBERT J. BLENDON,
CRAIG A. HILL, CATHERINE HOFFMAN,
DIANE ROWLAND, MARTIN FRANKEL,
DREW ALTMAN

Four years ago, in the presidential campaign, in major medical journals and medical associations, in the media, and in civic groups, our nation was engaged in a great debate about the best way to provide health insurance coverage to all Americans. By contrast, these debates have been conspicuous by their absence in this election year.

The health system reform debate was marked by some controversy about whether there was a health insurance crisis at all.[1] On one side were those who said that most of the uninsured could get care when they needed it, a view that was expressed in a commentary in the *Wall Street Journal* in 1994 that noted that "these [uninsured] citizens are not denied health care" and only 1 in 5 uninsured (about 3% of the population) cannot obtain affordable insurance.[2] On the other side were those who claimed that many of the uninsured faced major barriers to needed health care services and experienced health and economic consequences because of these barriers.

While the political urgency of these concerns has subsided, we know that gaps in insurance coverage remain for a sizable number of Americans—recent estimates indicate that approximately 40 million people in the United States were uninsured in 1994 (oral communication, B. Katherine Swartz, PhD, April 23, 1996, regarding unpublished data from analyses of March 1995 *Current Population Survey*); another 29 million are underinsured.[3] Reports of public opinion surveys have noted that support for reform was driven in large part by anxieties about access to and cost of medical care among both insured and uninsured persons.[4-6]

Prior research has documented decreased access to health care services, and increased burdens of economic hardship, ill health, and mortality that the uninsured and underinsured experience.[7-9] In the midst of the health system reform debate, media reports about this research were frequently augmented with vignettes illustrating the consequences of access and financial problems for individuals and families. While vignettes can add a valuable qualitative dimension to quantitative estimates of problems, they are not randomly selected and may illustrate extreme, rather than average, consequences. Verbatim responses are common in the development of sample surveys, but in larger-scale surveys, structured and coded responses are preferred to minimize cost and increase analytic power.

Now that the politically charged health system reform debate has subsided, we return to the basic questions that marked that discussion. What problems do uninsured and insured people have in getting and paying for medical care in today's changing health care system? How many Americans are affected? How severe are their problems and their consequences? We sought to answer these questions by using a combination of quantitative measures of access to health care and personal qualitative accounts in a recent survey of Americans to determine who has experienced problems getting medical care and paying for it.

❖ Data and Methods

The survey design and instrument were developed by research staff of the Harvard School of Public Health, the Henry J. Kaiser Family Foundation, and the National Opinion Research Center (NORC) at the University of Chicago. NORC conducted the survey by telephone from February 22 to April 27, 1995. A random adult respondent (aged 18 years or older) was selected in each household, with no substitution if that person refused or could not be contacted. At least 16 attempts were made both to select the random adult in each household and to interview the person selected.

In all, 3993 interviews were conducted. All respondents were asked to respond to a common battery of health status, health services utilization, and demographic questions. Interviewers used computer-assisted software that prompted the survey questions, which were read to the respondents; responses were then typed into the computer. Among all respondents, a subgroup of 1234 (31%) reported experiencing at least 1 of 3 core problems in the past year: an episode of being uninsured (unweighted n = 596), a time when they did not get medical care that they thought they needed (unweighted n = 636), or a problem in paying medical bills (unweighted n = 606). Respondents with the 3 core problems of interest were interviewed at greater length in topic-specific modules to explore the nature and consequences of their experiences. Among respondents reporting 1 of the 3 core problems, interviews averaged 19 minutes; other interviews averaged 4 minutes.

At the close of the interview, respondents were asked to describe the consequences of their experiences using an open-ended item: "I would like you to tell me in your own words what happened to you as a result of the problems you have experienced. We are especially interested in the consequences of your [insert: not getting medical care that you thought you needed / time without insurance / problems in paying medical bills] on, for example, your physical or mental health, your family relationships, your employment or your household finances." The responses were coded for content in areas of health, employment, family, and financial consequences. Coded and illustrative verbatim responses are reported here. Edits to the verbatim responses are indicated in brackets and were used only to protect respondent identity or correct typographical errors. Where they appear, verbatim responses were selected at random with substitution for cases where responses were unintelligible or missing.

To ensure conformity with known distributions in the national population, the data are weighted to adjust for age, race, sex, region, education, and marital status, as well as for household size.

The response rate, calculated as complete interviews at all telephone numbers known to be households and not known to be businesses, was 52%. In NORC's experience in recent years, this rate is about average for random-digit-dial telephone surveys with random respondent selection. The margin of sampling error for a sample of 3993 people is approximately ±1%, and increases for smaller subgroups of the sample (eg, a maximum of ±3% for 1234 people, ±4% for 600 people, and ±10% for 100 people).

❖ Results

Among all 3993 respondents surveyed, 18% of adults said that there was a time in the past year when they did not get medical care that they thought they needed, and 16% said they had a problem in the past year in paying medical bills. Nineteen percent indicated that they were without health insurance either at the time of the survey (12%) or at some point in the year prior (7%). Throughout this article, people who were uninsured at the time of the survey are combined with people who were uninsured for some part of the year prior to the survey; this group is referred to as the "uninsured."

Uninsured and insured respondents reported significantly different experiences. The uninsured were 4 times more likely than the insured to report an episode of needing and not getting medical care and 3 times more likely to report a problem in paying for medical bills. Differences between the uninsured and the insured are also observed in key health and demographic measures.

The Uninsured

Who Are the Uninsured and Why Don't They Have Insurance?—The findings of this survey confirm many things we know about the uninsured from prior research. The general demographic profile is similar, with about 70% of the uninsured saying that they were employed during at least part of the time they were without coverage. Of these, approximately 40% worked for employers who provided coverage to at least some employees.

Cost and the lack of employer-provided coverage are the principal reasons for being uninsured. Political rhetoric to the contrary, very few Americans are uninsured by choice. Fewer than 1 in 10 of the uninsured said that they did not want or need health insurance coverage or just did not think about getting it.

More than half (59%) of the uninsured said that this was the first time in the past 5 years that they had been without insurance coverage; 40% reported other periods of being without insurance.

Difficulties in Getting Needed Care.—Forty-five percent of the uninsured and 11% of the insured report a time in the year prior to the survey when they needed care and could not get it. Among all survey respondents, episodes of not getting needed care were reported by about 25% to 35% of people with a higher burden of illness (defined as self-reported fair or poor health or disability). Barriers to care are amplified among the uninsured— 75% of those in poor health and 54% of those in fair health said that there was a time in the past year when they experienced this problem.

How often does getting needed care present an obstacle for the uninsured and for what symptoms are they delaying care? About half of the uninsured (49%) reported 1 episode; the remainder indicated that there were multiple occasions. Of those who did not get needed care, 60% said that it was for a "specific medical problem" (actual text of question); 17% needed preventive care (defined as "checkups, immunizations, cancer screening"); the remainder said that both types of care were needed.

We asked respondents to describe the medical symptoms they had at the time they needed and did not get medical care. Seventy percent of the uninsured said that their symptoms were either "very serious" or "somewhat serious" at the time they could not get care.

For the overwhelming majority of the uninsured, cost and insurance reasons are the predominant reasons for not getting needed medical care. Fifty-one percent said that they could not afford to pay, 25% said that they had no insurance at the time, and the remainder indicated other reasons. Only 2% said that they didn't think that their symptoms were serious enough to warrant getting care.

Approximately half (52%) of uninsured people who said that there was a time when they needed care and did not get it tried to get help from a medical professional for the problem they described to us; 75% were successful. At the time of the survey, 50% of uninsured respondents who said that there was a time when they did not get needed care in the past year (representing about 1 in 4 of uninsured adults surveyed) said that they still had either "pain or disability" as a result of the medical problem or problems they reported.

Problems in Paying Medical Bills.—Lack of health insurance coverage may be associated with lower utilization of health services, but it sometimes leaves uninsured people who do need and use medical care with substantial out-of-pocket medical costs. While 12% of people with health insurance coverage had a problem in paying medical bills in the year prior to the survey, more than one third (36%) of people without health insurance reported this experience. Just as uninsured persons in fair or poor health are more likely than the insured to have difficulty in obtaining care, 48% of those in fair health and 67% in poor health told us that they had problems in paying medical bills in the year prior to the survey.

Because it is difficult to obtain such information from respondents with unaided recall, out-of-pocket medical expenditures were broadly measured (>$1000, >$5000). Among the uninsured who reported problems in paying bills, 49% said they paid more than $1000 out of pocket for medical bills in the year prior to the survey; 8% paid more than $5000. Among all adults surveyed, 34% paid more than $1000 out of pocket; 4% paid more than $5000.

At the time of the survey, two thirds (67%) of the uninsured who had problems in paying medical bills still owed money for those bills; 70% owed less than $1000, 22% owed $1001 to 5000, 5% owed $5001 to $20,000, and 2% owed in excess of $20,000. Forty-four percent of the uninsured with problems in paying bills have been contacted in the past year by a collection agency.

It is a commonly held assumption that the uninsured can get free or charity care if they need it. Only 37% of the uninsured who reported problems in paying medical bills said that they had received medical care "for free or for a reduced charge" in the previous year.

Consequences of Core Problems for the Uninsured.—Among the uninsured with problems in paying medical bills (but not in getting care) 67% say the consequences were "very serious" or "somewhat serious"; a significantly higher proportion (79%) of those with difficulty in getting needed care point to serious consequences. People who are uninsured and report both problems (about 5% of all adults surveyed and 28% of the uninsured) are distinguished from the general adult population in several ways—they are more likely to rate the consequences of their experiences as serious, they are sicker, more likely to be female, and to have higher out-of-pocket expenses for health care.

Coding of all the verbatim responses demonstrated that while 37% of the uninsured report virtually no consequences of their problems, others mention problems ranging from major health conditions such as heart disease, cancer, and diabetes (16%); problems in paying for food or shelter (6%); employment difficulties (10%); or stress, worry, or fear (22%). Nearly half (42%) of those uninsured who also had difficulty in getting care or in paying medical bills reported a major health condition.

The Insured

We have seen that a number of the health and health care problems studied here disproportionately affect uninsured people. However, the sheer magnitude of people in the United States who have health insurance means that even if a small proportion of the population experiences difficulty, millions of people are affected.

Difficulties in Getting Needed Medical Care.—Eleven percent of insured adults in the United States reported a time in the year prior to the survey when they could not get medical care that they thought they needed. As in the uninsured population, problems in getting needed care are disproportionately high among insured people in fair or poor health.

When asked to rate the severity of that medical problem as they perceived it at the time, 60% (compared with 70% of the uninsured) said that they thought their problem was either very or somewhat serious when they could not get care.

Among the uninsured, cost and lack of insurance coverage predominated among reported reasons for not getting needed medical care. One in four (25%) insured respondents also said that they could not afford to pay for care; 1 in 10 (11%) said that their problem was not serious enough to warrant care. An additional 20% of insured respondents report a variety of problems with insurance coverage, including denial of insurance claims, perceptions of respondents and their physicians that certain services would not be covered, and services used that were not covered by insurance. Approximately 10% reported structural barriers to care such as transportation problems, difficulty in getting time off from work, and problems in getting appointments.

Problems in Paying Medical Bills.—A previous study conducted in 1992[7] found that 19% of Americans reported problems in paying medical bills and 75% of those had insurance. In this study we found that 58% of people with problems in paying medical bills were insured for the whole year prior to the survey, while another 14% who were insured at the time of the survey had had no insurance for some part of the previous year. Twenty-eight percent were uninsured at the time of the survey. These findings underscore the value of considering the dynamics of health insurance coverage over time and of not relying solely on point-in-time measures of coverage in analyses.

We asked insured respondents who had problems with medical bills why their health insurance did not cover the cost of their care. Among more than a third of respondents (38%), costs were part of copayments, deductibles, or coinsurance. Other reasons included services costing more than insurance covered (21%), services not covered by insurance (16%), and care from a provider outside the plan (5%). Only 1% reported exclusion because of a preexisting condition, an unmet waiting period for coverage, or failure to get proper approvals from insurance.

Consequences of Core Problems for the Insured.—As already noted, the proportions of insured people who report difficulty in getting needed medical care and/or in paying medical bills are significantly lower than in the uninsured population. However, if we translate these proportions into approximate numbers of adults in the United States, about 28 million had insurance that was inadequate to guarantee freedom from access and cost burdens. This is approximately the same number as the estimated number of the underinsured reported in 1995.[4] Respondent ratings of the severity of the consequences of their financial and medical care difficulties demonstrate that, as in the uninsured population, majority of insured people who report these problems see them as severe: 75% said the consequences of problems paying bills were serious, and 62% of those with problems getting care noted serious consequences. Among the insured who have both problems, 86% said there were serious consequences—a proportion that does not differ significantly from the uninsured.

❖ Comment

This survey's findings bring us back to central questions raised during the failed health system reform effort. Do we have a crisis in the US health insurance system? How big is the problem? How many people are affected? How serious are the consequences?

As described at the outset of this article, in one view, virtually all the uninsured in America can get all the health care services they need. In another view, virtually all without coverage are at risk for tragedy. This study's findings challenge both extreme views. On one hand, the notions that only 3% of the uninsured do not have access to affordable insurance coverage and most do not have problems getting care when they need it[2] are pure speculation; the majority of the uninsured cite cost as the principal reason they do not have insurance coverage and approximately half of the uninsured reported difficulty in getting needed care and/or in paying for medical bills in the course of a year. The overwhelming majority of this group rate the consequences of their problems as serious.

On the other hand, the uninsured are a minority of Americans, and about half of them reported that they did not experience problems in getting or in paying for medical care in the year prior to the survey. Results shown here point to the fact that while many people in this group worry about the future, and we may speculate about their plight in the event of a major accident or illness, about half of the uninsured in America are not experiencing difficulties in obtaining medical care.

Among the insured, approximately 1 in 6 people (some 28 million adults) have insurance policies that do not protect them from problems in getting needed medical care or in paying medical bills. The cost-sharing requirements of health plans generate out-of-pocket expenditures that are unaffordable for some Americans.

From these findings, some might legitimately conclude that, even adding the experiences of the uninsured and insured, difficulties with access to needed medical care and the affordability of medical bills affect a minority of the US population and need not be of broader societal concern. Others might conclude that even though these problems affect a minority of Americans, it is a minority of millions of people; 1 in 4 insured or uninsured adults surveyed means that approximately 50 million adults are affected. The 70% who say that their problems are serious translates into about 34 million people. Problems in getting needed medical care affect about 17 million uninsured adults and 17 million insured adults in America, and problems in paying medical bills are reported by 13 million uninsured and 17 million insured Americans.

Other dimensions of the findings reported here could also be troubling. First, although similar numbers of insured and uninsured people report difficulty in obtaining medical care and paying for it, those without health insurance face disproportionate burdens. Second, aspects of our health care system are especially challenging to negotiate for uninsured and insured people who are sick. People in fair or poor health, people with major chronic illnesses, and people with disabilities are disproportionately represented in every problem area studied—health insurance, getting needed care, and paying medical bills. One in 6 of the uninsured noted in verbatim responses about consequences of these problems that they had a concurrent major illness.

Is there a crisis in our health care system? The voices of the people that we surveyed give life to the statistics and tell us a story of millions of individual crises in getting and in paying for health care each year. Are the crises of this minority a crisis for our society? That is a question this study will not resolve.

❖ About the Authors

Karen Donelan, Sc. D., is Professor, Department of Health Policy and Management, Harvard School of Public Health, Boston.

Robert J. Blendon, Sc.D., is Professor, Department of Health Policy and Management, Harvard School of Public Health, Boston.

Craig A. Hill, Ph.D., is with the National Opinion Research Center at the University of Chicago.

Catherine Hoffman, Sc.D., is with the Henry J. Kaiser Family Foundation, Menlo Park, California.

Diane Rowland, Sc.D., is with the Henry J. Kaiser Family Foundation, Menlo Park, California.

Martin Frankel, Ph.D., is Professor, Department of Statistics, Baruch College, City University of New York.

Drew Altman, Ph.D., is with the Henry J. Kaiser Family Foundation, Menlo Park, California.

REFERENCES

1. Swartz K. Dynamics of people without health insurance: don't let the numbers fool you. *JAMA*. 1994; 271:64–66.
2. Stelzer IM. There is no health care crisis. *Wall Street Journal*. January 25, 1994;section A:12.
3. Short PF, Banthin JS. New estimates of the underinsured younger than 65 years. *JAMA*. 1995;274:1302-1306.
4. Henry J. Kaiser Family Foundation/Commonwealth Fund/Harris poll. Storrs, Conn: Roper Center for Public Opinion Research; January 31, 1992.
5. Henry J. Kaiser Family Foundation/Commonwealth Fund/Harris poll. Storrs, Conn: Roper Center for Public Opinion Research; August 6, 1993.
6. Blendon RJ, Donelan K. Public opinion and efforts to reform the U.S. health care system: confronting issues of cost-containment and access to care. *Stanford Law Policy Rev.* Fall 1991;3:146-154.
7. Blendon RJ, Donelan K, Hill CA, Carter W, Beatrice D, Altman D. Paying medical bills in the United States: why health insurance isn't enough. *JAMA*. 1994;271:949-951.
8. Weissman JS, Epstein AM. *Falling Through the Safety Net: Insurance Status and Access to Health Care.* Baltimore, Md: Johns Hopkins University Press; 1994.
9. Henry J. Kaiser Family Foundation: *Uninsured in America: Straight Facts on Health Reform.* Menlo Park, Calif: Kaiser Family Foundation; April 1994. Report 1004.

❖ Medicare Analysis
Preserving and Strengthening Medicare

Marilyn Moon and Karen Davis

Medicare has opened the door to health care and greater economic security for the nation's elderly and disabled populations. It has contributed to improved health and quality of life for millions of vulnerable Americans. Without Medicare, many of the program's chronically ill beneficiaries would quickly exhaust their financial resources.

Yet changes are dictated by the projected insolvency of the Medicare Hospital Insurance (HI) trust fund by 2002, rapid growth in Medicare outlays in an era of federal budget deficits, and the looming retirement of the baby-boom generation. Medicare now faces two problems (brought on in part by its own success): continuing to ensure access to care and financial security for beneficiaries while stemming unsustainable cost growth.

Grappling with the necessary choices will be extraordinarily difficult. Yet a reexamination of Medicare affords an opportunity for creative restructuring of the program to meet the growing health and long-term care needs of an aging population, while being cognizant of competing demands for the nation's health care and budgetary resources. In this paper we argue that it is possible to build on the strengths and current structure of the Medicare program, while at the same time undertaking long-term changes to ensure its fiscal soundness. We offer pragmatic suggestions on how to improve the program while recognizing the substantial fiscal responsibilities ahead.

❖ Strengths of The Medicare Program

Medicare has many strengths that should be retained, including some of the basic principles on which the program was founded.

Universal social insurance. Medicare provides universal health insurance coverage to nearly all persons age sixty-five and over and those who are permanently and totally disabled for two years or more. Because of Medicare, a far higher percentage of the elderly population (98 percent) have insurance coverage than any other population group. By offering a uniform benefit package and ready access to most health care providers, Medicare has achieved its goal of offering mainstream medical care even for the sickest and poorest members of the covered groups. There are, at present, few opportunities to discriminate against individual beneficiaries, thus assuring truly universal coverage.

This universality contributes to the program's low administrative costs—disenrollment occurs primarily because of death. Medicare does not advertise; it does not pay commissions to a sales force; it does not pay profits to shareholders. Yet it uses private entities to perform functions when it can do so economically. It contracts with private insurers to pay claims. Health care services are provided by private hospitals, physicians, and other health care providers. Medicare also offers private health maintenance organizations (HMOs) to beneficiaries, with the requirement that HMOs return any excess profits to beneficiaries in the form of improved benefits.

Medicare's universality has increased public support for the program and has eased the public's anxiety about unpredictable medical expenses in retirement. It has corrected the private market's failure to provide basic health insurance to a high-risk population. Finally, along with Medicaid, Medicare has tilted benefits toward lower-income recipients.

Medicare's risk pools. One of Medicare's strengths is its sharing of risks across a large population group. With thirty-seven million beneficiaries, Medicare is the largest risk group for health insurance in the United States. Effectively, costs for chronically ill eighty-five-year-olds are averaged in with those of healthy seventy-year-olds, making insurance less expensive than it would be if these eighty-five-year-olds were insured in the private market by a company that covered a much smaller number of persons. In addition, once a commitment has been made to treat all beneficiaries alike, the costs associated with underwriting and differentiating risks are forgone.

Medicare's discounts. While Medicare has been criticized for not promoting managed care alternatives for its beneficiaries aggressively enough, the program is itself similar to a preferred provider managed care plan. Medicare sets prospective prices for hospitals and physicians at a substantial "discount" from usual charges. Medicare's physician payments, for example, average 68 percent of the physician fees paid by private health insurance plans.[1] All providers are permitted to enroll, and physicians who agree to take "discounted" payments as payment in full become participating physicians. This has worked remarkably well; 92 percent of all Medicare physician services are now paid on this basis.[2] Even when compared with formal preferred provider organizations (PPOs)—now the fastest-growing type of managed care in the United States—Medicare's payment levels are much lower.[3] Medicare's payments to hospitals also are lower than the fees paid to hospitals by private insurers. Medicare has already achieved the discounts that are just now helping to hold down premiums for private insurers.

❖ Short-Term and Long-Term Problems

Medicare faces two sets of financing problems. The first and more immediate is driven by high health care costs. The second is the demographic problem of a declining ratio of workers to retirees. The second problem will become severe when the baby-boom generation begins to become eligible for Social Security after 2010. Solutions for these two problems are likely to differ, but both need to be part of the debate about Medicare's future.

In the current debate attention has focused on the near-term insolvency of the HI (Part A) trust fund. Part A is financed by a dedicated payroll tax, and its revenues and outflows are tracked by means of the trust fund. The most recent report on the status of this fund indicates exhaustion of its balance by 2002.[4] That is, without any policy changes, the trust fund's balance will drop rapidly from now until 2002. Actuaries have indicated that it will take $147 billion to keep the fund solvent until 2002.

This deficit is an artifact of the nature of Medicare financing. The Supplementary Medical Insurance (SMI) trust fund (Part B) is financed by premiums and general revenue contributions. It does not face insolvency because it has an unlimited draw on the federal treasury. The real issue, however, is not the solvency of the HI trust fund. If it were, its solvency could be assured by measures such as shifting Medicare home health benefits from Part A to Part B, which would make the HI trust fund solvent for nearly five more years; or increasing the payroll tax rate by 0.65 percent on both employers and employees, which would make the HI trust fund solvent for another twenty-five years; or adding general revenues as a source of financing the balance of HI outlays, which would make the trust fund solvent indefinitely as it does for the SMI trust fund.[4] The HI trust fund originally was established to protect the Medicare program and to ensure that its revenues would not go to other government programs. The importance of the HI trust fund deficit today is much like that of the federal debt ceiling: It helps instill fiscal discipline and requires explicit policy choices periodically regarding Medicare spending and revenues needed to support it.

The real issue is the rate of growth of Medicare outlays—Part A and Part B—and the tax resources the nation is willing to commit to support Medicare. Because of Medicare's size, no discussion of balancing the federal budget or changing tax rates is complete without examining whether to devote either more or fewer resources to Medicare. In fact, every year, Medicare has been a major focus of budget reduction efforts. While many of these efforts have focused on reducing payments to providers, some also have affected beneficiaries. As part of the 1994 budget reduction efforts, Medicare was cut by $56 billion over five years.[6]

Medicare faces an even more serious financial crisis in the longer term in relation to the aging of the baby-boom generation and the changes that will occur as a result in the age distribution of the population. There will be fewer contributors to the system and more beneficiaries drawing from the system, making it very expensive to fund the program on a pay-as-you-go basis. At that time, Americans will need to decide how large a Medicare and Social Security program to support. Rational discussions concerning these changes need to begin immediately, although action can be deferred.[7]

❖ Vouchers And Managed Care: Promise And Concerns

In a difficult federal budgetary climate, capping the federal budget obligation for Medicare is an attractive policy option. Two types of proposals are receiving serious consideration: turning Medicare into a voucher program and increasing incentives for beneficiaries to join a wider array of managed care plans. These options represent mechanisms for capping budget outlays, shifting financial risk to individuals or health care providers, and creating incentives for individuals and providers to control costs.

While there are different types of voucher and managed care proposals, vouchers essentially cap the federal budgetary contribution and let beneficiaries choose their own private health insurance or managed care plan. If the premium for the coverage exceeds the amount of the voucher, the beneficiary pays the difference.

Most Medicare managed care proposals differ from vouchers in two important respects: (1) Only managed care plans that meet Medicare standards would qualify (with a fall-back fee-for-service option available directly from Medicare); and (2) Medicare would continue to set or negotiate a capitated payment rate. Managed care plans would not be permitted to charge beneficiaries more than Medicare's payment rate.

Vouchers would provide more choices for beneficiaries but also would shift more financial risk to individuals. Under the managed care proposals, most financial risk would be shifted to managed care plans or health care providers, although beneficiaries might have higher premiums depending on their choice of plan. Therefore, although vouchers and managed care proposals have some similarities—and hybrid proposals can have features of each—the philosophy behind the two approaches and their mechanisms for saving costs are actually quite different.

Vouchers

Advocates of a private-sector approach to financing health care for Medicare enrollees argue for a system of vouchers in which eligible persons would choose their own health care plan from among an array of private options.[8] For example, beneficiaries might be able to opt for higher deductibles or coinsurance in exchange for coverage of services such as prescription drugs or long-term care. In addition, since many Medicare enrollees now supplement Medicare with private insurance, this approach would allow beneficiaries to combine the voucher with their own funds and buy one comprehensive plan. They no longer would have to worry about coordinating coverage between Medicare and their private supplemental plan. Moreover, persons with employer-provided supplemental coverage presumably could remain in the health care plans they had as employees.

Competition among plans to attract enrollees might help to lower prices, but it also seems likely that there would be considerable nonprice competition. As a consequence, the only certain way for Medicare to reduce costs under a voucher scheme would be to fix the payment level and its rate of growth over time (presumably with appropriate adjustments for risk).

To the government, this option offers the appeal of a predictable rate of growth. For example, the federal government could set the vouchers to grow at the same rate as that of gross domestic product (GDP) or some other factor. Most importantly, this option would achieve major cost savings. The "price" of offering choice to enrollees might be a voucher set at 90 or 95 percent of the current level of government spending per enrollee. Furthermore, by capping the rate of the benefit's growth, vouchers shift the risk to the beneficiary if the cost of coverage exceeds the voucher amount.

If a plan is not successful in holding down health care costs and Medicare's contribution is fixed, the most likely response would be to raise enrollees' required supplemental contribution. This would effectively be an indirect premium increase on beneficiaries.[9] Advocates of vouchers argue that consumer opposition to paying higher prices would force insurers to hold down costs and that the potential for higher costs therefore would be a good thing. Opponents claim that both consumers and insurers would lack the clout to achieve such cost controls.

How successful is the private sector likely to be in holding down costs, compared with the current Medicare program? First, private insurers almost surely will have higher administrative overhead costs than Medicare has. Insurers will need to promote their plans. They will face a smaller risk pool that may require them to make more conservative decisions regarding reserves and other protections against losses over time. They will not have the advantage of Medicare's scale and governmental authority in imposing steep provider price discounts. In addition, these plans are expected to return a profit to their shareholders. All of these factors will work against private companies' performing better than Medicare.

On the other hand, private insurers may be able to develop effective new cost containment schemes. They may be able to adapt to changing circumstances more readily than the public sector can, and they would not be subject to political opposition. By combining coverage of services that Medicare now covers with coverage of other medical care such as preventive services, drugs, and long-term care, the private sector may be able to find better ways to package and deliver care. But with Medicare payments already at the low end of the scale, the real challenge will be whether the private sector can truly manage the care that beneficiaries use.

Regulation would be needed to require insurers to take all comers and to guard against adverse selection. The program is most likely to be problematic in this regard if it is voluntary. Also, adverse selection would be more likely if Medicare enrollees were free to supplement their vouchers to enhance their coverage. Insurers may consider persons with the most to spend on certain types of supplemental coverage to be the best risks.

The most serious potential problem with vouchers is that the market would begin to divide beneficiaries in ways that would put the most vulnerable—those in poor health and with modest incomes—at particular risk. If voucher programs or other types of specialized plans such as medical savings accounts (MSAs) skim off the healthier, wealthier beneficiaries, many Medicare enrollees who now have reasonable coverage for acute care costs, but who are the less desirable risks, would face much higher costs. The result could be a two-tier system of care in which families with modest incomes would be forced to choose less desirable plans.

On balance, vouchers offer less in the way of guarantees of continued protection under Medicare. They are most appealing as a way to cut indirectly but substantially the federal government's contributions through erosion of the comprehensiveness of coverage that the private sector offers. The burdens of making the tough choices and assuming the financial risks would be borne by beneficiaries. Further, the federal government's role in influencing the course of our health care system would be substantially diminished. For some, this is a major advantage. But the history of Medicare is one in which the public sector has often played a positive role, first by insuring persons largely rejected by the private sector and then by leading the way in many cost containment efforts.[10] The most troubling aspect of this option is the likelihood that the principle of offering a universal benefit could be seriously undermined.

Managed Care Plans

Rather than creating vouchers that effectively put enrollees at risk, Medicare could move to a system of expanding the types of managed care plans that can participate in Medicare, and providing incentives for beneficiaries to join these plans. Medicare could continue to set standards for plan participation, set or negotiate capitated rates, and share some of the risks. Medicare beneficiaries now may enroll in qualified HMOs, but the more loosely organized PPOs and point-of-service plans are not available under the program.

In a well-managed, high-quality capitated system, patients receive better continuity of care. Patient records and information can readily be shared within the organization, and thus services are better coordinated. Physicians have no incentives to prescribe unnecessary tests or procedures because they add to the cost of care. They do, however, need to perform good diagnostic and preventive services to reduce use of the big-ticket items such as hospitalization.

It is important to look closely at how managed care may hold down the costs of care, particularly in relation to Medicare beneficiaries. The private sector has been seeking ways to hold down health care spending, particularly in comparison with traditional indemnity insurance plans, using essentially four types of tools: (1) lowering administrative costs, in part by streamlining management and minimizing paperwork; (2) paying doctors and other providers lower fees in exchange for promises of high patient volume; (3) directly managing patient care, for example, by setting strict rules on hospital length-of-stay, offering financial incentives and imposing penalties to control the use of tests and referrals to specialists, and requiring that patients use network providers or pay a large copayment if they go outside the system; and (4) marketing products so as to attract good risks—that is, persons who are less likely to be high users of health care services.[11]

Managed care savings for Medicare beneficiaries may not be the same as those for private employees who are moved from generous indemnity plans into managed care, because Medicare already is a relatively low-cost plan. Even more important, advocates of the privatization of Medicare presume that growth rates can be lowered year after year, so we need to consider whether these savings are sustainable over a long period of time.

Administrative savings may prove problematic for Medicare. First, Medicare's administrative costs are low compared with those of most managed care plans. Moreover, if private plans compete for Medicare business, their marketing and advertising costs will be substantial. For-profit HMOs on average have a 14 percent differential between their premiums and medical care outlays, split between profits and administrative costs.[12] Start-up costs for new entrants into this market and even for those adding Medicare patients to existing covered populations may be high as well. For example, who will pay for the reserves necessary to ensure that private plans are on sound financial footing? Adding five or ten million new insured lives in the private market will pose major capitalization needs. New plans thus are not likely to save a lot from administrative advantages compared with the traditional Medicare program, particularly in the early years.

Similarly, many managed care plans can be very attractive to private employers because of the discounts they receive from providers, which can result in lower premiums. Medicare, however, already has obtained discounts in the form of administered prices that are usually well below what private insurers pay, and even below what managed care plans pay.[13] It will be difficult for private plans to drive a harder bargain than Medicare already has. The likely exception is in areas in which there is excess capacity and managed care plans are wringing out that excess capacity by forcing providers to bid against each other at rates well below costs. But some of these deep discounts likely cannot be sustained over time, and it is not clear whether this approach to eliminating excess capacity will result in closing the lowest-quality or least-needed hospitals and physician services.

One area in which managed care may be able to improve upon Medicare is in truly managing patient services. Private plans not only can provide closer oversight, but they also can be more arbitrary and prescriptive than a national public program like Medicare can be. This means that, particularly in some areas such as home health and hospital outpatient services, private plans could control the use of services more effectively than Medicare now does. Although Medicare certainly could do better under its current structure, private plans can exclude problematic providers or restrict their behavior in ways that Medicare is not able to do. However, although Medicare is limited by due process requirements and other legal restrictions, these restraints are not all bad. They help to guarantee access to the system to all patients and providers. Further, private contractors are not likely to be concerned about the impact on society of their behavior, while Medicare should and will be held accountable.

Older and disabled beneficiaries represent a unique patient type, and many managed care firms have not been eager to move into this market. Older patients with multiple health problems may need to see a specialist regularly, for example, when many managed care plans seek to limit such contacts as much as possible. Such cost containment strategies might be less cost-effective for the Medicare population, and thus other arrangements might be needed. It will take time for new entrants into this market to develop the expertise to deal effectively with this population.

Because performance varies widely among managed care plans, consumers must be aggressive advocates for their own care. The barriers to care that HMOs and others establish to discourage overuse may be intimidating, particularly for the very old or frail. It may be easier for HMOs to establish barriers to the use of needed services than to manage care on a case-by-case basis. Further, the restrictions on choice implicit in such a system are viewed negatively by many Medicare beneficiaries.

Finally, health care costs for Medicare beneficiaries are very unevenly distributed. Some elderly persons enjoy good health and rarely use health care services. Others are seriously disabled and require extensive treatment. In 1993, 10 percent of Medicare beneficiaries accounted for 70 percent of outlays, or an average expenditure of $28,120 per person. This is contrasted with $1,340 per person for the 90 percent of Medicare beneficiaries with the lowest outlays.[14] Understanding this variation is particularly important in any discussion of expanding capitated managed care coverage under Medicare. If capitation payments are not appropriately adjusted for health status, over- or underpayments can be quite serious. Plans can make a considerable profit at a capitated rate of $4,000 or even $3,000 if they can avoid enrolling those beneficiaries who are in the most costly 10 percent.

❖ Building On Medicare's Strengths

At present, too little attention is being focused on how to improve the functioning of the basic Medicare program, as opposed to departing radically from its basic structure. The goal should be to preserve genuine choice for all Medicare beneficiaries of type of health care delivery system while guaranteeing high-quality care at a reasonable cost to both beneficiaries and taxpayers. Fee-for-service care has the disadvantage of creating incentives for too much care at too high a cost; capitated managed care has the disadvantage of creating incentives for too little care of substandard quality. Providing a genuine informed choice of both options for beneficiaries may counter the harmful consequences of either one. Even if Medicare moves dramatically toward offering private plans, a fee-for-service component will likely remain for the foreseeable future.

Major issues for improving Medicare include (1) improving Medicare's fee-for-service option; (2) expanding Medicare managed care choices while assuring quality; (3) minimizing the difficulties posed by risk selection; and (4) determining what financial contribution Medicare beneficiaries and taxpayers can reasonably be expected to make.

Improving the fee-for-service option. Medicare's greatest strength as a social insurance program is the efficiency of its fee-for-service option. It has low administrative costs and low provider payment rates. It could be characterized as a PPO that takes any willing provider that meets quality standards. Its hospital prospective payment system (PPS) has built-in incentives for shortening hospital stays and lowering the cost of hospital care. Its system of physician payment promotes primary care and penalizes increased use by pegging future price levels to performance in meeting spending targets. These payment systems have markedly slowed the growth in Medicare hospital and physician outlays since their introduction in 1983 and 1992, respectively. They are a largely unsung success story.

Where the fee-for-service option falls short is the adequacy of its benefit package, the difficulty of coordinating benefits with Medicaid and private supplemental coverage, and its lack of oversight in the use of some services. The first two problems create complexity and confusion among beneficiaries and providers. Consequently, Medicare restructuring options should include the following: (1) a merging of Medicare Part A and Part B to simplify financing and administration; (2) creation of two standardized Medicare benefit packages—the current package with a unified deductible and a ceiling on out-of-pocket costs, and a comprehensive package that covers current services with little or no cost sharing and prescription drugs; (3) beneficiaries who prefer the comprehensive benefit package would pay an additional premium to cover the differential cost; beneficiaries who prefer private supplemental coverage or who have retiree health benefits could select the basic benefit package; others who prefer the simplicity and/or premium of the comprehensive Medicare benefit package could elect it; and

(4) federalization of Medicaid supplemental acute care coverage for Medicare beneficiaries; Medicare cost sharing and premiums for poor and near-poor Medicare beneficiaries would be financed from federal general revenues and administered jointly with Medicare.[15]

Improving Medicare's fee-for-service environment also requires attention to further cost containment activities, particularly its payment and oversight activities. In some cases, Medicare could adopt innovations from the private sector. Changes could include expansion of prospective payment methods to include all Medicare benefits, including consideration of spending targets that link future prices to performance in controlling outlays; use of sophisticated computer techniques for profiling use of services, thus identifying outliers and possible abuse; establishing and applying strict principles for appropriateness of care; and selective contracting of some services, building on the concept of centers of excellence.

Since home health and skilled nursing home services have been the most rapidly growing portion of Medicare, savings could be sought in this area. Prospective payment methods have worked remarkably well for physician and hospital services and should be developed for home health, skilled nursing facility services, outpatient hospital services, clinical laboratory services, and durable medical equipment.

Consider the example of home health services. Costs for such services are reimbursed up to a ceiling, but we do not know, for example, how long each visit lasts, how many separate services are provided at one time, or even how many services patients with various characteristics are receiving. The available data suggest that home health side services provided by proprietary agencies are where much of the explosive growth is occurring. New standards and prospective payment or other reforms in payment policy are needed, and careful assessment of the provision of services through profiling of providers and beneficiaries is in order. It may be necessary to place specific limits on particular types of visits or for particular diagnoses. While a high copayment could be very expensive for the frailest elderly and disabled persons, a nominal payment per visit might be appropriate, at least for home health aide services. In sum, there is much that Medicare can and should do to improve its oversight of home health care services. But this would require considerable new administrative efforts, and perhaps even an increase in administrative costs.[16]

Medicare also could adopt innovations from the private sector, such as high-cost case management, to generate efficiencies in the treatment of very expensive illnesses such as cancer, and perhaps in chronic care; and selective contracting with providers for particular types of services, particularly those for which outcomes improve when large numbers of procedures are provided at one center. Enforcement of appropriateness-of-care standards is now possible with sophisticated computer programs for profiling service use.[17] Many of these techniques could be readily adopted by Medicare with some investment in the necessary tools and training.

Expanding Managed Care Options

Medicare now permits federally qualified HMOs and state-accredited competitive health plans to enter into risk contracts. Plans may make a profit on their Medicare beneficiaries, but only to the extent to which they make a profit on non-Medicare enrollment. Additional savings must be returned to beneficiaries in the form of improved benefits, reduced cost sharing, or reduced premiums.

Currently, 9 percent of Medicare beneficiaries belong to HMOs. Surveys and focus groups indicate that more beneficiaries would be willing to join managed care plans if their current physicians belonged to such plans and if their out-of-pocket costs were lower than they now are under Medicare and any supplemental coverage.[18] As managed care grows in the private market, more physicians will participate in such plans, and more beneficiaries would be able to enroll without changing their current physician arrangements.

Medicare could take several steps to expand its managed care options. It could include PPOs and point-of-service plans that meet quality and fiscal soundness standards and provide either the basic or comprehensive benefit package. It could inform Medicare beneficiaries of all managed care plan options available in their geographic area, provide beneficiaries with information on which to base an informed choice, and have beneficiaries enroll annually in either Medicare's fee-for-service option or a managed care option. Finally, Medicare could allow beneficiaries to receive all or a portion of the savings generated when they enroll in a managed care plan with premiums below those of Medicare's fee-for-service option.

Minimizing Risk Selection

The primary problem with expanding Medicare's managed care options is the potential for risk selection—healthier persons will enroll in managed care plans, while less healthy persons will elect the fee-for-service option. Given the extreme variability in health care spending among Medicare beneficiaries, there is great leeway for plans to select relatively healthier beneficiaries for whom capitated rates exceed true costs. If managed care plans succeed in attracting and retaining relatively healthier Medicare beneficiaries, Medicare will overpay for those who enroll in managed care plans, while continuing to pay the full cost of the sickest Medicare beneficiaries who are unattractive to managed care plans. Medicare HMOs can switch to a fee-for-service method of payment from a capitated risk contract if they experience adverse selection, or they can encourage sicker patients to return to Medicare's fee-for-service system (since Medicare allows monthly disenrollment).

Several approaches may help to minimize adverse risk selection: (1) regulation of marketing, enrollment, and disenrollment practices with Medicare managing the enrollment process and providing standardized information on plan choices; (2) adopting quality standards to ensure that chronically or seriously ill patients get appropriate specialty care; and (3) requiring all managed care plans to enter into risk contracts and requiring health care providers to choose between participation in Medicare managed care plans and participation in the Medicare fee-for-service option.

The most fundamental way to eliminate risk selection is setting capitation rates to reflect the risk of enrolled populations. However, we do not do this well now, and there is as yet no consensus on how to solve this problem. The current method of paying HMOs for Medicare patients is seriously flawed. Thus, even if enrollment were to expand more markedly, it is unlikely that the program would save money. In fact, it might even cost the program money. A recent study found that the actual cost of serving Medicare beneficiaries who enroll in HMOs is 5.7 percent more than Medicare would have paid for these same beneficiaries had they been covered under Medicare's fee-for-service option.[19]

There are several options that might improve the current system: setting a national capitation rate with geographic cost-of-practice adjustment, rather than the current complex procedure of basing capitation rates on fee-for-service costs in a given geographic area; setting the national capitation rate at 90 percent of the fee-for-service rate, rather than 95 percent, based on the extent of risk selection that now seems to be occurring; excluding the allowance for graduate medical education and disproportionate-share payments from managed care capitation rates; limiting the profit on Medicare HMO enrollment to a fixed rate, such as 2 percent, rather than the profit on non-Medicare enrollment that is now allowed; adding health status measures or proxies to the current Medicare capitation formula, using the best techniques available; designing explicit capitation payment rates for selected prevalent chronic conditions; and dividing payments into a basic capitation rate for low-cost patients and a new payment system for high-cost or special-needs patients. For example, once a patient exceeded a cost threshold (such as $5,000 of health care expenses in a given year), the capitation rate would no longer apply; instead, Medicare could place these patients in a separate special-needs plan with case management. Given the uncertainties surrounding these and other options, demonstrations or gradual implementation seems appropriate.

Financing Options

These improvements may not generate substantial savings over the long term. They represent program improvements and should be considered on their merits apart from their savings potential. Yet their extensive uncertainties make them an unreliable foundation on which to ensure the future fiscal soundness of Medicare. Thus, additional financing options need to be discussed.

There are two basic alternatives for financing Medicare benefit payments: direct beneficiary contributions and taxes. Ultimately, this is a public policy choice that the nation must make. There is no one right combination of financial responsibility between beneficiaries and government. Informed debate, however, can be enhanced by a complete identification of options and by careful analysis of their implications.

If beneficiaries are asked to pay more, some options would be more equitable than others. Consider cost-sharing changes. While cost sharing makes theoretical sense as a means for controlling the use of services. In practice it often results in less use of services mainly by low-income families.[20] Higher cost sharing would likely have only an indirect effect on most Medicare beneficiaries because they often have additional supplemental insurance that would insulate them from the direct impact. In addition, Medicare coinsurance and deductibles represent a complicated collection of mismatched requirements, some of which could be increased and some of which should be decreased. For example, the Part A hospital deductible ($716 per spell of illness in 1995) is very high by any standards, while the annual Part B deductible ($100) is quite low. Hospital and skilled nursing coinsurance are also unreasoanbly high. It makes sense to rearrange this cost sharing along more rational lines, with perhaps a small net increase.[21]

Medicare premiums could be increased, and this would be a reasonable way to require higher contributions if special efforts are made to protect low-income beneficiaries. In particular, the qualified Medicare beneficiary (QMB) and the specified low-income Medicare beneficiary (SLIMB) programs should be moved from Medicaid into Medicare.[22] This would likely improve low program participation rates. In addition, the eligibility cutoffs could be raised if premiums go up to ensure that moderate-income families would not be hit too hard. Savings from a premium increase should be more than sufficient to both reduce federal spending and cover the QMB program. This is one of the more promising areas for higher beneficiary contributions.

An income-related portion of a premium increase also could be considered, but there are practical implementation problems that may render this a less desirable initial step.[23] Implicitly, Part A already has an income-related premium via the taxation of Social Security benefits, a portion of which is dedicated to the Part A trust fund. This element could be retained rather than eliminated, as some have suggested.[24] Other ways in which Medicare beneficiaries could be asked to contribute more include the full taxation of Social Security benefits, or forgoing a portion of cost-of-living increases in Social Security benefits.[25]

It seems likely, however, that the fiscal soundness of Medicare can only be guaranteed as the baby-boom generation reaches retirement if the program's tax base is improved. To be dynamically sound, payroll tax revenues need to be supplemented with other sources of revenues that grow with the aging of the population, such as premiums paid by beneficiaries, especially if income related. By merging Parts A and B, a single trust fund could be established to receive payroll taxes, premiums, and general revenue contributions. If the fiscal discipline that the HI trust fund helps to instill is viewed as desirable, general revenues could be limited to a fixed percentage of total revenues or a fixed rate of increase over time.

In the current political climate it is tempting to rule out tax increases, but the United States has among the lowest tax rates of any industrialized society, and opinion polls indicate strong support for preserving Medicare benefits.[26] Some revenue options may make more sense in the context of broader reforms, such as coverage of uninsured persons and long-term care services. A value-added tax, for example, has high administrative costs and makes sense only if substantial revenues are to be generated.

One of the most basic long-term issues that must be considered is the extent to which the costs of retired persons are borne by current workers. By the year 2030 under current projections, there will be two covered workers for every Social Security beneficiary (the current proportion is 3.3 workers to one beneficiary).[27] The cost of Social Security and Medicare per worker could be staggering. The age for Social Security eligibility is gradually being increased to sixty-seven; Medicare could do the same. The difficulty, however, is that those who have retired involuntarily because of limited job opportunities or health reasons can take Social Security at age sixty-two, but at reduced actuarial rates. Medicare now has no such option, and many early retirees become uninsured and are at great risk.[28] If the Medicare retirement age were increased, consideration would need to be given to permitting early retirees to purchase Medicare on a subsidized basis, particularly given the lack of access to individually purchased insurance.

❖ Conclusion

What should be preserved is the essential role that Medicare plays in guaranteeing access to health care services and protecting beneficiaries from the financial hardship that inadequate insurance can generate for our nation's most vulnerable elderly and disabled people. No American should become destitute because of uncovered medical bills, nor should anyone be denied access to essential health care services. Medicare is a model of success. It should not be hastily jettisoned in an ill-conceived and short-sighted effort to obtain federal budgetary savings. Instead, a full array of options needs to be carefully analyzed, critiqued, and debated.

❖ About the Author

Marilyn Moon, Ph.D., is Senior Fellow of the Urban Institute, Washington, D.C.

NOTES

1. Physician Payment Review Commission, *Annual Report to Congress, 1994* (Washington: PPRC, 1995).
2. Ibid.
3. S. Zuckerman and D. Verrilli, "The Medicare Relative Value Scale and Private Payers: The Potential Impact on Physician Payments," Urban Institute Discussion Paper (Washington: The Urban Institute, 1995).
4. Board of Trustees, HI Trust Fund, *Annual Report* (Washington: HITF, 1995).
5. Karen Davis, "Medicare Solvency and Financial Security for Beneficiaries," testimony before the Senate Budget Committee, 3 May 1995; and June E. O'Neill, directors. Congressional Budget Office, "The Financial Status of the Medicare Program," testimony before the House Ways and Means Committee, 2 May 1995.
6. Summary of conference agreement on H. Con. Res. 67, prepared by staff of the Senate Budget Committee, 22 June 1995.
7. Just as the 1983 amendments set into law changes in the age of retirement that do not even begin to take place until 2000, it is important to signal to younger Americans what they can expect from these programs in terms of level of support, age of retirement, and level of tax contributions, for example.
8. S.M. Butler, R.E. Moffit, and J.C. Liu, "What to Do about Medicare," The Heritage Foundation Backgrounder 1038 (26 June 1995); and S.M. Butler and R.E. Moffit, "The FEHBP as a Model for a New Medicare Program," *Health Affairs* (Winter 1995):47–51.
9. M. Moon, "The Special Health Care Needs of the Elderly," in *Strategic Choices for a Changing Health Care System*, ed. S. Altman and U. Reinhardt (Chicago: Baxter, forthcoming).
10. M. Moon, *Medicare Now and in the Future* (Washington: Urban Institute Press, 1993): and K. Davis and D. Rowland, *Medicare Policy: New Directions for Health and Long-Term Care* (Baltimore: The Johns Hopkins University Press, 1986).
11. M. Moon and J. Mulvey. *Endorsements and the Elderly: Protecting Promises, Recognizing Reality* (Washington: Urban Institute Press, forthcoming).
12. Group Health Association of America, *HMO Industry Profile*, 1994 ed. (Washington: GHAA, 1994).
13. Zuckerman and Verrilli, "The Medicare Relative Value Scale and Private Payers."
14. Authors estimates based on data from Health Care Financing Administration, *Medicare: A Profile* (Washington: U.S. Government Printing Office, February 1995).
15. A voluntary long-term care insurance supplement financed by an income-related premium might be another option that could be considered as well. Davis and Rowland, *Medicare Policy*. Although offering two standardized Medicare benefit packages has considerable appeal to allow beneficiaries to opt for just one simple public program, there is the danger that sucker beneficiaries will opt for comprehensive benefits while healthier beneficiaries will select basic coverage. If so, premiums will need to be risk adjusted—encountering the same methodological problems that managed care options create. Some limits on shifting between options might need to be imposed as well. See M. Moon, "Adding a Long Term Option to Medicare," in *A Call for Action, Supplement to the Final Re-*

port, The Pepper Commission (Washington: U.S. GPO, September 1990); D. Rowland and B. Lyons. *Medicare's Poor* (Baltimore: Commonwealth Fund Commission on Elderly People Living Alone, 1987); and Moon and Mulvey, *Endowments and the Elderly.*

16. Internal Medicare will find it difficult to adopt new techniques for improving oversight of administrative budgets are severely cut in the future.

17. J Ratner, *Medicare: Rapid Spending Growth Calls for More Prudent Purchasing.* Pub. no. GAO/T-HEHS-95-191 (Washington: U.S. General Accounting Office, June 1995).

18. Frederick/Schneiders, Inc. "Analyses of Focus Groups concerning Managed Care and Medicare" (Prepared for The Henry J. Kaiser Family Foundation, May 1995).

19. J Hill et al., *The Impact of the Medicare Risk Program on the Use of Services and Costs of Medicare Final Version* (Princeton, NJ: Mathematica Policy Research, 1992).

20. J Newhouse, *Some Interim Results from a Controlled Trial of Cost Sharing in Health Insurance* (Santa Monica, Calif.: The RAND Corporation, 1982).

21. Moon, *Medicare Now and in the Future.*

22. Ibid. These programs are likely to be at considerable risk if Medicaid becomes a block grant or even if states are given more discretion concerning coverage and eligibility.

23. Davis and Rowland. *Medicare Policy.*

24. Marilyn Moon, "Taxation of Social Security Benefits," testimony before the House Ways and Means Committee, 19 January 1995.

25. Moon and Mulvey. *Entitlements and the Elderly.*

26. *Kaiser/Harvard/KRC, National Election Night Survey* (Menlo Park, Calif.: The Henry J. Kaiser Family Foundation, November 1994).

27. *1995 Annual Report of The Board of Trustees of the Federal Old-Age and Survivors Insurance and Disability Insurance Trust Funds* (3 April 1995).

28. Karen Davis, "Uninsured Older Adults: The Need for a Medicare Buy-In Option," testimony before the House Ways and Means Subcommittee on Health, 12 June 1990, and Marilyn Moon, "Expanding Medicare Coverage to the Near-Elderly," testimony before the House Ways and Means Subcommittee on Health, 19 March 1991.

❖ Medicaid and Long-Term Care

THE KAISER COMMISSION
ON THE FUTURE OF MEDICAID

Medicaid is the nation's primary insurer for long-term care services. Medicaid covers about 1 million of the 1.5 million people in nursing homes and provides more than half of nursing homes' total revenues. Medicaid devotes 35% of total program spending for long-term care (in institutions and in the community), on behalf of about 8% of the program's beneficiaries.

❖ Medicaid's Role

Medicaid Coverage for Long-Term Care

- ❖ More than one-third (35%) of Medicaid spending goes to long-term care.
- ❖ Of the $44.2 billion Medicaid spent on long-term care in 1993, more than half (59%) was for care in nursing facilities, 21% was for care in intermediate care facilities for the mentally retarded (ICFs/MR), 15% was for home- and community-based care, and 5% was for mental health services.
- ❖ The elderly account for 58% of Medicaid's spending on long-term care. The remaining 42% goes to the blind and disabled, slightly more than half of which is for persons with mental retardation and developmental disabilities residing in ICFs/MR.
- ❖ Medicaid spending accounted for 52% of total national health spending on nursing homes and 13% of total spending on home care.
- ❖ Federal Medicaid law specifies the kinds of services that states must or may cover:
  - • Institutions. Medicaid requires states to cover nursing facility care to individuals ages 21 or over. States have the option to cover nursing facility care to individuals under age 21 and ICFs/MR. Virtually every state covers ICFs/MR, serving 140,000 people during 1995. Medicaid does not pay for care in mental institutions for persons between 21 and 65 years old, and does not pay for room and board in residential facilities (board and care homes or assisted-living facilities) that may provide long-term care services.
  - • Home- and community-based care. Medicaid requires states to cover home health services for any individual eligible for nursing home

care. States have the option (used by 29 states) to cover personal care. Under waivers subject to approval by the Secretary of Health and Human Services, all states have developed programs designed to target a specific mix of home- and community-based services (often including personal care) to distinct population groups or limited geographic areas.

Qualifying for Medicaid Long-Term Care

❖ As for other Medicaid services, people are entitled to Medicaid long-term care services if they fall into Medicaid's covered population categories and

- satisfy asset and income requirements, or
- become medically needy by "spending down" to these levels.

❖ In general, people who qualify for SSI as aged, blind, or disabled; have incomes at or below the SSI benefit level (in 1995, $5640 for an individual, $8460 for a couple); and have assets below approximately $2000 (approximately $3000 for couples) are automatically entitled to Medicaid benefits.

❖ Children qualify for Medicaid based on their own (rather than their parents') income and resources if they remain in institutions for longer than one month. States may apply the same eligibility rules to children with disabilities living at home for children who would be eligible if they resided in an institution (as long as the home care costs do not exceed what Medicaid would have paid had the child been institutionalized).

❖ Many nursing home residents receiving Medicaid are not poor until they need nursing home care. In 36 states, people whose assets are less than a specified level (in general, $2000) can qualify for Medicaid as medically needy if the cost of nursing home care exceeds their incomes (that is, if they "spend down" their incomes). States may also cover nursing home residents using a special income standard—up to 300% of the SSI benefit. In the 15 states that use only this standard, however, people whose incomes are too high to qualify but too low to pay nursing home costs are not eligible for Medicaid.

❖ Estimates are that 10% to 23% of persons entering nursing homes as private-pay patients "spend down" their assets to become Medicaid patients. Concern has been expressed that, despite prohibitions, elderly people are transferring assets to avoid spending down. However, the asset levels of elderly people likely to need nursing home care are typically low to begin with and recent legislation (OBRA 1993) has made the transfer of assets to become Medicaid-eligible more difficult.

Financial Responsibilities of Nursing Home Residents

❖ People receiving Medicaid in nursing homes must contribute all their income to the cost of care, retaining only a modest monthly allowance for personal needs. The minimum allowance is $30 per month; the average for all states is $45 per month.

❖ Since 1989, Medicaid has protected spouses of nursing home residents from exhaustion of assets and income in paying for nursing home care. Because most nursing home residents are not married, only about 176,000 people (11% of Medicaid nursing home users) receive these protections during the year.

❖ Spousal protections do not include Medicaid coverage for the spouse at home; rather, they assure that the spouse of a nursing home resident retains sufficient resources on which to live. In addition to the house itself, the spouse at home may retain half the couple's assets, subject to a minimum of about $15,000 and a maximum of about $75,000 (depending upon the state). Spouses at home may also retain up to $1870 per month to cover housing and other costs of maintaining a home.

Paying for Nursing Home Care

❖ States determine the rates they pay for nursing home care, subject to federal rules. Most important, the Boren Amendment requires that states' payments to nursing homes be "reasonable and adequate to meet the cost incurred by efficiently and economically operated facilities." The nursing home industry has used this amendment in court successfully to challenge state efforts to limit nursing home payments.

❖ Nursing home reforms enacted in OBRA 1987 included requirements that the rates states pay nursing facilities take into account the costs of compliance with quality standards.

❖ Under Medicaid law, nursing homes cannot charge residents or the adult children of residents amounts in excess of the Medicaid payment rates.

Quality of Long-Term Care

❖ By law and regulation, Medicaid establishes quality standards for participating providers.

❖ In OBRA 1987, the Congress adopted comprehensive nursing home reforms regarding quality of care, to be effective as of October 1990. Standards that nursing homes must meet to participate in Medicaid address such areas as the scope of services provided, levels and qualifications of staff, residents' rights, and nursing homes' physical environment. Assurance of compliance with standards involves an assessment of care residents have actually received. Regulations to enforce compliance are now being implemented.

❖ Research comparing post-OBRA 1993 to pre-OBRA 1990 nursing home care found reductions of 50% in dehydration among residents, 31% in hospitalization rates, 29% in the use of indwelling urinary catheters, and 25% in the use of physical restraints. In addition, the research found increases of 37% in the use of behavior management programs, 30% in the use of hearing aids, and 12% in the use of antidepressants and psychological therapy for residents with symptoms of depression.

❖ Policy Issues

Legislative changes in the Medicaid program have been proposed that affect both the federal dollars available to finance services and the federal requirements for the operation of state programs. These changes would have significant consequences for access, cost, and quality of long-term care for people in need of service.

❖ Spending constraints. Proposals under discussion would establish limits on the growth of federal support for state expenditures for medical assistance, including long-term care. The impact of spending limits depends on how restrictive they are relative to growth in the numbers of people needing service and growth in the cost of services per beneficiary. Limits also affect how much states invest to draw down or match federal dollars.

Proposals differ in the kinds of limits they would impose. A *block grant* limits federal dollars provided to states, without regard to growth in either factor. A *per capita cap* limits growth in federal dollars per person served, allowing expenditures to rise with increases in eligibility. Under either approach, the tighter the limit, the more limited the resources available to provide protection for long-term care. Different states would be differentially affected, depending upon the current status of their long-term care programs.

❖ Entitlements to defined benefits vs. block grant flexibility. Current Medicaid law entitles people who satisfy eligibility criteria to a defined set of benefits, including long-term care services. A block grant approach would repeal the Medicaid statute and eliminate the entitlement. Decisions as to whom would be covered for which services would be left to the states. Resource constraints could require states to make difficult choices among different populations in need of long-term care.

❖ Flexibility in delivery and payment. Either as modifications to current Medicaid law or as matters of state discretion under block grants, legislative action could change many policies toward the delivery of and payment for long-term care.

• Covered services. States could gain greater flexibility to use federal funds to finance services outside the nursing home, including home- and community-based services (for which waivers are now required) and residential care facilities or state mental institutions (now financed with state funds). However, resource constraints could mean more limited access to some types of services now covered.

- Patient and family responsibility. Nursing homes might be newly allowed to charge residents amounts above program payments (including lump sum payments as a condition of admission or continued stay); or to seek extra payments from a nursing home resident's family.

- Provider payment. Boren amendment requirements on state payments to nursing homes might be repealed, likely reducing rates paid for publicly financed patients. This change could affect these patients' access to care. Access problems become more likely if, in addition, prohibitions on financial screening and other discriminatory practices affecting prospective nursing home residents are also repealed.

- Quality standards. Federal nursing home standards, along with standards for other providers, like ICFs/MR and home health agencies, could be eliminated. Short of elimination, nursing home standards could be modified to reduce each resident's guarantee to services and other protections and to shift primary responsibility for standards enforcement from the federal government to the states. Lower payment rates may also have an impact on quality of care.

- Managed care. States would have greater flexibility to rely on capitation and managed care for long-term care along with other Medicaid services. In addition, states might be granted authority to manage Medicare funds on behalf of dual eligibles or to channel medical and long-term care assistance through private health plans receiving Medicare capitation payments. To date, long-term care has not generally been included in Medicaid managed care. Only Arizona includes comprehensive long-term care services, including nursing home care, in a statewide program.

❖ Summary

As the nation's chief source of financing for long-term care services, Medicaid plays a vital role in the lives of those in need of care in nursing homes, intermediate-care facilities for the mentally retarded, and home- and community-based settings. Recent legislative efforts to limit federal Medicaid spending and reduce federal requirements on state programs have significant implications for people who rely on Medicaid for long-term care services. Substantial financial constraints, coupled with increased state flexibility in delivering and paying for care, could affect access to and quality of long-term care services. In the future, states are likely to face serious challenges and difficult choices in balancing the needs of the multiple groups that rely on Medicaid for health and long-term care.

❖ About the Author

The Kaiser Commission on the Future of Medicaid, Washington, DC, is headed by Diane Rowland, Sc.D., Chair Senior Vice President, The Kaiser Family Foundation, and Executive Director, The Kaiser Commission on the Future of Medicaid.

REFERENCES

American Health Care Association. *Facts and Trends: The Nursing Facility Source Book* (Washington, D.C.: American Health Care Association, 1994).

Congressional Research Service. *Medicaid Source Book: Background Data and Analysis* (Washington, D.C.: Congressional Research Service, January 1993).

Hawes, Catherine. Memorandum to Mary Harahan, Deputy to the Assistant Secretary for Disability, Aging, and Long-Term Care Policy, U.S. Department of Health and Human Services, on the preliminary results of a study on the use of restraints in nursing homes. Durham, North Carolina: Research Triangle Institute (September 26, 1995).

The Kaiser Commission on the Future of Medicaid. *Medicaid and the Elderly* Policy Brief (Washington, D.C.: The Kaiser Commission on the Future of Medicaid, September 1995).

The Kaiser Commission on the Future of Medicaid. *Medicaid Expenditures and Beneficiaries: National and State Profiles and Trends, 1984–1993* (Washington, D.C.: The Kaiser Commission on the Future of Medicaid, July 1995).

❖ Medicaid 1115 Demonstrations: Progress Through Partnership

BRUCE C. VLADECK

States often have been leaders and innovators in many aspects of public policy. The paper by John Holahan and colleagues in this volume of *Health Affairs* highlights a continued interest by researchers and policymakers in one particularly notable arena of state innovation: recent state reforms in the delivery of health care services.

The federal government also provides leadership by supporting programs that test innovations in health care delivery and financing. The Medicaid program is a prime example of this federal strategy of demonstration and testing. The joint federal/state program that provides health care to the poor, disabled, and chronically ill, Medicaid today serves nearly thirty-four million people and spent an estimated $146 billion in fiscal year 1994.

State and federal interests in restructuring Medicaid programs have converged at a time when the health care reform debate continues but consensus remains elusive. Medicaid, built on a foundation of shared federal/state responsibility and financing, is both an optimal and a logical area for reform and demonstration. The very structure of Medicaid—in which individual states have considerable discretion, within broad federal parameters, over whom they will cover, what services they will cover, and how they will pay for those services—has always encouraged substantial variation and "natural" experimentation across the states. More formal Medicaid experimentation also has been part of the program, although in the past it has been constrained by administrations fearful that demonstrations of new services would lead to demands for new public expenditures.

❖ A Key To Innovation

The failure of Congress to enact comprehensive health care reform legislation has meant that the lion's share of work in the area of overall delivery system reform is now being undertaken as Medicaid demonstration programs. The most important of these programs, the so-called 1115 waivers, are authorized under Section 1115 of the Social Security Act.[1]

The general 1115 research and demonstration authority, enacted in 1962, actually predates the Medicaid program. Section 1115 allows the secretary of health and human services to waive, in the context of projects that test innovative methods of achieving program goals, certain regular requirements of Social Security Act programs, such as Aid to Families with Dependent Children (AFDC) and Medicaid. In the Medicaid program, 1115 demonstration authority allows states to demonstrate, within certain parameters, a variety of innovative concepts in health care financing and delivery. The projects "waive" applicable federal regulations covering such factors as statewideness; the amount, duration, and scope of services covered; eligibility definitions; and reimbursement methodologies.

The Health Care Financing Administration (HCFA) both solicits Medicaid demonstrations to test specific concepts and reviews proposals submitted by states on their own initiative. In either case, proposals are reviewed to assure innovation, feasibility, and conformity to federal laws and requirements. The review process emphasizes assuring budget-neutral financing and positive results for beneficiaries. HCFA staff also provide a range of technical assistance to help states apply successfully.

Through 1115 demonstrations, state Medicaid agencies can implement changes in their programs related to coverage, eligibility requirements, payment methods, and benefit packages for a limited time to see if the changes will achieve certain objectives. The 1115 authority is broad: It allows tests in limited geographic areas of a state or in an entire state; among defined groups of beneficiaries or for all beneficiaries; and including only a few specified services or entire systems of care. The demonstrations permit states to experiment with their current Medicaid programs when changes appear to improve the program in some way and when the results might benefit other state programs.[2]

Since Medicaid began in 1965, some eighty 1115 demonstration waivers have been granted. More than thirty have been approved since 1993, and fifteen were pending as of February 1995. Approvals include eight welfare reform 1115 demonstration waivers approved during the Clinton administration. These totals represent more waivers than were approved under the two previous administrations combined.

❖ The Past Is Prologue

Many components of today's health care financing and delivery systems have their roots in 1115 demonstration projects. Over the past several decades nearly two-thirds of the states have taken advantage of 1115 demonstration authority, and a number of these projects broke new ground. Although it is beyond the scope of this Perspective to detail all 1115-generated innovations, the following examples highlight some of their contributions that have had lasting value.

Past Demonstrations

(1) Georgia, South Carolina, New York, Connecticut, and other states tested ways of providing home or community-based services two decades ago, when nursing home care was the only alternative for most dependent frail and chronically ill patients. Their findings resulted in the

enactment of the Medicaid home and community-based program waivers that have been used by all states.

(2) Some early demonstrations focused on facilitating implementation of the Early and Periodic Screening, Diagnosis, and Treatment (EPSDT) program. Many of these projects tested ways of improving access to care for young children that are now standard practice in many areas. In the early 1970s, for example, 1115 demonstration waivers permitted EPSDT services to be provided in schools and day care centers. School-based projects were particularly effective in achieving high participation rates, and many states have expanded Medicaid funding in school settings.

(3) Managed care for Medicaid populations is a common theme in most health care reform proposals. The majority of 1115 demonstration proposals submitted during the past two years have embraced the use of managed care arrangements. The seeds for today's efforts were sown two decades ago in 1115 demonstrations to test the effectiveness of alternative delivery systems and to develop techniques for monitoring and controlling care delivered in managed care settings. Later, demonstrations in the early 1980s focused on developing large systems of competitive managed care plans for Medicaid beneficiaries. One of the oldest and best known of these demonstrations took place in Arizona, which sponsored the first statewide Medicaid managed care program in 1982.

Current 1115 demonstrations continue to build upon the themes of earlier demonstrations. Several widely discussed 1115 demonstrations created Medicaid managed care programs to expand access to care for poor and uninsured persons in Oregon, Ohio, Tennessee, and other states. But not all current Medicaid demonstrations deal with managed care for the traditional Medicaid AFDC populations. Several address ways of expanding access and coverage to targeted populations, such as the disabled.

Current Demonstrations

(1) Ohio recently received approval to implement a managed care program that includes acute care, mental health services, and capitation of drug and alcohol treatment. The demonstration also is expected to extend coverage to an estimated 400,000 Ohioans living below the poverty line. (2) Postpartum family planning and preventive reproductive services will be made available for five years to a specific group of pregnant women in Maryland and South Carolina, who otherwise would lose eligibility after delivery. (3) Oregon anticipates that savings generated by expanding the use of managed care and using a "priority" list to determine covered conditions and treatments will finance the coverage of an additional 120,000 previously uninsured residents. (4) Several ongoing projects improve access for specified populations, including pregnant substance abusers and disabled persons. New York, South Carolina, and Oregon, for example, are developing programs to improve access to care for pregnant substance abusers.

❖ Future Directions

We have learned many lessons in our three-decade partnership with states. The key outcome is that we have developed better ways to deliver and finance care. We have expanded access to care and have developed innovative methods to deliver health services to millions of poor, disabled, and previously uninsured Americans. The conventional wisdom has been that Medicaid is not a vehicle for change or innovation, but it can be and has been. The process has been accelerated, and the credit for this change and for our accomplishments must be shared by the states and the federal government. Future efforts must build on the foundations of innovation and partnership that have been developed between governors and Washington. Some of the necessary links from the past to the future are described below.

Avoid Homogenized Health Policy

Future health policy must continue to strive toward carefully balancing the need to treat states similarly and equitably and the need to consider their individual needs and circumstances. The cookie-cutter approach to national health policy will not work. One size and one shape simply do not fit all, and we must be flexible in our approach.

Not all 1115 demonstrations are statewide reforms, but all of them are customized to build on the diversity inherent in each state and each Medicaid program. In some sense, it is inaccurate to speak of the Medicaid program as one program. The differences are so significant among states that there are really more than fifty Medicaid programs, counting the territories and the District of Columbia.

Continue to Streamline the Process

A major lesson emerging from our long-standing partnership with states is how we can all work together to reduce the administrative burden associated with demonstration waivers. Through collaborative efforts, 1115 demonstrations have on average been processed more than 50 percent faster than similar waivers have in the past. This in itself has been quite an undertaking, since these proposals are far-reaching and complex.

Consumer and Provider Views

We must make sure that the views of consumers and providers are sought and considered when states undertake major changes in Medicaid. This does not presume that all program beneficiaries and providers can or should be happy with a proposed change—it is human nature to question change and cling to the status quo. But the process for designing and implementing change should be open and available for all to review.

Recently promulgated requirements for states to provide public notice and solicit public comment before they submit a proposal to HCFA for review should greatly facilitate such public input.

Facts and Finances

Long-standing and appropriate federal policy dictates that 1115 demonstrations not cost more than what would have been spent under the traditional Medicaid program. Despite the potential limitations the fiduciary obligations pose, the states and HCFA have developed innovative ways to significantly expand access to care and service delivery. For example, the recent 1115 statewide expansions in Oregon, Ohio, Hawaii, Tennessee, Rhode Island, Kentucky, and South Carolina will make health care available to more than a million previously uninsured persons. These demonstrations were approved within the past two years, and evaluation contracts were recently awarded to determine how the projects are implemented. Increased access to care and innovation can be accomplished without breaking federal and state budgets or bankrupting providers. We have been able to cover new populations in new ways while reducing aggregate Medicaid spending.

Foster Innovation

The 1115 demonstrations were created because often good ideas must be tested to determine their real-world effects. That is our approach in the Medicaid program. We will try to develop synergies among demonstrations and share the results with the health care community. We are developing a guide to help states prepare their proposals and speed up the process. And we are publishing a monthly status report on 1115 demonstrations in the *Federal Register* to share information with the health care community about innovative ideas that have been approved.

Leadership and Vision

In health care, as in all areas, we must envision a bigger picture of where we are going and what must be done. Our past can be a guide to the future. Medicaid has evolved from a program primarily serving women on welfare to a complex system covering a range of health issues and populations: women, children, the chronically disabled, and elderly persons in nursing homes. That evolution resulted from vision and leadership: identifying unmet needs and having the courage to address them. That evolution also resulted from new thinking. As Albert Einstein observed, "The significant problems we face cannot be solved at the same level of thinking we were at when we created them."

Vision and leadership also mean taking risks. The future cannot rest on the status quo. We must continue to anticipate threats and opportunities, initiate change, and become learning organizations. Investments in people and technology must continue to improve service to beneficiaries and program performance. We need to recognize mistakes and be flexible enough to change strategies when necessary.

HCFA's vision for the future is to provide equal access to the best health care. This cannot be done alone. It will require a continued partnership with states and others to make the vision a reality.

❖ Conclusion

Finding solutions to the complexities of tomorrow's health care system and our nation's health care needs will require even more innovation and collaboration with the states. This relationship has been extremely fruitful, and the list of accomplishments is long. It includes improving quality; expanding access to the uninsured and new populations with special needs; upgrading the efficiency and effectiveness of our programs; and reducing aggregate Medicaid spending levels. The 1115 demonstrations have provided the flexibility to experiment with change. Results have been used to make key policy decisions concerning Medicaid and welfare reforms.

As we approach the thirtieth anniversary of Medicaid, it is appropriate to renew our commitment to communication, collaboration, and experimentation with the states. It is a productive partnership on which to build for the twenty-first century.

❖ About the Author

Bruce Vladeck is administrator of the Health Care Financing Administration.

NOTES

1. Medicaid also grants "program" waivers for home and community-based care and managed care under Section 1915 of the Social Security Act. These waivers are not discussed in this Perspective.
2. The 1115 waiver authority also extends to demonstrations for welfare reform. There are two kinds: demonstrations requiring only Medicaid waivers, which are administered by HCFA, and demonstrations requiring Title XIX (Medicaid) and Title IV-A (welfare) waivers.

❖ Academic Medical Centers Under Siege

JEROME P. KASSIRER

The future viability of academic medical centers is threatened. These institutions have flourished since the 1960s, even managing to survive the shift toward prospective payment over the past decade, but many are now in danger of becoming seriously compromised. In battles for the rapidly expanding number of managed-care patients, and in vigorous competition with nonacademic hospitals, teaching hospitals and their faculty-practice plans are being forced to negotiate bargain-basement rates of payment. In fact, they are often forced to price services below cost. In response to these pressures, many have reduced the number of faculty members and other personnel.[1] At present, only a dozen or so academic medical centers are losing money,[2] but if many of them are unable to maintain their financial well-being in the next several years under accelerated pressures to reduce costs, the consequences to the future of medicine in this country could be grave.

The impending threat to academic medical centers is part of the fallout of the past year's national debate on health care reform. Most of us expected that Congress would approve some kind of legislation favoring managed care and large integrated systems of care, but partisan squabbling and pressure from lobbyists eroded our legislators' resolve. Even without governmental intervention, however, managed-care plans have proliferated and more and more employers have forced employees into them. At a frenzied pace, both managed-care organizations and hospitals are acquiring ambulatory facilities, physicians' practices, nursing homes, and rehabilitation facilities in an attempt to be part of an integrated "system" of care. Physicians, faced with the loss of a growing number of patients to managed care, are more or less reluctantly joining open-panel and staff-model health maintenance organizations.

Although academic medical centers are now competing with managed-care plans, their missions are quite different. Managed-care organizations, particularly those owned by investors, are required only to apply existing knowledge to routine patient care. Academic medical centers, on the other hand, also create new knowledge, develop and assess new technologies, evaluate new drugs, educate medical students, train tomorrow's physicians, and care for the sickest patients. The costs of these programs, as well as other factors (for example, local economic and demographic variables), make academic medical centers some 30 to 40 percent more expensive than nonacademic hospitals.[3]

Managed-care companies, for-profit or not, are particularly concerned to minimize their expenses. They often try to attract a relatively healthy population of patients, and they tightly regulate the number and specialties of their physicians and the cost of the care they deliver. As a result of these efforts, their premiums are lower than those of traditional indemnity insurance. Because academic medical centers, given their broad responsibilities, cannot compete with nonacademic institutions in price, they are used as little as possible by managed-care organizations. In consequence, many academic institutions are overbedded, underused, and in turmoil.

In my view, we must support the special functions of the academic medical centers. Their educational and research products are our investment in the future. Under most of the health care bills that were introduced in Congress over the past year, supplementary funds derived from a tax on all health insurance premiums were to be set aside to sustain academic medical centers in the future. Nonetheless, as Iglehart points out elsewhere,[4] many argued that the amount was insufficient, and at present it is not clear what the level of support will be in the next year or two. Because the academic medical centers benefit all of us (and in particular managed-care organizations, which use their educational and research products directly), their added expense should be borne broadly. Insurance companies should not be allowed to reap the benefits of the academic centers without paying the price. Unless they make a substantial voluntary commitment to support these essential medical center programs, a premium tax on the insurance companies is probably an appropriate funding mechanism.

In return for such support, however, there must be a substantial quid pro quo. The academic medical centers should not be permitted to use educational goals as an excuse not to deal with inefficiencies and excessive costs. They will have to upgrade their clinical and financial information systems and control their processes of care far more tightly. They will have to minimize the cost of their most complex and specialized care without sacrificing quality. Many will have to trim their faculties and staffs even further and refrain from unnecessary expansion. In addition, they must no longer blind themselves to the kind of training most needed by physicians employed by managed-care organizations. They must train more primary care physicians and fewer specialists, and they must be more alert to the training that best suits a primary care physician. More attention to how to use diagnostic tests appropriately, more focus on cost-conscious decision making, more training of generalist physicians in "specialty" medicine, and more investigation of the outcomes of physicians' therapeutic recommendations might go a long way toward an accommodation with managed care. As shown by Rogers et al.[3] as well as by Iglehart's analysis,[4] many academic medical centers have already made progress in adjusting to the new environment. But all of them must do more: their survival is likely to depend on it.

There are cogent reasons to expect that managed-care organizations, particularly those owned by investors, can well afford to help support academic medical centers. As massive changes are made to the delivery system under managed care, money is being shifted around without a major effect on the overall cost of our health care system. Whereas we once spent more money than necessary on testing, treatment, and administrative services, we are now replacing these inessential expenses with others, including millions of dollars for marketing, vastly inflated salaries of managed-care executives, and payments to insurance company stockholders.[5,7] Imagine what could be done if there was no such waste.

Our academic medical centers are the envy of the world. But new, powerful market forces that divert money away from direct patient care into business profits impern their critical missions. We must not let these unintended consequences of our inconclusive national debate on health care devitalize institutions that we have nurtured for decades.

❖ About the Author

Jerome P. Kassirer, M.D., is the Editor of the *New England Journal of Medicine*.

REFERENCES

1. Critical data about academic health centers: survey report. Washington, D.C.: Association of Academic Health Centers, 1994.
2. Council of Teaching Hospitals' Survey of Hospitals' Financial and General Operating Data. 1988–1993. Washington, D.C.: Council of Teaching Hospitals, 1994.
3. Dobson A, Coleman K, Mechanic R. Analysis of teaching hospital costs. Fairfax, Va.: Lewin-VHI, 1994.
4. Iglehart J. Rapid changes for academic medical centers. N Engl J Med 1994;331:1391-5.
5. Rogers MC, Snyderman R, Rogers EL. Cultural and organizational implications of academic managed care networks. N Engl J Med 1994; 331:1374-7.
6. Winslow R. HMO juggernaut: U.S. Healthcare cuts costs, grows rapidly and irks some doctors. Wall Street Journal. September 6, 1994T, A9.
7. Blumenstein R. The pitch for patients: once considered taboo, hospitals are now aggressively using ads to compete. Newsday. April 18, 1994:C1.

❖ Chapter 9
Managed Care, Mergers, and the Role of Corporations

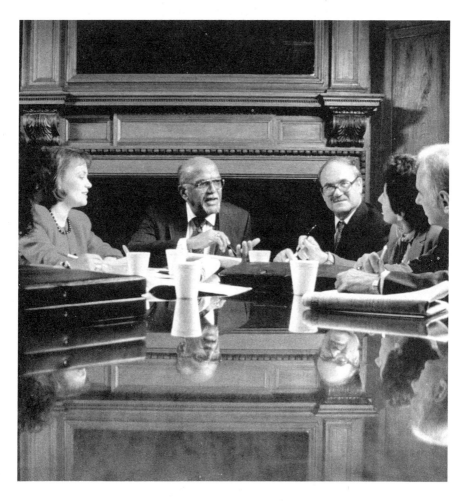

The rapid restructuring of health care in the 1980s and its acceleration in the 1990s may be attributed to the increasing pressures for cost containment from both industry and government, the growing awareness of the large number of uninsured Americans (approaching 16-20 percent of the population), the inability of more and more middle class workers to change jobs without adverse health insurance consequences, growing coverage problems for consumers with pre-existing conditions, a looming federal deficit, and the absence of national health insurance, among other difficulties. The failure of the Clinton health reform plan in 1994 set off a new round of reform, this time by the private insurance market. Managed care has revolutionized the financing, structure, and delivery of medical care and with it, there has been another wave of mergers, consolidation, and concentration in the health insurance market as the for-profit industry has gained a larger and larger market share of power and wealth.

Alain C. Enthoven and Richard Kronick make an important contribution to the dialogue with their article, "Universal Health Insurance through Incentives Reform." Dr. Enthoven, a founder of the principles encompassed in the managed competition model, continues to be a key theorist in the health care reform debate. In this analysis, included in chapter 9, Enthoven and Kronick propose "comprehensive reform of the economic incentives that drive the system." They include a diagnosis of the paradox of excess (health care spending) and deprivation (lack of insurance coverage) as well as a clear and detailed discussion of the basic principles embraced by managed competition and how this model addresses economic incentives.

Enduring issues of cost and quality have new import under managed care as the HMO enrollment of Americans climbs. In this chapter, Harold Luft offers a set of proposals, adapted from the automobile industry including patient satisfaction and safety ratings, to address these cost and quality concerns. John Rother explores consumer protection issues outlining three generations of approaches focused on: (1) individual treatment decisions; (2) insurance related practices of HMOs (e.g., marketing and risk selection); and (3) health plan performance aimed at the financial arrangements and incentives driving HMO behavior. The third generation approach is essential, Rother suggests, including the examination of physician financial incentives, appropriate utilization, and regulation.

The transformation of health care from a merit good to a market good and the growing strength of commercial investor interests in the medical market are described in this chapter by Allan W. Immershein and Carroll L. Estes as a commodity transformation that presently is expressed through increasingly rationalized and profitable product lines. A major byproduct of these changes is a shift both in tax status and institutional "logic" of health care entities from nonprofit (democratic culture based on principles of serving human needs) to proprietary entities (with practices based on principles of profit and growth), raising an old set of questions about the role of the state, charity care, and access to health care.

Several additional recommended articles could not be included in this chapter due to space limitations. James C. Robinson (1996) explores "The Dynamics and Limits of Corporate Growth in Health Care" asking whether bigger is better in terms of efficiency, consumer interests, innovation, competition, and potential anti-trust violations.

Patrick Bond and Robert Weissman (1997, forthcoming) show that "the costs of mergers and acquisitions" in the health industry raise profound questions of oligopoly pricing and political power across-the-board in which there is little role for patients in making the critical choices concerning their care in an article included in chapter 9.

In the area of mental health and managed care, Boyle and Callahan (1996) address the ethical issues concerning managed care in mental health contrasting them with those of the fee-for-service (FFS) system. Chief among the debatable issues are the roles of these two types of delivery systems in expanding or limiting access to, and in addressing the use/misuse and rising costs of mental health services. Additional concerns are about quality and adverse effects on the provider-patient relationship in mental health service delivery. Responding to Boyle's and Callahan's presentation, Schlesinger (1996) raises a compelling ethical question related to "the ends toward which the health care system being managed ought to be directed," contending there is neither a balanced assessment nor adequate evidence to support Boyle and Callahan's positive conclusions about managed care in mental health since "morally relevant differences in the outcomes associated with managed care" are insufficiently treated. Surles (1996) raises the level of analysis to deal with the *interface* of organizations managing care and consumers and patients in behavioral health programs, the under-funding and state variations in mental health services, and erosions in the larger health care system affecting the economically and socially disadvantaged.

While the recent literature, as reflected in this chapter, resounds the growing concerns about managed care, the limits it places on consumer choice, the high profits for proprietary health plans, growing provider dissatisfaction, and ethical issues, there is also a significant potential for managed care to place a greater emphasis on population health than is true in fee-for-service plans and to control costs while improving quality. Although these potential benefits of managed care are yet to be realized, they must be carefully considered in the current spate of legislation, particularly at the state level, to turn back to indemnity insurance and fee-for-service medicine.

❖ Universal Health Insurance through Incentives Reform

ALAIN C. ENTHOVEN AND RICHARD KRONICK

❖ The Paradox of Excess and Deprivation

American national health expenditures are now about 13% of the gross national product, up from 9.1% in 1980, and they are projected to reach 15% by 2000, far more than in any other country. These expenditures are straining public finances at all levels of government. At the same time, roughly 35 million Americans have no health care coverage at all, public or private, and the number appears to be rising. Millions more have inadequate insurance that leaves them vulnerable to large expenses, that excludes care of preexisting conditions, or that may be lost if they become seriously ill. The American health care financing and delivery system is becoming increasingly unsatisfactory and cannot be sustained. Comprehensive reform is urgently needed.

❖ Diagnosis

The etiology of this worsening paradox is extremely complex; many factors enter in. Some factors we would not change if we could (e.g., advancing medical technology, people living longer). We emphasize factors that are important and correctable.

First, our health care financing and delivery system contains more incentives to spend than to not spend. It is based on *cost-unconscious demand.* Key decision makers have little or no incentive to seek value for money in health care purchases. The dominant open-ended fee-for-service (FFS) system pays providers more for doing more, whether or not more is appropriate.

Contrary to a widespread impression, America has not yet tried *competition* of alternative health care financing and delivery plans, using the term in the normal economic sense; i.e., *price* competition to serve cost-conscious purchasers. When there is price competition, the purchaser who chooses the more expensive product pays the full difference in price and is thus motivated to seek value for money. However, in offering health care coverage to employees, most employers provide a larger subsidy to the FFS system than to health maintenance organizations (HMOs) thereby destroying the incentive for consumers and providers to choose the economical alternative. Many employers offer no choice but FFS coverage. Others offer choices but pay the whole premium, whichever choice the employee makes. In such a case, the HMO has no incentive to hold down its premium; it is better off to charge more and use the money to improve service. In many other cases, employers offer a choice of plan, but the employer pays 80% or 90% of the premium or all but some fixed amount, whichever plan the employee chooses. In all these cases, the effect is that the employer pays more on behalf of the more costly system and deprives the efficient alternatives of the opportunity to attract more customers by cutting cost and price.

Health care is as much a component of American goods and products and services as are raw materials. The U.S. spends eight times more than many of its international competitors on health care.
—Richard D. Lamm, Governor of Colorado, 1975–1987

The rational policy from an economic point of view would be for employers to structure health plan offerings to employees so that those who choose the less costly plans get to keep the full savings.

The second major problem is that our present health care financing and delivery system is not organized for quality and economy. One of the main drives in the present system is for each specialist to exercise his or her specialty, not to produce desired outcomes at reasonable cost. In a system designed for quality and economy, managed care organizations would attract the responsible participation of physicians who would understand that, ultimately, their patients bear the costs of care, and they would accept the need for an economical practice style. Data would be gathered on outcomes, treatments, and resources use, and providers would base clinical decisions on such data.

There are too many beds and too many specialists in relation to the number of primary care physicians. A high-quality cost-effective system would carefully match the numbers and types of physicians retained and other resources to the needs of the population served so that each specialist and subspecialist would be busy seeing just the type of patient she or he was trained to treat. We have a proliferation of costly specialized services that are underutilized.

The third major problem area is "market failure." The market for health insurance does not naturally produce results that are fair or efficient. It is plagued by problems of biased risk selection, market segmentation, inadequate information, "free riders," and the like. Insurers profit most by avoiding coverage of those who need it most. The insurance market for small employment groups is breaking down as small employers find insurance unavailable or unaffordable, especially if a group member has a costly medical condition.

Fourth, public funds are not distributed equitably or effectively to motivate widespread coverage. The unlimited exclusion of employer health benefit contributions from the taxable incomes of employees is the second-largest federal government health care "expenditure," trailing only expenditures for the Medicare program. While providing incentives for the well-covered well-to-do to choose even more generous coverage, this provision does little or nothing for those (mainly lower-income) people without employer-provided coverage.

In brief, powerful *incentives* that shape behavior in the health care system and that influence the distribution of services point the system in the wrong direction: services too costly for those who are covered, and the exclusion of millions from any coverage at all.

❖ Our Proposal

We propose a set of public policies and institutions designed to give everyone access to a subsidized but responsible choice of efficient, managed care (HMO, preferred provider insurance plans, etc.). *We propose comprehensive reform of the economic incentives* that drive the system. We propose cost-conscious informed consumer and employer (or other sponsor) choice of managed care so that plans competing to serve such purchasers will have strong incentives to give value for money. We also propose a strategy of *managed competition* to be executed by large employers and public sponsors (explained below), designed to reward with more subscribers those health care financing and delivery plans that offer high-quality care at relatively low cost. The goal of these policies would be the gradual transformation of the health care financing and delivery system, through voluntary private action, into an array of managed care plans, each competing to attract providers and subscribers by finding ways to improve the quality of care and service while cutting costs. We propose restructuring the tax subsidies to create incentives to cover the uninsured and to encourage the insured to be cost conscious in their choice of plan. We propose the creation of public institutions to broker and market subsidized coverage for all who do not obtain it through large employers. We favor substantial public investments in outcomes and effectiveness research to improve the information base for medical practice and consumer/employer choice.

The rise and growth of competition is surely one of the most significant developments in the health care sector in the last decade.
—Lawrence D. Brown, University of Michigan

Public Sponsor Agencies

The Public Sponsor, a quasi-public agency (like the Federal Reserve) in each state, would contract with a number of private-sector health care financing and delivery plans typical of those offered to the employed population and would offer subsidized enrollment to all those who do not have employment-based coverage. Except in the case of the poor, the Public Sponsor would contribute a fixed amount equal to 80% of the cost of the average plan that just meets federal standards. The enrollee would pay the rest. (The 80% level was chosen to balance two incentives. First, we wanted the subsidy level to be low enough so that there would be room for efficient plans to compete by lowering prices and taking subscribers away from inefficient plans. Second, we wanted the subsidy to be high enough so that the purchase of health insurance would appear very attractive even to those who expect to have no medical expenses.) To the enrollee, the Public Sponsor would look like the employee benefits office.

In the case of the poor, we propose additional subsidies. People at or below the poverty line would be able to choose any health plan with a premium at or below the average and have it fully paid. For people with incomes between 100% and 150% of the poverty line, we propose public sharing of the premium contribution on a sliding scale related to income.

Public Sponsors would also act as collective purchasing agents for small employers who wished to take advantage of economies of scale and of the ability of Public Sponsors to spread and manage risk. Small employers could obtain coverage for their groups by payment of a maximum of 8% of their payroll.

Today, a substantial part of the money required to pay for care of the uninsured comes from more or less broadly based state and local sources, including employers' payments to private hospitals for bad debt or free care and direct appropriations from state and local governments to acute-care hospitals. In our proposal, federal funds (the sources of which are described below) would be the main source of support for the Public Sponsors. These funds would be supplemented by funds from state and local sources.

Mandated Employer-Provided Health Insurance

For better or worse, we have an employment-based system of health insurance for most people under age 65 years. It can be modified gradually but not replaced overnight. Most employers and employees agree that health care will be included in the compensation package. This is responsible behavior; if one of the group gets sick, the group pays the cost. Some employers and employees do not include health care in the package. The effect is irresponsible behavior; if an employee becomes seriously ill, these employers and employees count on someone else to pay. They are taking a "free ride." It is hard to justify raising taxes on the insured to pay for coverage for the employed uninsured unless those uninsured are required to contribute their fair share.

The existence of Public Sponsors would give all employers access to large-scale efficient health care coverage arrangements. However, in the absence of corrective action, the availability of subsidized coverage for un-insured individuals would create an incentive for employers to drop cov-erage of their employees. This would create additional expense for the Pub-lic Sponsor without compensating revenue. To prevent this, our proposal requires employers to cover their full-time employees (employers would make a defined contribution equal to 80% of the cost of an average plan meeting federal standards and would offer a choice of health plans meeting federal standards).

Premium Contributions from all Employers and Employees

Many people who are self-employed, who have part-time or seasonal work, or who are retired and under age 65 years do not have enough attachment to one employer to justify requiring the employer to provide coverage.

We propose that employers be required to pay an 8% payroll tax on the first $22,500 of the wages and salaries of part-time and seasonal em-ployees, unless the employer covered the employee with a health insurance plan meeting federal standards. Self-employed persons, early retirees, and everyone else not covered through employment would be required to con-tribute through the income tax system. An 8% tax would apply to adjusted gross income up to an income ceiling related to the size of the household. The ceiling would be calculated to ensure that households with sufficient income paid for approximately the total subsidy that would be made avail-able to them through the Public Sponsor.

The proceeds of these taxes would be paid by the federal government to the states, on a per-person-covered basis, for use by Public Sponsors in offering subsidized coverage to persons without employment-based cov-erage.

This tax would be at the federal level because individual states might be deterred from levying such a tax by employer threats to move to a state without the tax.

Limit on Tax-Free Employer Contributions

We propose that Congress change the income and payroll tax laws to limit the tax-free employer contribution to 80% of the average price of a comprehensive plan meeting federal standards. The average price of a qualified health plan in 1991 might be roughly $290 per family per month. As a condition of tax exemption, employer health plans would be required to use fixed-dollar defined contributions, independent of employee choice of plan, not to exceed the limit, so that people who choose more costly health care plans must do so with their *own* money, not with that of the taxpayer or employer.

The purposes of this measure are two-fold. First, it would save the federal budget some $11.2 billion in 1988 dollars. This money could be used to help finance subsidies for the uninsured comparable to those received by the employed insured. Second, making people cost conscious would help enlist all employed Americans in a search for value for money in health care, would stimulate the development of cost-effective care, and would create a market for cost-effective managed care. Thus, this tax reform is defensible on grounds of both equity and efficiency.

Budget Neutrality

The Congressional Budget Office has estimated the effects of our proposal on coverage, costs, and the federal budget and has found that our proposed new revenues would equal the added outlays. We have not done a state-by-state analysis, but, in the aggregate, required state and local contributions appear to approximately equal outlays for care of the uninsured.

Managed Competition

The market for health insurance does not naturally produce results that are fair or efficient. It is plagued by problems of biased risk selection, market segmentation, inadequate information, etc. In fact, the market for health insurance cannot work at the individual level. To counteract these problems, large employers and Public Sponsors must structure and manage the demand side of this market. They must act as intelligent, active, collective purchasing agents and manage a process of informed cost-conscious consumer choice of "managed care" plans to reward providers of high-quality economical care. Tools of effectively managed competition include the annual open-enrollment process; full employee consciousness of premium differences; a standardized benefit package within each sponsored group; risk-adjusted sponsor contributions, so that a plan that attracts predictably sicker people is compensated; monitoring; surveillance; ongoing quality measurement; and improved consumer information.

Outcomes Management and
Effectiveness Research

As Ellwood and Roper et al. have pointed out, there is a poverty of relevant data linking outcomes, treatments, and resource use. Although such data are costly to gather, they constitute a public good, and their production ought to be publicly mandated and supported. Combined with the incentives built into our proposal, such data could be of great value to providers and patients seeking more effective and less costly treatments. Without incentives for efficiency, such data are likely to have little impact on health care costs.

Mutually Supportive Components

We recognize the propensity of the American political system to seek minimal, incremental change. Some components of our proposal would be viable and helpful on their own. However, we believe that effective solution of the problems of access and cost requires a comprehensive strategy, and the merits of the combined package exceed the merits of the individual components.

❖ Will It Work?

Our confidence that a reasonably well-managed comprehensive reform plan along these lines can be made to work rests on two propositions.

First, efficiently managed care does exist. It is possible to improve economic performance substantially over the non-selective FFS, solo practice, third-party intermediary model.

Second, people do choose value for money. Our limited experience with even attenuated price competition in employment groups such as federal employees, California state employees, and Stanford University suggests that, over time, people do migrate to cost-effective systems.

In recent years, the main inhibitor of the growth of HMOs has been the employer contribution policies we have discussed; that is, most employers do not structure their health plan offerings in such a way that the employee who chooses the most economical plan gets to keep the savings. Nevertheless, some nonprofit HMOs have been growing rapidly through the 1980s.

❖ Comprehensive Reform That Relies on Incentives Is Preferable to Direct Government Controls

One alternative to the system we have proposed is a system like Canada's, in which the government is the sole payer for physician and hospital services. While Canada's system has evident strengths, there would be major difficulties in successfully adopting or implementing it in the United States. First, it would require a political sea change to adopt such a system here. . . . Second, government regulatory processes tend to freeze industries and often penalize efficiency. The Canadian system is not as frozen as it might be because proximity to the United States exposes Canadians to our innovations. If American medical care were also entirely financed and regulated by the government, the negative effects of regulation would likely loom larger.

A second alternative would be to leave the financing of health insurance for the employed population in the private sector but to have the government regulate physician and hospital prices for all payers. It is possible to imagine a political compromise in which such a system could be adopted—in the midst of a recession, providers might agree to accept all payer price controls in exchange for an employer mandate, and employers might acquiesce to a mandate in exchange for price controls—but it is hard to imagine that such a regulatory structure could be effective over time in promoting quality or economy.

Finally, administrative costs in the present system are high and increasing. We believe administrative costs would be greatly reduced under our proposal. After a competitive shakedown, there would be relatively few managed care organizations in each geographic area. Everyone would get coverage through large group arrangements. Eligibility determination would be simple in a system of universal coverage. Today, the best managed care organizations do not bill patients for services. Providers are paid by health plans in simplified ways using prospective payments for global units of care. In a system with relatively few managed care organizations competing to serve competent sponsors and cost-conscious consumers, payers would not have to attempt to micromanage the delivery of care because providers would be at risk. Administrative costs and the "hassle factor" would be much lower than they are today. However, the most important economies would be in the effective organization of the process of care itself.

Over time, we would expect slowed growth in the price of the average health plan and continuing improvements in efficiency comparable to those in other competitive industries.

❖ About the Authors

Alain C. Enthoven, Ph.D., is Marriner S. Eccles Professor of Public and Private Management in the Graduate School of Business, Stanford University.

Richard Kronick, Ph.D., is in the Department of Community and Family Medicine, University of California, San Diego.

❖ Modifying Managed Competition to Address Cost and Quality

Harold S. Luft

The concept of managed competition emphasizes cost and quality comparisons among alternative health care delivery systems. This calls to mind competition within an area amongst Kaiser Permanente, a highly integrated group practice with its own physicians and hospitals; perhaps a few health maintenance organizations (HMOs) comprising large multispecialty group practices; a relatively broadly based individual practice association (IPA); and perhaps an open-ended fee-for-service option. Plans would offer uniform benefits to minimize risk selection based on differential coverage, and contributions would be fixed, so that marginal differences in premiums would be paid with after-tax dollars. Premium differences would reflect efficiency and perhaps "style of practice," and measures of quality would ensure comparable performance along important dimensions of outcomes.

❖ The Current California Marketplace

The California marketplace in the mid-1990s reflects this idealized model of managed competition only partially. After many years of employers' offering choices of health plans, but contributing so much that employees were not encouraged to engage in price-conscious decision making, several major employer sponsors have begun to change their policies. The California Public Employees Retirement System (CalPERS) (the sponsor of health benefits for state employees and those of many other public agencies) began with the requirement that all health plans offer enrollees a uniform benefit package. State budget pressures forced the contribution offered by CalPERS so low that most plans now require some employee copayment. (Recent reductions in premiums, however, have reduced some of this sensitivity). The University of California (UC), which for years had followed the CalPERS model, also forced uniform benefit packages and now sets its contribution at the level of the lowest-cost HMO, rather than the average of the largest plans. The falling contribution level has now made several long-term low-cost HMOs, including Kaiser in northern California, have net out-of-pocket premiums.

In some ways, the private market is closer to President Bill Clinton's 1994 proposal, which encouraged collective purchasing of health benefits by groups of employers, than it is to Alain Enthoven's approach, which envisioned more individualistic purchasing by employers.[1] Not all of the

334

developments in California, however, are moving toward the model of managed competition. In particular, California is far from the ideal of having differing health plans compete on the basis of quality. The HMO market there has been consolidating, and four large plans now account for 66 percent of total enrollment.[2] Kaiser is still the largest single health plan and retains its unique integrated nature, although it has some point-of-service options in parts of the state to allow more enrollee choice. Many of the large IPA/network-model plans contract with groups of physicians organized either in formal medical groups, such as the Palo Alto Medical Clinic or Friendly Hills Healthcare Network, or less formal IPAs that include otherwise "unrelated" physicians.[3] More importantly, the provider networks offered by many of these HMOs are often identical, or nearly so, especially in terms of primary care providers.

The implications of this similarity in delivery systems are not yet clear. Given the uniformity in benefits and providers among plans, one would expect price-sensitivity to be far greater than it has been in the past. This seems to be the case. A recent study by Thomas Buchmueller and Paul Feldstein of plan switching by UC employees in 1994 indicates much greater price-sensitivity than was observed in earlier studies.[4] Not surprisingly, this extreme price-sensitivity has led health plans to cut their premiums in the past few years for employers such as UC, CalPERS, and the Pacific Business Group on Health (PBGH). These pressures on premiums are then translated into reduced capitation payments to the contracting provider groups; there has not been a corresponding reduction of profits by the health plans.[5] Lower capitation payments obviously create strong incentives for increased efficiency by providers, and there are many stories, but little published evidence, of how plans are changing the ways in which they structure and deliver care.

It is unclear, however, to what extent the current dynamic is encouraging improvements in quality and patient outcomes through a "reengineering" of medical care. In the standard model of marketplace competition, firms that develop better ways of producing a product or service at lower cost with comparable quality would gain market share by lowering their prices. The current managed care market in California makes it difficult for this to take place. Suppose that a medical group is able to improve its efficiency and can absorb reductions in capitation payments without jeopardizing quality of care. Because people sign up with a health plan, rather than a medical group, and copayments and premiums are the same regardless of which medical group one uses within a plan, there is no way for the plan to channel enrollees to this group. At the same time, less efficient medical groups are faced with the same lower capitation rates and have to cut their costs through whatever means are available. This may mean reducing provider fees, restricting the pool of available physicians, skimping on quality, or attempting to avoid high-cost cases.

❖ Risk Adjustment In A Competitive Environment

Influences on Selection. It has long been recognized that biased selection is likely to occur whenever people have a choice of health plans.[6] The question of risk selection becomes far more problematic in a highly competitive atmosphere of multiple options. Consumers are encouraged to choose among a set of alternative health plans, which differ primarily in terms of their "style" of health care delivery, perceived quality, and premium, since benefit packages have been made standard. If persons have differing needs for medical care, perhaps because they have certain illnesses rather than because they prefer certain types of treatment, they may seek to enroll in, or avoid enrolling in, certain plans. Thus, for example, someone with a difficult-to-diagnose illness may seek a health plan that is affiliated with a major teaching hospital. Likewise, such persons may avoid health plans that have limited panels of subspecialists or that subtly restrict coverage of certain services, particularly since uniform benefits are required only by some of the largest employers.

These influences on selection are more subtle than the classic approaches of insurance underwriting and preexisting condition clauses. Health plans can avoid high-risk enrollees by not contracting with providers known for specializing in certain high-risk conditions.[7] More stringent protocols for referring patients to subspecialists, thereby encouraging them to switch to another plan in the next open season, are even more difficult to detect. Such selection strategies may not even be conscious decisions on the part of health plans or their contracting medical groups but may merely reflect natural variability in setting practice parameters. Even if they reflected internal policies, it would be difficult for patients or regulators to detect these strategies or to determine who is responsible for them.[8]

Effect of Biased Selection on Health Spending. The problem of biased selection across health plans is of crucial importance because of the extremely skewed distribution of medical expenditures. The top 1 percent of the population in terms of expenditures accounts for 30 percent of all medical care costs, while the bottom 50 percent accounts for only 3 percent of expenditures.[9] This distribution is far more skewed than, for example, expenditures among the hospitalized population for which the diagnosis-related group (DRG) mechanism was developed when Medicare instituted prospective payment. (Obviously, the DRG system need not be concerned about the vast majority of the population that incurs no hospital expenses in a given year.) Moreover, with roughly 470 DRG categories, Medicare still incorporated an outlier payment system to reduce the risk for those hospitals with very expensive cases. Congress also included a teaching hospital subsidy partially to account for unmeasured severity-of-illness differences in referral centers.

Adjusting for Risk. The risk adjustment task required of DRGs is simplified by the fact that it is essentially a retrospective payment. The only risk is that associated with variability in costs within a DRG after accounting for outlier payments; the mix of cases across DRGs is determined after the fact. (Even this overstates the task, since some provider-controlled treatment decisions, such as whether to care for a back problem medically or surgically, lead to different DRGs.) Hospitals are not given a fixed prospective budget based on their expected case-mix. In contrast, health plans are paid a fixed premium that must incorporate the expected variability in the occurrence of illness, the nature of those illnesses, and the variability in costs in treating specific types of conditions.

Addressing risk differences across health plans is a difficult problem, conceptually and empirically. At a conceptual level, some health plans could legitimately argue that if they do their job well, they will reduce the incidence of certain conditions, and adjusting payments based on their occurrence will penalize them for undertaking effective prevention programs. For example, a health plan might institute a program to instruct its members how to lift heavy items safely and simultaneously encourage its physicians to use restrictive criteria for the diagnosis of back pain. Over time, the educational program may reduce the incidence of acute back problems. However, people with chronic back problems also may switch to other health plans. It would be difficult to have an objective measure of whether the lower costs attributable to back problems in the plan are due to its prevention program or to its restrictive access to care, yet one would like to encourage the former and not the latter.

Implementation of a risk adjustment approach also is difficult, even if the conceptual problems can be addressed or set aside temporarily. The difficulty arises partly from the fact that, because a very small proportion of cases accounts for a substantial fraction of the expenditures, enormous numbers of enrollees are needed to observe enough cases in the very high cost categories. Most researchers have had to ignore these high-cost cases, assuming that there will be a reinsurance or similar mechanism.[10] Although this allows a focus on the vast majority of cases and the assessment of alternative approaches for risk-adjusting the "usual" problems, it leaves open an important loophole in the process. For example, in our analysis of 5,000 Bank of America employees, representing more than 10,000 persons, forty-nine subscriber units had expenses of $50,000 or more. Although the expense above $50,000 accounted for approximately 20 percent of the total expenditures of this population, the very small number of high-cost cases makes it impossible to detect a pattern of selection, let alone develop a reasonable set of "DRG-type" values for specific conditions.

In a highly competitive environment, with the absence of appropriate adjustment, adverse selection can have a substantial negative impact on plans' profitability. Likewise, favorable selection can lead to unwarranted profits. Plans are forced to make investment decisions and set premiums in advance based on little information; the effects of selection can affect those decisions and plans' ability to implement them. Moreover, yearly premium cycles and strategic pricing behavior by competitors may force out of business (or make vulnerable to takeover) some well-run plans that happen to experience adverse selection for a year or two.

Risk adjustment approaches in the Medicare program rely on an enormous underlying population of enrollees in a fee-for-service system with uniform benefits. (This is not entirely true because the presence of various Medigap plans has a substantial effect on patient incentives, but Medicare chooses to ignore this effect in setting risk factors for DRGs or HMOs.) For employed populations, the problem is that, until recently, most large employers had tailor-made benefits and plan designs, which limit the ability to pool fee-for-service data. To the extent that enrollees were in HMOs, the effects of unique practice patterns and the potential for biased selection were already incorporated in their data. Moreover, within an HMO, data often do not exist in simple claims-type fashion because it is a highly integrated plan like Kaiser and does not rely on such payments, and even when such data do exist, internal pricing may bear little relationship to resource use. In other situations, the plan pays the medical group a capitation rate and often gets little or no information from it.

Major California purchasers are beginning to address issues of risk adjustment, with varying levels of sophistication. For example, UC examines the demographic profile of various HMOs to determine whether differences in risk can explain why some premiums are higher or lower than others, but it does not take this into account in whether the "low bid," which determines the contribution rate, should be adjusted for risk differences. In contrast, The Health Insurance Plan of California (The HIPC) requires its health plans to quote age- and family structure-specific premiums, thereby eliminating a major aspect of risk differentials. In the future, adjustments will be made for differences in sex and number of dependents. In addition, a list of high-cost conditions has been identified, and health plans with disproportionately few such cases will pay those with disproportionately many such cases to bring risk differences into an approximate balance.[11]

This discussion of the problems associated with biased selection is intended to be cautionary. From a policy perspective, we must be aware of the need to adjust for risk differences and to not simply "assume" that an adequate mechanism exists or will be available in time for its effective use. Instead, efforts must be undertaken to develop and test various approaches to addressing these problems.

❖ Assessing Quality Of Care

The second major requirement of managed competition is adequate measures of quality, so that consumers can assess their health plan choices. Again, there are both conceptual and logistical problems in the collection and presentation of quality-of-care measures. Arnold Epstein notes many of the difficulties in the development and use of various types of "report cards" to assess quality of care.[12] In terms of health plans, the current focus is on the Health Plan Employer Data and Information Set (HEDIS), a collection of measures developed by health plans and purchasers. Roughly fifty of the approximately sixty-five measures in HEDIS 2.5 relate to overall use of services, finance, and plan management; the remainder focus on access, satisfaction, and quality. Even the latter measures are of questionable relevance, because they address narrow issues, such as rates of screening for certain conditions, and only a handful examine outcomes, rather than measures of process. It is important, however, to keep the HEDIS measures in perspective. They represent the first major attempt to collect on a uniform basis indicators of performance from health plans for comparative purposes. The limitations of HEDIS are far less important than the fact that HEDIS exists at all.

Limitations of Report Card Data. Given that newer and more complete versions of HEDIS and similar reports will be developed, there are still major problems, which relate largely to the conceptualization of these quality indicators as tools to help consumers choose among health plans. An analogy is the assessment of automobiles. Measures of consumer satisfaction with cars developed by J.D. Power and Associates track a wide variety of consumer perceptions regarding performance, dependability, and dealer responsiveness. Power surveys roughly 800,000 automobile owners a year, with a response rate of 38–42 percent.[13] The large sample size assures relatively stable estimates for most measures, but the low response rate suggests that there may be a loss of representatives, with those feeling more positive or more negative likely to reply. Furthermore, as the quality of automobiles has improved and the defect rate has fallen, this sample may be too small to detect significant differences across models. In addition, the National Highway Traffic Safety Administration runs "crash tests" to determine the safety of various vehicles under controlled conditions, and the Insurance Institute for Highway Safety documents injuries and accidents of cars in use.

The analogies to health care are straightforward and revealing. The principal advantage of the HEDIS model is health plans' ability to collect from their own administrative and medical records information on the types of services used, immunizations received, and the like. Such information is even more valuable if it is made conditional on various factors, such as the proportion of people with diagnosed hypertension whose condition has been corrected by use of appropriate medications. While the HEDIS data are collected and reported by the health plans, the PBGH requires that these records be audited by an independent group.

The analogue to crash tests is information on how well plans perform with respect to specific outcome measures in selected circumstances, such as inpatient mortality among patients undergoing coronary artery bypass graft (CABG) surgery without other open-heart procedures, after adjusting for various clinical risk factors. Just as the crash test data provide only information on safety in head-on crashes, these measures provide useful information on the performance of a plan in selected high-profile areas but little information on performance in other areas. For example, we found little correlation in risk-adjusted outcomes across California hospitals for CABG surgery and percutaneous transluminal coronary angioplasty (PTCA), even though the two are substitutes for one another and CABG surgery is sometimes required on an emergency basis after PTCA has been attempted.[14] Despite these limitations, some health plans are requiring this type of data from their contracting hospitals. Blue Cross sent out a Request for Proposals last summer requiring hospitals' risk-adjusted rate for infant mortality, inpatient deaths after acute myocardial infarction, mortality after CABG surgery, and cesarean section rate.

One might argue that overall injury and fatality data would be the most useful safety information in the purchase of cars, yet more careful consideration reveals the importance of self-selection and risk adjustment. Some models of cars are driven more than others; some are used primarily on highways, while others are used mainly in suburban car pools. Without careful adjustment for differential risk, the highway accident data may be quite misleading. Similarly, extensive and complex risk adjustment would be needed to develop valid measures of broad-based outcomes such as birth outcomes, hospitalization rates, work-loss days, and overall health status, or even the narrowly focused HEDIS measures. For example, a health plan with a high proportion of well-educated enrollees might have an easier time achieving a high rate of mammograms.

Data Collection Issues. The PBGH and CalPERS have been at the forefront of undertaking enrollee satisfaction surveys. These survey data are limited, however, because potential enrollees want to know the performance of plan providers in their local area, not the plan as a whole. Thus, it is noteworthy that UC is undertaking a survey of enrollees in its own plan (UC Care) and will sample enrollees at each campus.

As one attempts to develop more locally defined measures, the ability to get solidly based assessments of quality, particularly using clinically based outcomes rather than satisfaction measures, is constrained by small sample size. Experience with developing risk-adjusted measures of patient outcomes for California hospitals suggests that many hospitals have too small a patient volume to develop stable estimates of their outcomes with just a year or two of data.[15] Yet relying on multiple years of data to develop stable estimates blunts the incentives to improve performance.

The experience of the California Hospital Outcomes Project also highlights some of the logistical problems in developing valid and reliable measures of clinical quality of care. This project was designed to use routinely collected discharge abstract information to reduce the data collection burden on hospitals. Unfortunately, this means that data are not due at the state agency until six months after the end of the calendar year, and it takes nearly another year for the data to be edited, returned to the hospitals for cleaning, and then made available for the development of outcomes measures. The cleaning and editing process is crucial, since it is fairly easy for hospitals to be assigned markedly better or worse outcomes because of coding errors and inconsistencies. In the past, when information was collected primarily for statistical and research purposes, occasional errors could be tolerated as not having a major impact on overall results. However, as such information is put to use for the assessment of quality and then for contracting and other purposes, there is greater potential for mischief through erroneous coding.

Another issue is the validity and reliability of the measures being used as dependent and independent variables in the risk adjustment models. That is, even if the data are entered in an unbiased and reasonable way, do the resulting outcomes measures reflect true differences in quality? The California Hospital Outcomes Project has undertaken validation studies of its acute myocardial infarction mortality and diskectomy complication models. In each case, 1,000 charts were examined from randomly selected hospitals in a stratified sample emphasizing outlier institutions.[16] The study of acute myocardial infarction indicated that although coding was less than perfect, the errors appeared not to explain the observed differences in outcome rates. Although the addition of selected clinical measures not included in the diagnosis data improved the fit of the models, it made little difference in the overall results. Furthermore, there were observable differences in the process of care among low and high outlier hospitals that could account for the differences in outcomes. The findings from the diskectomy study were less encouraging. The outcome measure was complications based on reported diagnoses, and it was found that the coding of the diagnoses that entered into this measure was not sufficiently valid or reliable to continue focusing on those outcomes.

An alternative strategy is to use targeted data collection systems, such as those developed by New York State for its Collaborative Cardiac Services Study.[17] This approach allows far more flexibility in the development of clinically specific and scientifically based risk factors, microcomputer-based data entry and editing in the units responsible for the patient subpopulations, and more timely delivery of data. On the other hand, this approach has several problems in terms of applicability to a broader range of services than CABG and PTCA. For example, in New York CABG and PTCA services are available in only thirty-one of the state's nearly 200 hospitals, and data collection is targeted to a relatively small number of prospectively and well-defined cases. Even so, comparisons of the routinely collected and special data sets indicate that some hospitals do not capture data from all of the CABG and PTCA cases in the special data system.[18] Whether the omitted cases are a biased subgroup is still unknown. Applying this type of data collection to a broad range of medical conditions, in which the patient's diagnosis is often not determined until near the end of the hospital stay, would require retrospective data collection, and the system may be more efficient if it were made universal. However, universal data collection is expensive, and data for many of the relatively rare types of cases would never be useful in their own condition-specific models, yet may be impossible to exclude *a priori* because they may reflect complications or comorbidities in other more common conditions.

❖ Assuring Fair Payment And Improved Quality

One general approach to designing a policy is to carefully craft the proposal that, if implemented appropriately, would achieve the desired outcomes. Another approach, especially relevant to more market-based strategies, is to focus on developing those things necessary to avoid a disaster. In this context, much worsened patient care and the destruction of high-quality, well-meaning organizations would constitute a disaster. Inadequate attention to risk adjustment and quality measurement, along with inadequate tools and willingness to intervene by key players, increase the risk of such a potential disaster in a competitive strategy. Furthermore, cost pressures on employers are leading to attempts to control labor costs, often by substituting contract workers for regular employees. One oft ignored aspect of this shift is the lack of group insurance, especially large-group sponsorship to protect such workers and guarantee them health benefits. Thus, one must be careful, in assessing the overall performance of a managed competition strategy, to recognize that it may work well for those "inside" the system but be far worse for those "outside" it.

Two Sides of the Selection Problem.   The potential profits attainable by favorable selection may encourage aggressive behavior by "sharks" among the health plans in California. The wide range of tactics that can be used make it possible for such plans to eschew the most obvious and egregious underwriting approaches and thereby escape the types of regulation that might be imposed by the Department of Corporations. Instead, approaches to selection are likely to be subtle, and perhaps not even consciously designed to achieve favorable selection, but nonetheless result in unwarranted profits to health plans that are not particularly efficient. A simple example would be health plans' refusal to adjust capitation payments to provider groups with high-risk populations, thereby leading such groups to drop out of a plan and making the plan unattractive to high-risk patients.[19] The flip-side of the selection problem is even more worrisome. Health plans and provider groups that have structured themselves to take excellent care of high-risk patients—and have even designed creative, cost-effective practice protocols—may find themselves with a disproportionate number of such cases, and the resulting undercompensated costs may adversely affect their survival.

In the classic model of competitive markets, this would not be a major problem because those firms making such "errors" would go out of business and be replaced by others not making such mistakes. The real world of California's medical care system differs from such a classic market environment in many ways, the most important of which is the relatively small number of players, the high costs of entry, and the complexity of the market environment. The small number of players leads to strategic behavior that may be reflected in short-term underpricing to gain market share or overpricing, counting on slowly responding consumers to accumulate profits to fund expansion. Entry is difficult and risky and therefore attractive primarily to entrepreneurial firms that perceive profitable market niches and strategies. Caring for high-cost groups of patients under the current payment system, particularly if those patients do not have powerful sponsoring organizations, is not likely to occur merely as a market response. As the system is downsizing, providers are concerned about survival and are seeking new partners, some of whom may provide important synergies, others who may merely be the only available choice. Some health plans and providers are local, but others are national—and thus able to rely on deep pockets. For the latter, California is merely one of many market areas. Thus, there is little reason to believe that the most efficient plans would necessarily survive; in fact, biased selection would give short-run advantages to the least desirable plans.

The HIPC's Solution. There are some positive efforts on the horizon. As described earlier, The HIPC is implementing an approach this year (to affect next year's bids) to adjust for differential prevalence of high-cost cases among its health plans. This is a pathbreaking approach because it establishes a method to adjust for risk and will test the feasibility of its implementation. Furthermore, it does not rely just on risk adjustment methods applied to claims files, but rather uses the claims (or encounter) data to identify cases fitting a potential high-cost profile and then makes those records subject to audit. Although not a part of The HIPC's plan, such an approach also would allow the monitoring of the quality of care given to these patients. One should not make too much of this effort, however, because The HIPC is still quite small relative to the PBGH and other sponsors. Furthermore, the legislation establishing The HIPC requires all rates to be prospective, while the logic of a high-cost risk pool is to retrospectively make such payments reflect actual enrollment. Thus, a relatively technical legal issue may blunt the effectiveness of an otherwise very exciting demonstration. If the approach works and if it is adopted, perhaps with modifications, by the PBGH and other very large purchasers, then much of the advantage of selection in the realm of very costly conditions may be offset.

It is important to note some other important differences between The

HIPC and the PBGH. The HIPC is structured as an impartial purchasing pool to allow choice among a wide range of health plans. The PBGH is a coalition of large employers, often with their own complex choices of health options designed to serve a national labor force and accustomed to negotiating with plans. While some HMOs in California are offered by many PBGH employers, few are offered by all. Large employers' ability to selectively add and drop health plans gives them much more bargaining power, at least in the short run, than The HIPC or CalPERS has, both of which focus on choice by enrollees, rather than purchasers.[20] Although selective contracting has bargaining advantages, it complicates risk adjustment because selection will depend on the choices available to enrollees.

Pros and Cons of Disease-Specific Risk Categories. It is important to recognize, however, that substantial selection also might occur in more common, but nonetheless expensive, conditions such as diabetes, heart disease, and cancer. If health plans differ markedly in their mix of such patients—an empirical question yet to be examined—then more broadly based risk adjustments using methods such as ambulatory care groups and diagnostic cost groups may be needed. While such methods are not yet well developed for routine application in employed populations, much of the underlying work has been done. In particular, careful attention should be paid to the role of risk adjustment incentives vis-à-vis prevention incentives.

It will be important to examine how such risk adjustment approaches mesh with the development of various capitation and other managed care programs that focus on specific diseases. At one level, the creation of disease-specific risk adjustment categories will make it easier for a health plan to contract with specialized groups to care for patients. This could be highly beneficial if these groups develop specialized expertise and protocols that allow more cost-effective and higher-quality patient care for complex problems. The concentration of patient volume, while it may or may not increase quality, will make it easier to collect data to track outcomes. However, fragmentation of care may cause major problems in treatment management. At the very least, the development of specialized programs will force a more careful consideration of risk adjustment for payment and for outcome measurement.

As care shifts to the outpatient setting, and the need for data for risk adjustment and quality assessment becomes more pressing, some of the limitations of the current approach to data collection in California become clearer. Although the statewide collection and public release of extensive hospital discharge abstract information by California was at the cutting edge in 1982, substantial limitations in the data set are beginning to hamper its usefulness. Unfortunately, in California all significant changes to the discharge abstract, including requirements for new variables, require legislation. Thus, the California Healthcare Association (formerly the California Association of Hospitals and Health Systems) has been able to prevent the collection of even basic physiological variables, such as blood pressure on admission. Likewise, the California Medical Association has been able to block the collection of license numbers for attending and operating physicians, and the collection of data on major procedures done on an outpatient basis. Each of these types of data is collected in other states. If these data were to be collected in California, along with a detailed code for the patient's health plan (usually the first piece of data collected on arrival at the hospital), then the state could assure uniform coding and editing of the data and pay for the development of clinically appropriate risk adjustment models.

Just such an approach has been initiated by the PBGH and the California Office of Statewide Health Planning and Development (OSHPD) with respect to CABG surgery. CABG surgery was one of the first procedures considered for analysis using discharge abstract data, but it was rejected for two reasons. Although it is commonly done, has high mortality for a surgical procedure, and has been shown to be highly variable across hospitals, it is performed only in 30 percent of California hospitals and thus was deemed of lower priority for a statewide report. More importantly, published studies from New York suggest the importance of certain clinical risk factors not included on discharge abstracts, so any results were likely to be challenged by clinicians as invalid. While stymied in its attempts to add data to the abstract, the OSHPD is collaborating with the PBGH in an experiment for hospitals to voluntarily collect clinical data for all CABG patients using state-of-the-art data collection protocols. Cooperation can be encouraged by the PBGH's ability to require that its health plans only contract with hospitals making data available to the effort.[21] Data collection is scheduled to begin in 1996, with a goal of releasing the first reports in mid-1997. Various payers, such as the PBGH, and health plans then could apply the risk adjustment methodologies to their own patients or providers to assess differences in outcomes. Clinicians also could use the findings to identify the best practice models and thereby improve their patient care processes. The PBGH also is creating incentives for health plans to improve their quality and enrollee satisfaction. A proportion of their total premiums is placed at risk and made available if the plans meet certain quality goals. Although the dollar amount is relatively small, the message concerning the importance of improved performance is clear.

❖ A Crucial Role For Government

The underlying concept behind managed competition is that consumers should be able to make cost-conscious decisions in choosing health plans. Health plans should be forced to compete on the efficiency with which they care for their enrolled population and not have to worry about risk selection. All plans should provide a reasonable level of quality of care. There may be differences in style and convenience, just as truly unsafe cars are not allowed to be sold, but there may be a wide range in design, comfort, and handling. This ideal model does not exist in California, and there is little reason to believe it will evolve naturally. On the other hand, important efforts by the PBGH, CalPERS, and The HIPC are moving in the direction of creating a more level playing field and keeping at least part of the focus on quality as well as cost.

It is important to remember, however, that not all managed care enrollees are well-educated employees in large firms. Many are elderly Medicare beneficiaries, and, increasingly in California, many are being forced into managed care plans. Particularly for these persons, risk adjustment and a guarantee that a reasonable minimum level of quality of care is maintained will need to be a public responsibility. This does not necessarily mean that government has to microregulate plans, particularly if some of the larger, more flexible private entities can do the job for their own enrollees. It does mean, however, that government as the sponsor for these enrollees must establish the mechanisms for quality assurance and must hold the plans responsible.

Government also has a crucial role in the collection of information needed to develop reliable and valid measures of quality. Legislation is needed to assure confidentiality of patient data, yet this crucial concern should not be a reason for health plans to avoid accountability. Public requirements for data submission can lead to much simpler and less expensive data collection because a single setting would collect and process all of the raw data and then make these data available to qualified organizations for their own assessments of risk and quality. Although the joint PBGH/OSHPD effort is exciting, it is not clear that the particular approach that works for CABG patients will be broadly applicable to all patients. The vast majority of hospitals with CABG patients are large facilities that have for several years been using data collection protocols designed by the Society of Thoracic Surgeons. Gaining the cooperation of smaller hospitals and those not threatened by the loss of PBGH patients, perhaps because they represent local monopolies, may require government efforts. Again, the actual collection and processing can be done under contract to private firms, but universality of collection must be assured by a public entity.

California is among the leaders in competition among managed care plans. In this role, it is beginning to explore the range of tools needed to truly implement managed competition among these plans. How well it is able to develop and implement these tools is likely to determine the viability and attractiveness of this approach as a policy option for the rest of nation.

❖ About the Author

Harold S. Luft, Ph.D., is Professor of Health Economics and Director, Institute for Health Policy Studies, School of Medicine, University of California, San Francisco.

NOTES

1. A.C. Enthoven, "Consumer-Choice Health Plan," *The New England Journal of Medicine* (23 March 1978): 650–658; A.C. Enthoven, "Consumer-Choice Health Plan," *The New England Journal of Medicine* (30 March 1978): 709–720; A.C. Enthoven and R. Kronick, "A Consume-Choice Health Plan for the 1990s," *The New England Journal of Medicine* (5 January 1989): 29–37; and A.C. Enthoven and R. Kronick, "A Consumer-Choice Health Plan for the 1990s," *The New England Journal of Medicine* (12 January 1989): 94–101.

2. J. Hillman, *GHAA's National Directory of HMOs* (Washington: Group Health Association of America, 1994).

3. J.C. Robinson and L.P. Casalino, "The Growth of Medical Groups Paid through Capitation in California," *The New England Journal of Medicine* (21 December 1995): 1684–1687; and B.N. Shenkin, "The Independent Practice Association in Theory and Practice: Lessons from Experience," *Journal of the American Medical Association* 273, no. 24 (1995): 1937–1947.

4. T.C. Buchmueller and P.J. Feldstein, "Consumers' Sensitivity to Health Plan Premiums: Evidence from a Natural Experiment in California," *Health Affairs* (Spring 1996): 143–151.

5. M. Hiltzik and D.R. Olmos, "Are Executives at HMOs Paid Too Much Money?" *Los Angeles Times,* 30 August 1995, A13.

6. G.R. Wilensky and L.F. Rossiter, "Patient Self-Selection in HMOs," *Health Affairs* (Spring 1986): 66–80; H.S. Luft, J.B. Trauner, and S.C. Maerki, "Adverse Selection in a Large, Multiple-Option Health Benefits Program," in *Biased Selection in Health Care Markets,* Advances in Health Economics and Health Services Research, vol. 6, ed. R.M. Scheffler and L.F. Rossiter (Greenwich, Conn.: JAI Press, 1985), 197–229; and J.L. Buchanan and S. Cretin, "Risk Selection of Families Electing HMO Membership," *Medical Care* (January 1986): 39–51.

7. S. Lehrman, "Health Plans Shutting Out Those Who Need Care the Most: AIDS Patients Feeling the Pinch of Managed Care," *The San Francisco Examiner,* 4 June 1995, A1.

8. D.R. Olmos and M.A. Hiltzik, "Family Prevails in Long Struggle with HMO," *Los Angeles Times,* 28 August 1995, A12.

9. M.L. Berk and A.C. Monheit, "The Concentration of Health Expenditures: An Update," *Health Affairs* (Winter 1992): 145–149.

10. J.C. Robinson et al., "A Method for Risk Adjusting Employer Contributions to Competing Health Insurance Plans," *Inquiry* (Summer 1991): 107–116.

11. The Health Insurance Plan of California, "Methods for Calculating and Applying Risk Assessment and Risk Adjustment Measures: Results of Simulation No. 2" (Sacramento: California Managed Risk Medical Insurance Board, September 1995).

12. A.M. Epstein, "Performance Reports on Quality—Prototypes, Problems, and Prospects," *The New England Journal of Medicine* (6 July 1995): 57–61.

13. N. Nauman, "A Powerful Force in the Auto Industry," *San Jose Mercury News,* 9 April 1995, 1D, 4D.

14. H.S. Luft, E. Hannan, and J. Wong, "The Effects of Variation in Provider Performance on Recommended Strategies for the Treatment of Ischemic Heart Disease" (Paper in progress).

15. H.S. Luft, P. Romano, and L.L. Remy, *Annual Report of the California Hospital Outcomes Project, Vol.*

1: *Study Overview and Results Survey* (1993).

16. P.S. Romano et al., "The California Hospital Outcomes Project: Using Administrative Data to Compare Hospital Performance," *The Joint Commission Journal on Quality Improvement* (December 1995): 668–682.

17. E.L. Hannan et al., "New York State's Cardiac Surgery Reporting System: Four Years Later, *Annals of Thoracic Surgery 58* (1994): 1852–1857.

18. E.L. Hannan et al., "Clinical versus Administrative Data Bases for CABG Surgery," *Medical Care* (October 1992): 892–907.

19. Lehrman, "Health Plans Shutting Out Those Who Need Care the Most."

20. Pacific Business Group on Health, "Negotiating Alliance Selection Results Are In—High Value HMOs with Medicare Risk Plans Win in 1996," *Pacific Currents* (January 1996): 5.

21. Pacific Business Group on Health, "PBGH Teams with State of California to Develop Hospital Mortality Reporting Program," *Pacific Currents* (January 1996): 2.

❖ Consumer Protection in Managed Care: A Third-Generation Approach

❖ JOHN ROTHER

The rapid expansion of managed care organizations has caught many consumer advocates trying to play catch-up in response to the sophisticated techniques that health maintenance organizations and other managed care plans use to lower their healthcare costs. The promise of prepaid healthcare seemed to be nonthreatening in such nonprofit, community-based movement is no longer growing. Instead, the rapid enrollment growth of for-profit plans, driven by the bottom line, has fueled the perception of many Americans that more aggressive consumer protection measures are necessary to safeguard the interests of the enrolled individual. Advocates have focused on three generations of consumer-protection issues.

❖ First Generation—Individual Treatment Decisions

Consumer advocates focused first on the more dramatic problems that HMOs have sometimes posed for the individual enrollee. The attention has been on the individual who wants treatment that the plan either does not cover or deems unnecessary. Because these issues often must be resolved quickly to avoid harm to the patient, and because the treating physician cannot be assumed to be the patient's advocate in these situations, there is a compelling need to establish appeals mechanisms that can resolve denial-of-treatment problems quickly and fairly.

Most HMOs today have internal mechanisms that, in effect, provide for a second medical opinion at the request of a member. Consumers have also advocated for external reviews by doctors not affiliated with the plan, to ensure objectivity. Medicare risk plans now have an established external appeals process, but the fact of life under capitation (payment of fixed amount per capita) is that some procedures and treatments of dubious or very marginal effectiveness will be discouraged or not covered, while others of untested efficacy will always be in the "gray zone" that may be covered under some plans and not under others. This situation is a function of the dynamic nature of medical knowledge, and consumers will always have to test the boundaries of coverage when they or a loved one are seriously ill.

So the first generation of consumer protection issues in managed care has been a response to the anxiety caused by the possibility of undertreatment. Undertreatment is the most easily dramatized concern and has the greatest human-interest potential, even if it is relatively rare. The press usually uses undertreatment as an example when it wants to raise questions or challenge the growth of HMOs. Shortsighted and ill-advised plan practices like physician "gag rules" and a lack of standard definitions and applications of emergency care, urgent care, or experimental treatment classifications have fed concerns about undertreatment.

This individual, case-by-case perspective also characterizes the earlier consumer protection approach to concerns about overutilization that led to the establishment of the Medicare Peer Review Organization (PRO) program. The original impetus of that effort was to review medical charts in order to find and sanction "bad doctors" who were exploiting Medicare's fee-for-service payment system at the expense of their patients and the tax payers. Consumer advocates were supportive of the program's initial focus on overutilization and on the risks that inappropriate care posed to individual patients.

There are, however, very serious limitations to case-by-case approaches to consumer protection. Per case, they are expensive, they often catch only selected problems, and they ignore the functioning of the rest of the health-care delivery system. They often do not lead to improved system performance even if the individual case is remedied. The PRO program was revised to respond to these shortcomings, and it no longer focuses on individual chart reviews. So, while the concern for the individual treatment decision is a necessary part of consumer protection efforts, it is clearly insufficient.

Medicaid managed care brings its own separate and urgent consumer protection issues. Separate because enrollment is not usually voluntary, and urgent because of the vulnerable nature of the Medicaid population, who have little financial or political clout to protect themselves. For this reason, I'll not try to address the special consumer protection needs of this population here, except to note that the rapid turnover of the Medicaid acute care population—turnover exceeds 40 percent per year—negates the usual incentives for managed care plans to perform with longer-term customer satisfaction or clinical outcomes in mind (Kaiser Commission on the Future of Medicaid, 1995).

❖ Second Generation—Insurance Practices and Risk Selection

A second generation approach for some consumer advocates has been to examine the insurance-related practices of HMOs, primarily marketing and risk-selection (Zelman, 1996). This approach reflects a focus not just on the treatment of the individual patient, but also on the impact that HMOs may have on the rest of the health insurance system—of particular interest to those who worry about the fate of the Medicare traditional indemnity program. Because it is widely assumed that Medicare HMOs are currently enrolling a healthier, younger segment of the

Medicare population, and because risk-adjusted payments today are an inadequate correction for the favorable selection of enrollees, marketing and risk segmentation (marketing to and selecting for inclusion a lower-risk segment of the population) are important areas of concern. These concerns may be more pronounced in Medicare because of the individual, rather than employer-based, marketing and enrollment process.

Indeed, the 1995 debate in Washington about the structure of Medicare "reforms" was striking in how many of the policy differences were based on risk selection issues. Risk selection takes place when the risk pool is distributed unevenly, so some plans face much greater expense than others. Most consumer organizations quickly saw the dangers posed by Medical Savings Accounts and private fee-for-service options in Medicare. Even the Medicare negotiations among the president, the Speaker of the House, and the Senate majority leader stalled, not so much over the total level of budgetary savings as over the issues of risk selection and the related threat to the future integrity of the Medicare risk pool.

For consumers, the potential for plans to select members based on risk leads to an unstable and inadequate set of insurance choices over time. The "gaming" of enrollment by plans sets up a different kind of competition than the competition to promote access and quality that most consumers would prefer. Plans can profit much more easily by enrolling healthier individuals and groups than they can by better managing the delivery of healthcare, so there is a strong temptation to market themselves only to the healthy.

Today, there is evidence that within Medicare, HMOs enroll new members who, on average, have substantially lower than average health expenses. This phenomenon may be inevitable in the early stages of HMO enrollment growth, since younger and healthier Medicare beneficiaries are more likely to be open to joining an HMO. The more serious problem is indicated by "disenrollment" of higher-cost individuals. If those most in need of health services leave the HMO, that could indicate a failure of the plan to meet the needs of the enrollee. It could also mean that costs are being shifted back to otherpayers, and thus the claimed advantage of risk plans in saving costs would be nullified. We need much more scrutiny of those sicker disenrollees to see if plans themselves are encouraging higher cost enrollees to leave or are failing to meet the medical or service needs of those enrollees.

Benefit and network design is also a key element in this competitive environment. One way to attract better risks is for plans to develop benefits and provide affiliations that will appeal to low-cost individuals but not to potentially higher-cost ones. Many plans emphasize preventive programs, for example, but not the specialists, services, or facilities important to chronically ill or disabled individuals.

The competitive dynamic that these practices create is problematic in two ways. First, the lack of incentive to recruit and serve the most medically needy people means that the plans do not reach the population that could benefit the most from well-coordinated and integrated healthcare arrangements. Since most of the dollars spent in the healthcare system today are spent on seriously or chronically ill people, risk selection also means that the potential budgetary benefits of managed care to the overall health system may never be realized.

Another concern of consumers is that risk selection sets up a competitive dynamic that could lead to a "race to the bottom." If plans are, in effect, rewarded for avoiding risk, their benefit designs and provider networks may be deliberately skewed to avoid being too attractive to higher-risk individuals. In the long run, this dynamic could well lead to inadequate benefit plans that are not designed to serve the needs of the sicker enrollee. Plans doing a better job of serving the more difficult and expensive individuals will be financially penalized because a disproportionate number of high-risk, expensive individuals will be drawn to them, and they will be forced to adjust benefits downward to protect themselves. This situation penalizes precisely those plans that do the best job of serving the full range of consumer needs in healthcare.

It should therefore be no surprise that consumer advocates are moving to a second-generation focus on risk selection as the long-term consequences of inadequate safeguards become clearer. But given the inevitability of growing managed care choices and consequent risk segmentation, how can consumers best be protected from these adverse consequences?

The first step is to structure the enrollment process to minimize deliberate selection practices. Medicare itself should conduct the enrollment and regulate the marketing of risk plans, as the Office of Personnel Management does for federal employees. Certain marketing practices, such as the use of agents, should not be permitted because of the practices' inherent potential for abuse. Second, we can try to more accurately adjust Medicare payments to plans to reflect the risk profile of their enrollees. Health status should be included as a factor in the adjusted payments. The use of outlier payments (extra payments for very expensive cases) or carve-outs (benefits paid for separately as an exception to prepaid care, usually for well-defined, expensive conditions such as mental health, substance abuse) might reduce some of the risk to plans and therefore the incentive for the plan to underserve those truly high-cost, riskier patients. Finally, it is essential to prevent manipulation of benefit design to accomplish risk selection. The lack or limitation of a pharmaceutical benefit, for example, can discourage those in need of high-cost drugs from enrollment in a particular plan if they have the choice of better coverage elsewhere. Again, the plans that do offer more generous coverage are then faced with adverse selection—that is, they will be the choice of more high-risk, expensive enrollees—when competing with plans that offer more limited benefits. To protect themselves, the better plans will be forced to cut back benefits. For this reason, a more adequate standard benefits package must eventually be required.

Even with such protections in place, however, problems will remain. For example, the plans may well enroll a fair cross-section of the population only to provide inadequate service or poor quality care. So the insurance-related concerns that focus on marketing abuses or risk selection are, like concerns about individual treatment decisions, a necessary but insufficient agenda for consumer protection. I believe that consumer advocacy must therefore broaden its scope to encompass a third-generation approach to deal with the issues of health plan performance.

❖ Third Generation—Health Plan Performance

If consumer advocates truly want to maximize value in healthcare, protest quality, and promote accountable and responsible health plans, they will have to expand their focus to include the factors that actually guide and limit health plan performance. This calls for a sophisticated assessment of plan structure and performance that takes into account such factors as physician financial incentives, appropriate utilization, consumer satisfaction, outcomes information, and the need for strong public and private regulation and oversight.

It may not be much of an overstatement to say that money drives behavior in organizations, so the third-generation approach to consumer advocacy has to look at the financial arrangements and incentives that drive behavior within the HMO. Central to this inquiry is the way the health plan compensates its primary care physicians.

Financial compensation usually underlies the behavioral norms for delivering care within the health plan. Reimbursement incentives influence the culture of the organization and, thus, everyone who works for it. These incentives set up an ongoing set of rewards and penalties for clinical providers. Expecting occasional, individual appeals or sanctions to affect behavior within the plan is like expecting a beach sandcastle to hold back the tide.

It is increasingly common for HMOs to "dump" risk to the physician level rather than to pay salaries to the physicians while accepting risk at the plan level. The practice of putting physicians at full financial risk for the costs of their own treatment recommendations (physician capitation) raises the stakes for consumer protection and also raises some difficult ethical issues for the physicians (American Medical Association, 1995).[1] Under physician capitation, the primary care physician accepts a monthly payment per covered plan member, then pays for the cost of tests, specialist referrals, and hospitalizations out of that monthly payment. In comparison, salaried physicians are presumably able to practice with the least regard to financial incentives, but even they are often paid bonuses based on the attainment of budgetary targets (Relman, 1988).

Physicians may want to accept risk in order to gain more money and more autonomy for themselves in their practice of medicine. But from the patient's perspective, the main question is. How strong is the financial pressure on the physician to underserve? If the physician group is relatively small and is at full risk, then the link between an individual treatment recommendation and the doctor's income may be direct and substantial enough to become a clear conflict of interest. If indicators of patient satisfaction and clinical quality are taken into account in determining a physician's compensation, then they may balance the other financial incentives satisfactorily. If the plan (or the physician's partners) simply use utilization data to identify outliers, then there is also less to worry about, so long as clinical decisions and practice styles conform to the latest guidelines.

Physicians paid on a fee-for-service basis are increasingly subject to a percentage "withhold" by preferred provider organizations or other forms of "managed care lite." The withhold has much the same impact on physician financial incentives as does capitation; it signals to the doctor that his or her expected income is possible only if certain utilization or budgetary targets are met. So, the healthcare consumer may soon face a medical delivery system in which, for better or worse, doctors are subject to a range of financial incentives that under some circumstances may not be in that individual's best interest. If program budgets are adequate, and the incentives light, then there may be little need for concern. But if the drive to cut costs becomes excessive, these tools are capable of creating serious conflicts of interest.

The most difficult and most worrisome situations involve high-cost treatments that are discretionary—that is, they are beyond the treatments indicated in practice guidelines for the patient's condition. Physicians who have accepted full risk for such a patient face a particularly direct ethical dilemma. How aggressive should their treatment recommendations be if high-cost aggressive treatment means a substantial negative effect on their income, and the net incomes of their partners? Disclosure of financial incentives in such situations is ethically required, but disclosure may not be sufficient by itself to protect the integrity of the physician-patient relationship.

Beyond these dramatic cases, however, lies the broader issue: What is it that we want to pay physicians, and plans, to do? What do we want them to be accountable for? What behavior do we want to reward? These are questions that consumer advocates must now address if they are to influence the direction our healthcare system will take.

For example, if we want plans to reach out to those segments of our population that are at greater risk and harder to serve, we will have to design and advocate for reimbursements that measure and reward such behavior. If we want to support "centers of excellence" that specialize in the treatment of a particular condition or disease, then we will need to become advocates for reimbursement arrangements that support access to such centers. If we want high clinical quality, then we have to measure and reward it through higher reimbursement and greater enrollment volume. If we want physicians to take the needs of the whole patient into account, and to be able to treat the whole person, then we must advocate for benefit designs and flexibility that permit and reward that kind of physician involvement.

Key to the attainment of goals for healthcare plans is the ability to measure performance (Epstein, 1995). Paul Ellwood has stated that organizations "are what they measure." Consumer advocates now need to pay close attention to what is being measured in managed care organizations. Is it what we most care about? Is it what we want plans to use as a basis for financial reward? If the only things that count in this new environment are what you can count, then consumers need to be clear about what counts with them. We need to know about how financial incentives and performance measures translate into quality patient care (Hillman, Pauly, and Kerstein, 1989).

These issues are difficult. Grappling with them requires a sophisticated knowledge of how capitated health plans function and how doctors and other providers within those plans behave. Also required is much more information and analysis than consumers may be used to, and it must be collected and presented on a provider, plan, and market-by-market basis, as well as nationally. For many individual consumers, this level of information will be overwhelming and functionally useless. Still, disclosure, while a necessary first step, is never going to be adequate by itself to assure good performance.

This analysis suggests the need both nationally and within specific healthcare "markets" to establish consumer protection organizations that can function as constructive participants in the necessary dialogue with plans and providers about how to improve healthcare coverage and services. Perhaps states can take the lead in making funding for these organizations available; perhaps the federal government could require that a small percentage of plan premiums be dedicated to such purposes. In any event, the need for an informed, sophisticated consumer advocacy network has never been greater.

Consumer advocates must now also focus on the need to establish an adequate regulatory and oversight infrastructure for managed care. Market-based purchasing decisions can promote good healthcare, but healthy competition can only work for the benefit of the consumer where there are clear, effectively enforced rules for competitive behavior (U.S. General Accounting Office, 1995). We are making a start on this structure already. The Health Care Financing Administration can exercise some oversight for Medicare enrollees, the National Committee on Quality Assurance can play a critically important role in both standardizing performance-related information and conducting accreditation reviews, and the PRO program is trying to monitor quality and resolve complaints within Medicare. But to date there is inadequate oversight in the states and local markets where the plans operate, especially for people under age 65. Where individual consumers need help is in making enrollment decisions and in dealing with problems once enrolled. National standards, combined with local oversight and enforcement, are necessary. Information alone, while necessary, will not be sufficient to protect most consumers.

Many large private employers have taken on the responsibility of assisting active employees in dealing with healthcare plans, but other large employers have reduced their employee assistance efforts. For employees of small and some large businesses, and for the self-employed and Medicaid and Medicare beneficiaries, accessible and effective remedies must be available to resolve problems. This is an urgent challenge for the consumer movement because of the speed and scope of the changes now occurring almost everywhere in healthcare insurance and delivery.

The dynamic character of the healthcare delivery system seems likely to continue for some years to come. Regional differences will continue to emerge, as will new organizational arrangements for financing care. If consumer advocates are to stay relevant to this process, they will need to expand their activities beyond concerns about individual treatment denials or risk selection. What is needed now is a third-generation approach to the behavior of these capitated healthcare organizations—an approach based on clearly stated systemwide goals for provider behavior and on the financial payments and incentives that support such behavior.

The promise of a new, more efficient, accountable, and more valuable healthcare system is incorporated in some of the managed care organizations that will soon provide healthcare coverage for most Americans. Without strong and informed consumer advocacy, that promise may never be realized. Consumer advocates must take up the challenge to engage health plans on their own terms—money and measurement—if the quest for a better healthcare system is to be fulfilled.[2]

❖ About the Author

John Rother is Director of Public Policy for the American Association of Retired Persons (AARP).

NOTES

1. The most thorough overall examination of ethical issues in managed care is found in Rodwin, 1993.
2. For good overviews of issues raised for consumers by managed care organizations, see also American College of Physicians, 1996.

REFERENCES

American College of Physicians. 1996. *Medicare Managed Care: How to En-sure Quality.* Task Force on Aging Report. Philadelphia.

American Medical Association (Council on Ethical and Judicial Affairs). 1995. "Ethical Issues in Managed Care." *Journal of the American Medical Association* 23: 4.

Epstein, A. 1995. "Performance Reports on Quality—Prototypes, Problems, and Prospects." *New England Journal of Medicine* 333: 57–61.

Hillman, A. L., Pauly, M. V., and Kerstein, J. J. 1989. "How Do Financial Incentives Affect Physicians' Clinical Decisions and the Financial Performance of Health Maintenance Organizations?" *New England Journal of Medicine* 321:86–92.

Kaiser Commission on the Future of Medicaid. 1995. *Medicaid and Managed Care: Lessons from the Literature.* Washington, D.C.

Relman, A. S. 1988. "Salaried Physicians and Economic Incentives." *New England Journal of Medicine* 319: 784.

Rodwin, M. 1993. *Medicine, Money and Morals.* New York: Oxford University Press.

U.S. General Accounting Office. 1995. *Medicare: Increased HMO Oversight Could Improve Quality and Access to Care.* Washington, D.C.

Zelman, W. 1996. *The Changing Health Care Marketplace: Private Ventures, Public Interests.* San Francisco: Jossey-Bass.

❖ From Health Services to Medical Markets: The Commodity Transformation of Medical Production and the Nonprofit Sector

ALLEN W. IMERSHEIN AND CARROLL L. ESTES

The changing constraints of nonprofit hospitals, and more generally of organizations in the nonprofit sector, have been widely noted (1–4). Services have become increasingly corporatized, privatized, and fragmented (5). The legitimacy of nonprofit status for medical care organizations has come under challenge (6–8). Organizational growth and the provision of services have become significantly deregulated, but the imposition of price and product controls (e.g., diagnosis-related groups, DRGs) has brought hospital financial management under new and different constraints (9, 10).

Concomitant with these changes, the language and logic of organizing medical care tasks have moved from providing medical services to marketing product lines. Our analysis examines this task transformation and its implications for transformation of the nonprofit sector and, ultimately, for the state. We contend that medical care tasks have undergone a two-stage transformation. The first transformation in the production of medical care tasks changed what had been a set of vaguely defined and largely unpredictable services supported by tenuous and variable funding managed in the nonprofit sector. They became more clearly routine and predictable services managed by an internal bureaucracy with stable funding from multiple sources, including that from the state, *but not* subject to external bureaucratic controls *or the logic thereof.* As a result of these changes in the organization and performance of medical care tasks, these services came to be viewed as potentially marketable goods attractive to capitalist enterprises, encouraging corporate entry into medical care delivery and promoting the development of multi-institutional and multi-facility systems (11).

The second and more recent commodity transformation of medical care tasks was constituted by a standardization of these tasks into product lines and payment schemes; that is, they became increasingly organized in terms of a capitalist logic, including resource control, management efficiency, product marketing, and fiscal accountability—organized toward profit-making. This transformation (*a*) undercut the claims of nonprofit hospitals to provide needed, yet otherwise unavailable "services," thereby also undercutting nonprofit claims of being worthy of tax protection by the state;

(b) challenged the political/institutional control by nonprofits over the hospital care arena as well as market control at the individual hospital level; and (c) required a shift in administrative management within nonprofit sector institutions, namely to organize by product and profit. Moreover, these changes further undermined legitimacy claims of those institutions as nonprofit entities as they altered relationships within the nonprofit sector with regard to task and fiscal management, and among institutions of the nonprofit sector and those of the capitalist sector and the state.

Ultimately, we suggest, this imposition of a capitalist logic on nonprofit sector organizations and the concomitant shift in administrative management—that is, the increasing development of an internal bureaucratic logic used to maximize resource management and capitalist accumulation—has come to allow a level of external review and state intervention/control that these organizations had for so long successfully avoided as part of their claims to nonprofit status.

Our discussion assumes that in capitalist democracies like the United States all institutions confront three institutional logics, which provide the legitimate (or illegitimate) legal models, ideological defenses, and potential economic resources. These logics are those of a capitalist economy, based on principles of accumulation and growth; a bureaucratic state, based on organizational survival and legitimation through claims to rationality; and a democratic culture, based on the principle of serving human needs defined and realized through autonomous participation in community life (12). "By a logic we mean a set of practices—behavior, institutional forms, ideologies—that have social functions and are defended by politically organized interests" (12, p. 11). So, under a democratic logic, individual rights and political participation are *claimed* as central to the community life of the society and take priority over bureaucratic rules or market rights. (See 12, especially pp. 11–13 for examples contrasting democratic, bureaucratic, and capitalist logics, and throughout for a presentation of these logics applied to aspects of the state; see also 13 for an application of this scheme to the nonprofit sector.) None of these logics is by any means exclusive to a particular institutional arena. For example, while the state is most often seen as the primary locus of bureaucratic development, corporate organizations in the capitalist sector use some elements of bureaucratic structure, such as for coordinating resource acquisition, production tasks, and product marketing (14).

More specifically for the argument here, key to nonprofit status becoming the dominant mode of early 20th century hospital development was the successful mustering by hospitals of claims to voluntarism and charity in the local community. By developing such claims to community purpose and participation, consistent with the above defined logic of democratic culture, hospitals could stave off government intrusion or competition from the development of government hospitals as unnecessary and unwanted by local communities. At the same time they could lay claim to "doing the public's business" and thereby claim quasi-public, or nonprofit, tax status. How such nonprofit organizations developed and changed according to differing logics for differing purposes over time is all important and will be a crucial point in the laying out of our argument.

Previous analyses (e.g., 15) cite the passage of Medicare and the unwillingness of the medical establishment to submit to public controls as the key elements in fostering corporate development in medical care. While not disagreeing, per se, we find both the transformation and the necessary explanation to be more complex. For an explanation of this historical transformation must account for (a) how public and nonprofit sector institutions, rather than capitalist sector institutions, came to be and continued to be the major source for provision of medical services in the first place, and how the commodity status of medical services came to be and continued to be obscured; (b) how and why institutions of the capitalist sector moved into (or were not kept out of) this arena at this historical moment; and (c) how, why, and to what extent the nonprofit hospital has become an institution that is largely indistinguishable from corresponding for-profit institutions.

To address these questions, that is, to assess the extent of these transformations, it is necessary to examine the changing relations between ideological claims and markets on the one hand, and the changing nature of work carried out within the hospital setting on the other. We argue that the transformations of how these tasks have been conducted internally, how they have been managed internally, and how they have become subject to external management (and by whom), have both been shaped by and affected broader ideological and market changes. That changing markets and ideology are restructuring the hospital industry is well known. Our analysis here will originate from the other pole of the dialectic, that of the commodity transformations of hospital tasks and the congruent structural changes in the nonprofit hospital sector.

❖ Hospital Tasks and Institutional Logics

Until the latter part of the 20th century, medical services delivery tasks have been "ill-defined," unstandardized, and lacking in clear specificity apart from the professional judgment of physicians (16). Neither having nor being required to seek clearly definable units of service to provide a consistent basis for payment, hospitals instead sought an open-ended payment for services, where available (17).

The uncertainty that historically characterized core hospital tasks has been typical of that for human service organizations more generally in both public and nonprofit sectors (18). These organizations differ from capitalist production organizations in that the core tasks of the latter are claimed to be, and have typically been regarded as, more well defined and measurable, and as having predictable and measurable outcomes (14, 19, 20). As such, successful task completion in production organizations is said to be evaluated according to efficiency criteria, which are in turn consistent with ac-cumulation in the capitalist sector. The question of measurability of tasks and predictability of outcomes in an organization is taken as important as a matter of capitalist logic for external monitoring, management, and/or investment. That is, such measurability and predictability are necessary for external control by investment capital.

By contrast, where tasks are not clearly specifiable nor outcomes pre-dictable, tasks cannot easily be subjected to efficiency criteria. By the same token, an organization conducting such tasks is not one whose activities can be easily structured under a logic of accumulation (except under special task and market conditions, as discussed below). Organizations whose tasks could not be organized under criteria of efficiency toward a goal of profit-making, but whose tasks were nonetheless understood to be responding to a need (if not a market), were largely developed in public or nonprofit sectors in keeping with the logic of a democratic culture (again, in contrast to capitalist or bureaucratic logics; see beginning arguments in the above discussion). Until recently, most medical and all human service organiza-tions could be characterized in these terms.

But the issue is not just the changing "nature" or "substance" of the tasks, though it is that. It is also a matter of who controls task definitions and how that control is maintained; similarly, who controls when, whether, and where the tasks are conducted, who judges the results (were they com-pleted successfully and what should be done next?), and—as a matter of market transaction—what payment is claimed and/or secured for task com-pletion. The changing (un)certainty with which tasks can be specified and conducted and their results evaluated (and by whom), and how those everyday judgments can be carried out as elements of market relations in the production of medical services—these are the central problems in ex-plaining the commodity transformations of medical care tasks.

The difference between physician production of tasks and hospital pro-duction of tasks is key to understanding the changes that have occurred. We begin by examining physician services as capitalist production.

❖ Physician Tasks and Capitalist Logic

Physicians, working mostly in solo practice, developed mo-nopoly control of medical services early in the 20th century (15, especially Part I, Chapt. 6; 21). While the medical services tasks conducted by phy-sicians were mostly ill-defined and open-ended, what allowed the organi-zation of these open-ended services under a capitalist logic (when they were not so ordered in the hospital) can be found in the level and character of task control in the (vigorously asserted) individualistic practice of physician services. Control and autonomy have of course been the central issue for defining professional status (16). Specifically, physician services were or-ganized by "visits," whether to the home of the patient or the office of the physician. The what/where/how/when of medical tasks performed by the physician were organized under the market unit of a "visit," all decided by physician judgment, for which the physician was directly paid. Although the level of uncertainty about the substance or outcomes of treatment/service tasks was high, because the tasks (of whatever sort) were not separate "tasks," but rather part of a "visit"—that is, the visit was the unit of labor/market transaction—and the physician determined the appropriate payment for that unit, then the uncertainties of the market could be almost completely controlled by the physician. (This logic also applied to small physician-owned, or proprietary, hospitals.) The later hallmark of "no interference in the doctor-patient relationship" was the core of maintaining stability in the original medical market transaction, capitalist independence of (petit bourgeois) physicians, and the exclusion of government as well as corporate "intrusion." This control, claimed as a matter of professional rights, would eventually come under significant challenge, as would physicians' position as capitalist entrepreneurs (22–25). But this gets us ahead of the argument.

❖ The Origin of Medical Services in The Nonprofit Sector

By contrast, original core public/nonprofit hospital tasks were largely custodial or supportive, requiring little sophistication and having little technical or technological support. The earliest hospitals in Colonial American society began as almshouses, places for the poor, that also became hospitals because of the number of sick among the poor (26, 27). They were places for people who had no one to care for them and, until the beginning of the 20th century, places where people died as often as they were cured. Since the services provided were largely to the poor and had unreliable outcomes, little payment was provided or expected in return; charitable support came from the local community.

Diagnostic and treatment capabilities were limited. Likewise, the course of an illness and/or treatment was of limited predictability. That is, we can say more generally that core hospital tasks were open-ended, lacking clear predictability in outcomes or specifiability of the relationship between treatment and outcome. Claims for payment were under the category of "hospital stay," typically defined by the number of days. Nor was payment assured, since hospital patients tended to be sicker and poorer than those treated at home. Moreover, treatments to patients and lengths of stay, to the extent they were specific, were decided not by the hospital but by the physician; that is, these tasks were not under hospital control. Consistent with our argument above, hospital tasks were not amenable to organization under a capitalist sector logic.

Instead, the conduct of medical services tasks since the beginnings of "scientific medicine" at the turn of the century and until fairly recently was seen by nonprofit hospitals as delivery of *services* in response to the needs of the community and as having a limited financial base from patient payments. Founded and operated by religious and other charitable organizations and by local communities (as public hospitals), these hospitals were thus deemed nonprofit entities and worthy of support by and protection of the state (17). As organizations of the nonprofit sector, hospitals have operated within an institutional logic that characterizes that sector as a whole. That is, they were entities that successfully claimed to exist not to make a profit but to serve community needs, needs that the state would otherwise have to respond to, and sometimes did. Of course, the definition of community needs by members of those local communities, as typically represented on hospital boards, meant that the definitions would themselves reflect, for example, patterns of stratification and/or exclusion. Stevens (17) has pointed out how much hospitals constituted vehicles for the visible demonstration of status and class differences. However these claims to serve community needs were constructed, a measure of their success was the response of the state to encourage and legitimate organizational tasks so conducted and accordingly to protect these organizations from taxation.

An initial but largely obscured variation in core hospital tasks was marked by the early successes of surgical procedures and the high visibility of these treatment results. The attraction of paying patients to community hospitals during the early decades of this century was coupled with clear demarcations between paying and indigent patients (the beginnings of two-tiered hospital care). Despite these resources and respective divisions, hospitals continued their ideological claims for charity status, based on their community orientation and the fact that any (capital) expansion could be accomplished only through outside, largely community (i.e., charity or foundation) support (17). Notably, however, while dependent on their local communities for expansion, at the same time hospitals controlled any local expansion by virtue of these very ties, the services they provided to local communities (and what Stevens (17) calls their function as repositories for community values), and the legitimacy thereby granted them by the local communities, as community and/or nonprofit hospitals.

Standardization of hospital tasks, at least theoretically possible for certain surgical tasks that produced clear and consistent results (and provided the basis for "marketing" of the hospital to those who could pay), was at the same time rejected by both doctors and hospitals. For example, E. A. Codman's attempt during the early part of the century (1913–1916) to establish an "end results" system that would analyze surgical results for their benefits to patients was rejected in favor of "standardizing the surgeon" (17, p. 77), thereby ensuring continued authority of the surgeon and eliminating an increased potential for external monitoring and control. Thus by controlling the *definition* of their core tasks, hospitals could market their (mostly surgical) successes to attract paying patients while claiming charity (nonprofit) status, and thereby control the flow of local resources, thus *essentially controlling the market and effectively denying its existence.*

❖ Technology and the Codification of Medical Service Tasks

A shift in the primary locus of medical care tasks to hospital settings (formerly managed by physicians in homes or offices), and the beginning codification of these tasks into identifiable units, were produced by the rapid expansion of hospitals and hospital technology after World War II and the corresponding growth of medical knowledge. Hospital growth during the period (roughly) 1946–1964, partially under the stimulus of Hill-Burton federal funding, was notably controlled at the local level. Where new hospitals were established, these entities developed under the same logic as existing facilities—that is, as community-based nonprofit organizations—and almost never competing with them.

A movement to an initial set of observable and potentially measurable hospital-based task outcomes emerged with the startling successes of new drugs, such as uses of antibiotics to produce "quick" cures, and the spreading availability of hospital-based technological equipment. Further, while the locus of medical expertise once resided solely in the person of the physician and in his judgment, now the locus of the "best" practice of medicine (core medical care tasks), although still under the direction of the physician, moved increasingly from the person of the physician to the technology of the hospital. That is, new medical diagnostic procedures and the treatment regimens indicated by them increasingly became focused around testing facilities and equipment available only in the hospital. Despite the shift in the locus of core medical care tasks, because the changes were perceived by physicians as the result of medical research conducted by physicians, they were regarded by physicians (and the public) as remaining under their definition and control.

Moreover, a significant portion of core medical care tasks were now performed by equipment whose use by technicians or physicians could be routinized, and whose results were measurable and predictable. Combined with the above-noted increasing potential predictability and measurability of treatment outcomes resulting from advances in drugs, treatment technology, and the concurrent development of medical research, the gathering and analysis of data on the course and consequences of treatment regimens promoted the codification and routinization of some of these regimens under the administrative control of hospital administrators or physician managers.

Medical care delivery tasks in the hospital were transformed into more well-defined and specifiable units of service as bureaucratic rules and a bureaucratic logic were increasingly used to control hospital operations.[1]

---

[1]As such, this transformation prefigured a proletarianization of physicians; but this delimiting of physician authority was itself initially delimited and obscured as such by continuing market entry control (of patients to hospitals) by these medical professions (25).

Notably, however, this imposition of bureaucratic logic was carefully circumscribed, developed only for internal hospital management, clearly not subject to external review or control by the state, and at most organized around ostensive goals of more efficient medical treatment, such as acquisition and use of latest available medical technologies, not around ones of economic efficiency. Although physicians in some instances had less direct control of these tasks, they supported and promoted most of these changes in a search for higher quality medical practice, which, as such, they still perceived themselves as controlling. In the name of better medicine, medical care delivery tasks were undergoing a movement in commodity form from open-ended services to potentially well-defined products. But this movement, like the emerging market, was ideologically and organizationally obscured.

The increase in employer-based health insurance and third-party reimbursement, predominantly Blue Cross, and the consequent routinization of billing, *could* have served as an external constraint to force *standardization* of all hospital diagnostic and treatment procedures. *Instead,* insurance payment was organized under an open-ended reimbursement for "usual, customary, and reasonable" charges, retrospectively defined by the hospitals (and doctors). That is, it was organized under the same logic of open-ended task conduct that undergirded the ideological claims to nonprofit status by hospitals. Further, following the community-based logic and control by hospitals, Blue Cross structured the fiscal and organizational management of health insurance with a community-based rating system under a state or regional, not a national, management structure (17).

Thus, despite increasing movement toward routinization and codification of significant core tasks under an internal hospital bureaucracy, hospitals still controlled how these tasks were defined and externally perceived. They thereby continued their ideological claims to nonprofit status, based on their charity/community orientation and rooted in the (supposed) nonstandardizability of the core medical service tasks they conducted. Absence of and resistance to external standards for monitoring fostered continued ideological success.

❖ State Intervention and the First Commodity Transformation

An essential impetus for transformation of both medical services and the nonprofit sector was provided by state intervention in 1965 with the establishment of Medicaid and Medicare as a (soon to be expanding) source of stable funding for the performance of increasingly specifiable medical care tasks. Ostensibly, Medicare was implemented in a fashion "without interference in existing arrangements of practice." It has been often noted, for example, that in so doing the federal government "surrendered direct control of the program," for example by lodging the reimbursement mechanism in existing arrangements, predominantly Blue Cross/Blue Shield organizations (15, p. 375; see also 28).

More generally we can say that Medicare was implemented under the organizational logic of tasks conducted by a nonprofit entity. That is, in keeping with existing patterns of practice, Medicare was implemented under a fiscal logic of open-ended service delivery and task management: cost-plus reimbursement that would be entirely determined by the hospitals and doctors receiving the payment. Such arrangements were likewise in keeping with the ideological claims made in the political arena by nonprofit hospitals in order to maintain their current market status.

However, while still in general keeping with this logic, two effective changes from existing arrangements made at the behest of hospitals had far-reaching implications. First, the choice of Blue Cross as the fiscal intermediary was intended to keep current payment mechanisms in place, but the provision of a national rather than local/regional fiscal base catapulted that organization to a national and *independent* status not answerable to the local community level, whose medically related institutional decisions, such as how to use funds, were still largely controlled by nonprofit hospitals (17). Second, the agreed upon patient cost-reimbursement schedules for the provision of (still) "open-ended" medical care tasks included capital assets depreciation, allowing significant direct expansion of capital assets and effective access by hospitals to capital markets for nonprofits (15).

It is well known that this produced a boom in hospital expansion, encouraged the further production of high-tech medical equipment, and was followed by the emergence of what soon would be called the medical-industrial complex (28; see also 22, 23, 29; for a recent review see 30). Significantly, however, and contrary to the extant nonprofit logic, Medicare and Medicaid monies, followed by private insurance monies, unlike those of Hill-Burton, were not allocated to local communities and thence to hospitals, but directly to any hospital providing medical care services under these programs. Where previously hospitals had controlled local expansion by virtue of their ties to local communities that effectively controlled and obscured local markets and monies and their use for potential expansion, now facilities development and market expansion could be based on economic and political considerations and funding sources *external* to the local community. Key to movement of corporate sector organizations into a theretofore hidden market of medical care services almost completely controlled by hospitals in the nonprofit sector was not just the availability of new funding for that enterprise, but the loss of local control of that funding—definition of when and where it could be used—by the nonprofit hospitals.

Local and regional health planning of the ensuing 15 years (following the 1974 Health Resources Development and Planning Act) could do little to stem that increasing loss of local fiscal control. Despite the fact that the administrative apparatus of health planning, the Health Systems Agencies (weak from the outset), were often dominated by local hospitals and physicians, the presence of business, health insurance, other community stake-holders, and—in some geographic cases—for-profit hospital representa-tives, eventually eroded the heretofore almost complete control by nonprofit hospitals and physicians of local health-related judgments (31).

The hospital arena of the 1970s—with a high demand market, a stable method of payment for those services, and an organization of services into definable units manageable under an internal bureaucracy, but whose def-inition could no longer be entirely controlled by existing nonprofit hospi-tals—thus became an attractive arena for direct capital/corporate invest-ment. Previous to this stage hospitals had been conveyors of capitalist production, such as high-tech equipment and drugs, fostering the growth of an attendant medical industry; at this point they became the locus for direct investment. With cost-plus retrospective reimbursement for services, hospitals faced few limits on services expansion and developed very rap-idly in both for-profit and nonprofit sectors.[2] That is, hospital operation could be funded under a nonprofit logic and at the same time—because of the funding arrangements—move significantly toward a capitalistic logic of accumulation, a transforming of medical care delivery from services to products.

❖ The Second Transformation and the Development of External Task and Market Controls

The implementation of the Medicare DRG system has pro-vided the logical and practical continuation to this process and reflects the second task transformation: a movement to unit task and price definition and to external (from physicians *or* hospitals) control of those unit prices, thereby partially controlling the definition of tasks—a movement from ser-vices to products. If the first transformation might be characterized as a movement of tasks from the physician's office to the hospital, a technolog-ical expansion of those tasks within the hospital, and thereby an organizing of these tasks into definable and measurable units within an internal hos-pital bureaucracy, the second transformation may be characterized as stan-dardizing these units across hospital organizations. That is, definition and measurement of tasks become issues not solely controlled by an internal hospital bureaucracy; they are now subject to external monitoring with con-sequent external task and price decision-making—decisions by purchasers of care as well as by providers.

---

[2]Among other effects these changes spawned new reform efforts, what Alford (32) character-ized as bureaucratic and market reformers, and resulted in almost two decades of debate over market versus regulatory alternatives for controlling hospital growth (for a discussion of how these earlier reform efforts relate to current ones, see 33).

With the increasing task complexity within the hospital came a greater technical sophistication required to manage the tasks therein. But these same capabilities for internal monitoring and management could be used for external market decisions. Thus not only could hospitals, especially non-profit hospitals, no longer be successful at obscuring the market and denying its existence, but they could no longer control the definitions of the tasks that constitute the core of the market. The actual conduct of medical tasks would still rest with the providers, but the specifications of which tasks should be carried out and when became subject to external price decisions and thereby to external scrutiny and control.

As such this transformation resulted in significant new potential power for the market sponsors of medical care (25), the newly deemed purchasers of care.[3] Importantly, however, the exercise of this power has been dependent upon a high level of technical expertise required to sufficiently monitor the substantive and fiscal complexities of the new medical markets (34). Moreover, indicative of the degree to which the power now vested in corporate (e.g., health insurance) or state technical bureaucracies is obscured, this new "regulatory" scheme and others like it have been successfully marketed and imposed under the rubric of a capitalist ideology, that of increased competition and prudent purchasing of care.

Correspondingly and more recently, the implementation of RBRVS (resource-based relative value scale) for physician payments constitutes a movement to unit price definition for physician services (35, 36). Ironically, and not simply coincidentally, the medical care tasks that initially brought greatest success, greatest visibility, and largest payment, surgical treatments, are those that are now seen as most codifiable, overpaid, and likely to come under greatest price control—to wit, the relative reductions in payments for surgical services.

It must quickly be noted, however, that the level of external control of medical services accomplished through codification and standardization of billing for medical care tasks reflected in RBRVS does not necessarily complete diagnosis and treatment standardization. Without narrowly specifiable and standardized diagnosis and treatment alternatives for given medical/surgical problems, variations in frequency (volume) and complexity of diagnoses and treatments are still at the discretion of physicians providing the services, as Wennberg (37) and others have suggested. Utilization review may be similarly understood as a means to standardize treatment provision, although it is more often used as a form of external billing control than as a form of (internal or external) quality control (38, 39).

---

[3]This shift of power, like the previous one, spawned a new round of reform efforts. These new efforts might be characterized in terms of cost-control reformers and inclusive access reformers, depending upon which set of problems and solutions are viewed as most significant, in turn dependent upon whether the interest of the purchaser or the provider of care is pursued (33).

Moreover, the establishment of the Agency for Health Care Policy and Research (AHCPR) with a mandate to promote patient outcomes research, while focused on a narrowly defined agenda relative to high-cost medical procedures, has sweeping implications. In keeping with the arguments here, the outpouring of funds for outcomes and appropriateness research through AHCPR will have the greatest impact on organizational (including billing) standardization for those diagnoses and treatments that can most easily be subjected to *task* standardization, that is, those medical tasks that can be clearly specified and have highly predictable outcomes, most often surgical tasks. Whether changes in practice patterns will occur as a result of changing internal task demands largely controlled by physicians, or of external fiscal demands controlled by purchasers of care, will likely have vast implications for the future overall performance of medical care tasks.

By our analysis, the imposition of cost controls by purchasers of care such as prospective payment, fixed price capitation schemes, contractual arrangements, discounting, and the establishment of DRGs/RBRVS for Medicare reimbursement by the state, all served to *stabilize* market arrangements and to impose limits on further market expansion by providers of care. As such, these actions constitute further impositions of capitalist logic upon the medical care arena and the nonprofit sector therein. Notably, state intervention in this circumstance (via DRGs) is not by virtue of typical state bureaucratic controls over process, but by market controls applied to the pricing of products.

Significant purchasers of care, such as large corporations, insurance companies, and the state, had not previously challenged providers of care over medical services profits, thus allowing uncontrolled expansion. The imposition of controls on these profits entailed the consequent imposition of efficiency criteria on commodity production, as typifies task management in the technical organizations of the capitalist sector, such as imposing measurement and control over, or forcing elimination of, tasks previously conducted under open-ended task organization—talking with patients, for example. Such controls involved the curtailment of medical care delivery tasks that provided little or no financial return.

Under force of these external constraints and internal conditions, medical service organizations of the nonprofit sector have moved to take on organizational structures and practices consistent with a capitalist logic and typical of other organizations within the capitalist sector (23). That is, they have become increasingly like their capitalist competitors (6, 8). Services are now "fragmented," where medical care tasks have been "unbundled" into individual commodity service units. The selection of which tasks would be offered in the "product lines" focuses (capitalist) logically on more profitable units. Service entry is more restricted with an obvious focus on payment ability and market control. Organizational structures are modified to control the flow of patients and dollars through horizontal and vertical integration, such as the development of multi-hospital systems (11) or the addition of home health care units as adjuncts to hospitals (40). In short, it is increasingly the case that medical service organizations of the nonprofit sector can no longer operate as they have in the past and in the manner by which they legitimated their nonprofit status. To wit, the second commodity transformation of medical care delivery tasks and the imposition of a capitalist logic upon the institutional organization of those tasks have required a transformation of the nonprofit sector.

❖ The Politics of The Second Transformation

The rapid expansion of medical care commodities and associated inflation of medical care costs produced an economic confrontation between medical care providers and purchasers of care that previously had been acquiescent partners in prior market arrangements (25, 38, 39). This expansion also produced a political confrontation. Since organizations in the nonprofit sector had been the significant providers of services, and since the state had fostered the growth of that sector under its protection and regulation, the state was equally subjected to that economic confrontation (1). Specifically, moving under a political/ideological banner of cost control, purchasers of care demanded that the state intervene (41, 42). Thus at the same time the state acted to withdraw its regulation and protection under the rubric of competition, it also imposed new and different regulations under the rubric of cost control.

Further, the entry of corporate capitalism not only challenged the status of the nonprofits controlling the medical arena, but confronted the state in its protection of organizations within that arena. As a capitalist logic could be imposed upon the delivery of medical services, no longer was it necessary that state protection be required (under the logic of democracy) to foster the delivery of needed services. With the imposition of a competitive ideology indigenous to the capitalist sector, the status of nonprofits, qua nonprofits, has become increasingly delegitimized.

Political movement has occurred in two basic and contradictory directions. Action initiated from the capitalist sector has been based upon recognition of the above-noted transformations and aimed toward corresponding state sanctions, that is, the removal of nonprofit status and state protection (8, 43). Action initiated from the nonprofit sector has been based upon denial of the transformation and aimed either toward reassertion of a specialized nonprofit role—the provision of services to indigents—and toward continued state support and protection of this role (44), or toward state intervention to provide or impose financing for services now provided by nonprofits to "uncompensated care" patients (30).

The state is forced to mediate between these conflicting sets of material and ideological interests in a fashion that has rarely been necessary before in the health care arena. As the nonprofit sector moves increasingly under a capitalist logic, the competition for market share among nonprofit (and other) medical care providers focuses primarily on those already "served" by medical care, resulting in greater class differences between those who are and are not served. As institutions of this sector are perceived as no longer responsive to the community needs they once assumed under a logic of democracy and nonprofit state protection, the satisfaction of those democratically asserted needs (i.e., needs for those who have no way to pay for medical care under the present system) must once again be assumed by the public sector, that is, the state.

Whatever the state response, it now is faced with traditional claims under the logic of democracy, that of providing services to those in need. The dramatic and rising proportion of the U.S. population denied access to health insurance approximates 37 million, and the political attention to legislative alternatives underscores the severity of this issue. Moreover, to the extent that the state, under attack and/or constraint from several sources, can no longer grant legitimacy to the ideological claims to service by those institutions in the nonprofit sector, neither can the state any longer ideologically defer to that sector's claims to meeting those needs on behalf of the state or the larger society. Put in other terms, the transformation of the nonprofit sector also has entailed the transformation of at least some elements of the state and state activity. For if the nonprofit sector can no longer fulfill its traditional functions under the logic of democracy, the state must assume those functions or find some other alternative. Such action will in turn further erode if not eliminate any remaining functions carried out in the nonprofit sector, such as residual charity care.

What those alternatives might be has been and will continue to be the focus of considerable national debate. State action might take the form of greater intervention in the financing and/or management of medical care on a national scale. Given the apparent limitations thus far of a market-driven medical care system under a capitalist logic to respond sufficiently either to market restraints or to community needs, some form of nationally authorized health management structure could be instituted to constrain and direct the system. The policy formation and implementation of such changes are constrained on the one hand by the capitalist logic that has undergirded present ideological debates and organizational structures, and on the other by the history of the state's intervention to meet democratically defined medical care needs by shifting/granting authority to the nonprofit sector rather than claiming that authority for itself. Because of these constraints a national health care bureaucracy, per se, is not likely. By the same token, little ideological or organizational history is available on which to build claims for the legitimacy of a single-payer system.[4]

---

[4]This is not to say that external histories or evidence, specifically the Canadian single-payer approach, might not be drawn upon to make arguments for reform. Rather the point is that such a model lacks a rich ideological or organizational history in the United States and is thus subject to attacks as being "foreign" to our experience and priorities and therefore not a "legitimate" alternative.

On the other hand, the recent movement in (geographic) state policy and in federal policy consideration to regional health purchasing cooperatives that foster "managed competition" can be seen as a means to accommodate both capitalist and nonprofit logics and ideologies, and to demonstrate the importance of state action—upholding the ideal of democracy in meeting the needs of the people while not violating presumptions of the marketplace. "Managed" competition could suggest both state management and capitalist competition. The response to the Clinton reform proposal was that under such a scheme the state, itself, would establish a national health insurance bureaucracy and, as such (and for other reasons), was explicitly rejected. But this is not the only possibility.

The state could grant authority and legitimation to independent health purchasing cooperatives that would "manage" competition in the public interest, as is happening in some (geographic) states. Under at least some versions of this scheme, these health purchasing cooperatives are nonprofit quasi-public entities that—under cost-containment provisions—would serve either to distribute (with appropriate guidelines and discretion) the flow of public and private dollars into medical care organizations and/or to legitimate insurance-industry control of this flow. The fiscal importance and legitimation function of these new organizations may be seen as a recasting at a broader organizational level of the democratic logic manifested in the earlier (especially pre-Medicare) performance of local nonprofit hospitals. In a sense such new arrangements would, after 20 years, finally "resolve" the health care crisis of the 1960s–1970s by providing the high-level coordination of services demanded by the bureaucratic reformers of that crisis (32, 33). Once again, rather than meeting democratically perceived needs itself, the state would do so by granting legitimate status to nonprofit organizations that organize and conduct the "necessary" activities to meet that need. In so doing, the state also shifts the legitimation deficit it has suffered from nonresolution of the health care crisis—and the health care battleground itself—onto a new entity, authorized by, but independent of, state administrative structures, per se. The state acts and simultaneously protects itself from the direct consequences (44). This process could in turn legitimate the continued expansion of control over providers by the insurance industry under so-called managed care models.

If arrangements such as these—some variation on managed care/managed competition models—simultaneously serve capitalist as well as nonprofit logics and ideologies, then most of the national and state health care debates must be seen as battlegrounds between purchasers and providers and as political occasions for working out the details of more stable market arrangements. Notably absent from the mainstream of the debates are voices from anywhere except purchaser and provider elites and/or sustained arguments about health as a social good rather than as a market commodity. Given long-standing anti-government ideologies and their use to combat most attempts at macro-reforms (31), and given, for example, the obvious success of such ideologies in characterizing market models in the Clinton health plan (i.e., market sponsors—health purchasing alliances) as big government, the likelihood of significant institutional change in health care resulting from Congressionally-based reforms must be considered extremely small. On the other hand, the continuing redefinition and standardization of tasks under managed care models could have significant long-term institutional consequences.

To wit, as suggested by our earlier argument, precisely those elements of task transformation that enabled greater capitalist development and control—the increasing medical task standardization, codification, and consequent external organization and management—will also allow greater intervention and control of these activities under whatever auspices that intervention may occur, including new nonprofit auspices or abdication to the private sector. Ironically, such changes, especially in the name of cost control, could result in the limitation and/or removal of the predominately market-related financial incentives and arrangements that fostered the importation of a capitalist logic to, and have undergirded the capitalist development of, medical care services for the past 25 years. It is more likely, however, that just as markets were secured and obscured by nonprofit hospitals half a century ago, so now the move to quasi-public or nonprofit organizations under managed competition will preserve and consolidate private insurance and thereby further institutionalize present market arrangements under a new rubric.

❖ About the Authors

Allen W. Imershein, Ph.D., is Professor of Sociology, and Associate Professor, Florida State University, Tallahassee.

Carroll L. Estes, Ph.D., is Director, Institute for Health & Aging and Professor of Sociology, Department of Social and Behavioral Sciences, School of Nursing, University of California, San Francisco.

REFERENCES

1. Estes, C., and Alford, R. R. Systemic crisis and the non-profit sector: Toward a political economy of the nonprofit health and social services. *Theory Society* 19(2): 173–198, 1991.

2. Estes, C. L., and Bergthold, L. The unravelling of the nonprofit sector in the U.S. *Int. J. Sociol. Soc. Policy* 9(213): 18–33, 1988.

3. Powell, W. W., and Freidkin, R. Organizational change in non-profit organizations. In *The Nonprofit Sector: A Research Handbook*, edited by W. W. Powell, pp. 180–194. Yale University Press, New Haven, 1987.

4. Ostrander, S. A., Langton, S., and Van Til, J. (eds.), *Shifting the Debate: Public/Private Sector Relations in the Modern Welfare State.* Transaction Books, New Brunswick, 1987.

5. Estes, C. L., and Wood, J. B. The

nonprofit sector and community-based care for the elderly in the U.S.: A disappearing resource? *Soc. Sci. Med.* 23(12): 1261–1266, 1986.

6. Estes, C. L., Binney, E. A., and Bergthold, L. The role of ideology and public policy: The delegitimation of the nonprofit sector. In *The Nonprofit Sector,* edited by V. Hodgkinson and R. Lyman, pp. 21–40. Jossey-Bass, San Francisco, 1989.

7. Herzlinger, R., and Krasker, W. S. Who profits from nonprofits? *Harvard Business Rev.,* January/February 1987, pp. 93–106.

8. Seay, J. D., and Sigmond, R. M. The future of tax-exempt status for hospitals. *Frontiers Health Serv. Manage.* 5(3): 3–39, 1989.

9. Gray, B. (ed.). *For Profit Enterprise in Health Care.* National Academy Press, Washington, D.C., 1986.

10. Gray, B. *The Profit Motive and Patient Care.* Harvard University Press, Cambridge, 1991.

11. Shortell, S. M., Morrison, E. M., and Friedman, B. *Strategic Choices for America's Hospitals.* Jossey-Bass, San Francisco, 1990.

12. Alford, R. R., and Friedland, R. *Powers of Theory.* Cambridge University Press, Cambridge, 1985.

13. Alford, R. R. The political language of the non-profit sector. In *Essays in Honor of Murray Edelman,* edited by R. Merelman. Westview, Boulder, Colo., 1992.

14. Thompson, J. *Organizations in Action.* McGraw-Hill, New York, 1967.

15. Starr, P. *The Social Transformation of American Medicine.* Basic Books, New York, 1982.

16. Freidson, E. *Professional Dominance.* Atherton, New York, 1970.

17. Stevens, R. *In Sickness and in Wealth.* Basic Books, New York, 1989.

18. Imershein, A. W., et al. Measuring organizational change in human services. *N. Engl. J. Hum. Serv.* 3(4): 21–28, 1983.

19. Meyer, J. W., and Rowan, B. Institutionalized organizations: Formal structure as myth and ceremony. *Am. J. Sociol.* 83: 340–363, 1977.

20. Meyer, J. W., and Scott, R. *Organizational Environments.* Sage, Beverly Hills, 1983.

21. Larson, M. S. *The Rise of Professionalism.* University of California Press, Berkeley, 1977.

22. McKinlay, J. Towards the proletarianization of the physician. In *Professionals as Workers,* edited by C. Derber. Oxford University Press, New York, 1982.

23. Navarro, V. *Crisis, Health, and Medicine.* Tavistock, New York, 1986.

24. Larson, M. S. Proletarianization and educated labor. *Theory Society* 9(1): 131–175, 1980.

25. Deber, C. Physicians and their sponsors. In *Issues in the Political Economy of Health Care,* edited by J. McKinlay, pp. 217–254. Tavistock, New York, 1983.

26. Rothman, D. *Discovery of the Asylum.* Little, Brown, Boston, 1971.

27. Shryock, R. *Medicine and Society in America: 1660–1860.* Cornell University Press, Ithaca, 1967.

28. Ehrenreich, B., and Ehrenreich, J. *The American Health Empire: Power, Profits, and Politics.* Vintage, New York, 1971.

29. Salmon, J. W. Organizing medical care for profit. In *Issues in the Political Economy of Health Care,* edited by J. McKinlay, pp. 143–186. Tavistock, New York, 1983.

30. Estes, C. L., Harrington, C., and Davis, S. Medical-industrial complex. In *Encyclopedia of Sociology,* Vol. 3, edited by E. F. Borgatta and M. L. Borgatta, pp. 1243–1254. Macmillan, New York, 1992.

31. Morone, J. A. *The Democratic Wish.* Basic Books, New York, 1990.

32. Alford, R. R. *Health Care Politics.* University of Chicago Press, Chicago, 1975.

33. Imershein, A. W. Health Care Politics—Revisited. Paper presented at the annual meeting of the

American Sociological Association, 1993.

34. Brown, L. D. Technocratic corporatism and administrative reform in Medicare. *J. Health Polit. Policy Law.* 10(3): 579–599, 1985.

35. Physician Payment Review Commission. *Annual Report to Congress.* Washington, D.C., 1988.

36. Lee, P. R., et al. The Physician Payment Review Commission—Report to Congress. *JAMA* 261(16), 1989.

37. Wennberg, J. Dealing with medical practice variations: A proposal for action. *Health Aff.* 3(Summer): 6–32, 1984.

38. Grogan, C. M., et al. How will we use clinical guidelines? The experience of Medicare carriers. *J. Health Polit. Policy Law* 19(1): 7–26, 1994.

39. Tannenbaum, S. J. Knowing and acting in medical practice: The epistemological politics of outcomes research. *J. Health Polit. Policy Law* 19(1): 27–44, 1994.

40. Bergthold, L., Estes, C. L., and Villanueva, A. Public light and private dark: The privatization of home health services for the aged in the U.S. *Home Health Serv. Q.* 11(4): 1–34, 1990.

41. Bergthold, L. *Purchasing Power in Health.* Rutgers University Press, New Brunswick, 1990.

42. Imershein, A. W., Rond, P. C., and Mathis, M. Restructuring patterns of elite dominance and the formation of state policy in health care. *Am. J. Sociol.* 97(4): 970–993, 1992.

43. U.S. Small Business Administration, Office of Advocacy. *Unfair Competition by Nonprofit Organizations with Small Business: An Issue for the 1980s.* Government Printing Office, Washington, D.C., 1983.

44. Imershein, A. W., and Rond, P. C. Elite fragmentation in health care: Proprietary and non-proprietary hospitals in Florida. *Soc. Sci. Q.* 70: 53–71, 1989.

❖ Chapter 10
Quality of, and Access to, Health Care Services

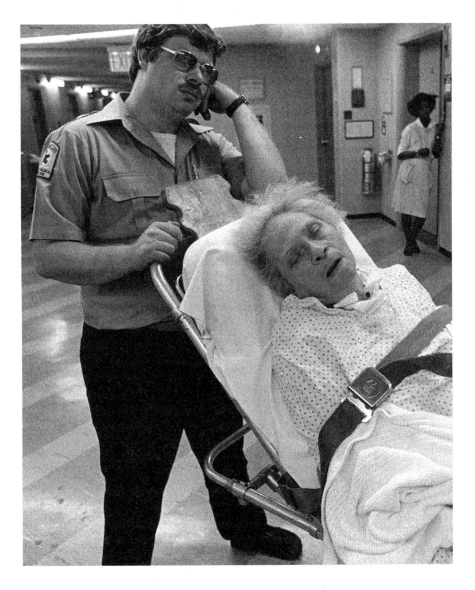

In the previous two chapters, we have addressed several critical access and cost issues emerging as the U.S. health care system undergoes unprecedented changes in the final decade of this century. We turn our attention now to specific concerns about the quality of, and access to, health care services in the United States. Initial studies of quality focused on the process of care and the structure of services provided. In recent years, however, policymakers and researchers have turned their attention to whether the care provided is appropriate and effective, and to identifying the specific outcomes of the services provided. Without outcome measures for increasingly complex therapies and treatments, it is impossible to determine whether or not specific approaches are cost-effective and, importantly, beneficial to patients. Previous emphasis on the process (versus the outcome) of health care services has rendered clinicians, patients, payers, and policymakers woefully uninformed about the efficacy, desirability, and cost-effectiveness of many health care procedures and services that are routinely provided.

The emerging managed care environment insists, as a structural mandate, on measures that concretely indicate the cost-effectiveness of care. In combination with knowledge about the efficacy of interventions and the skills needed to deliver care, the movement to contain costs requires prudent use of outcome data to inform the configuration of appropriate services. In the last edition of *The Nation's Health* (1994),we focused on the need to reduce uncertainty in medical care as much as possible while recognizing acceptable variations in professional practice and care. In this edition, we include papers that represent recent attempts to better define, describe, and measure the quality, appropriateness, and effectiveness of health care services under the increasing specter of constrained resources.

Robert H. Brook, Karen J. Kamberg, and Elizabeth A. McGlynn identify eight issues related to the "cost quality trade-off." To be certain, there were issues of the trade-off between cost and quality long before the current drive to managed care health services delivery systems. The authors are curious as to how the recently intensifying efforts to curtail the growth rate in medical expenditures might affect the balance of this trade-off. Although they have raised critical questions about this relationship within the context of medicine, these issues are also relevant to other health care disciplines and inclusion of this paper is intended to stimulate readers' inquiry as to the important questions facing health care professionals and policymakers on the eve of the 21st century. The authors have also included a succinct overview of the past 25 years of research on how health care system changes affect quality of care and health status and on past approaches to measuring quality of care. The authors address some of the pressing areas of information and action required to keep the issue of quality at the forefront of future policy debates.

The essay by David L. Sackett and his colleagues from the United Kingdom, Canada, and the United States, discusses the concept of "evidence based medicine" and again raises important issues relevant across health care disciplines. The overriding theme of this paper is the need to consider important and unique information about individual patients in light of research-based information about populations of similar patients and to make clinical decisions that reflect these considerations. As defined by the authors, "Evidence based medicine is the conscientious, explicit, and judicious use of current best evidence in making decisions about the care of individual patients" (Sackett et al., 1996, p. 71). Their presentation and discussion encourages thought-provoking consideration of how health care professionals in general might balance internal (patient-centered) and external (population-focused) evidence in formulating care decisions that are appropriate and effective and that result in increasingly better quality at the individual and system levels.

John Wennberg (1993), building on nearly twenty years of research on measuring variations in the health care experiences of populations, provides us with a cogent history and update on this valuable approach to addressing questions of quality, appropriateness, and effectiveness of health care. Wennberg's work and his presentation of future directions for similar study highlight the increasing importance of comprehensively documenting and describing the health care delivery system. His proposal to develop descriptive statistics of resource allocation and capacity is both timely and critical. Such information in conjunction with outcome measures will greatly enhance our abilities to accurately and adequately predict a reasonable balance to achieve optimum quality of services within specific fiscal constraints.

Also in chapter 10 included is Karen Davis' recent article in which she urges particular attention to finding practical mechanisms by which we can address the health care insurance coverage and access needs of the at risk population in light of the rapidly evolving market system that threatens to completely exclude them from any access to needed care.

Although they have not been included in this book because of space limitations, several recent papers add important dimensions to the discussion concerning quality of, and access to, health care. These papers are timely and raise a broad spectrum of continuing issues in the policy arena. We have included these references in the Recommended Reading list because of their importance. Friedman's (1995) informative paper describes the variety of issues in measuring and improving the quality of health care. In this comprehensive work, she provides an historical perspective on the evolution of the health care quality movement, addresses the conceptual issues that require attention in the definition and measurement of quality, identifies several current measures of quality in diverse settings, reviews possibilities for use of existing Medicare data sets and development of new data bases, and concludes with several suggestions for the future directions in the development and evaluation of quality measures. Other important articles on measuring and improving the quality of health care services are included in the issue of *Health Care Financing Review* (Summer 1995) in which this paper was originally published.

In a recent investigation that illustrates the comprehensive nature of health care services, Berk, Schur, and Cantor (1995) construct estimates of American's self-reported ability to access appropriate and needed health care services. Their findings support previous results that indicate approximately six percent of Americans believe they were unable to access needed medical and prescription drugs, eyeglasses, dental services, and mental health care or counseling. This research clearly documents the need to broaden our view of access to appropriate care to include the often neglected non-medically focused services that have quality-of-life implications and that may, indeed, affect the outcomes of other more routinely accessible medical and surgical services.

Appropriateness of care is also reflected in the study by Bindman and colleagues (1996) that investigated access to care for five chronic conditions and preventable hospitalizations in low-income communities. This research supports increasing overall access to care as a strategy to reduce the [costly] and questionably efficacious hospital admission of patients with chronic conditions to effectively receive care that may have been more appropriately provided on an outpatient basis and have eliminated the need for hospitalization altogether.

Uwe Reinhardt (1994), one of the nation's most distinguished health economists, compares the U.S. health care system with those of 23 other Western nations, with particular emphasis on costs of care and access to services. The greatest contrast is that most of these nations provide comprehensive, universal, first-dollar coverage for most major services. Another sharp contrast is that most consumers in these countries are much more satisfied with their health care systems than are consumers in the United States. Included in his article are a number of suppositions about how the European and Canadian systems and the U.S. system might be influenced in the coming years by economic events and public attitudes so that our system might begin to look more and more like theirs, while theirs begin to take on more of the characteristics of our market approach.

❖ Health System Reform and Quality

ROBERT H. BROOK, CAREN J. KAMBERG, AND ELIZABETH A. MCGLYNN

The US health care delivery system is changing rapidly, dominated mainly by the shift from fee-for-service to managed care medicine. What are the implications for the practice of medicine as a result of the shift from patient-based to population-based medicine? As resources directed to health care are reduced, how will the trade-off between cost and quality be altered? Will quality even remain on the agenda as health system reform proceeds?

Health services research over the past 25 years has produced many findings relevant to these issues. For example, losing or acquiring health insurance affects people's health; but if economic incentives are used to alter the amount of care consumed, then the use of clinically based tools is required to avoid the approximately equal decline in necessary and less-than-necessary care. To keep quality of care on the agenda, physicians should be provided both information about the use of specific health services in their geographic catchment area, and the variability of quality as a function of plan, hospital, and, where appropriate, physician. Physicians should also use tools and guidelines both to coordinate care and to determine what care is to be provided in a population-based, multiprovider managed care system. Information must also be made available to the public about the level of quality provided. Finally, to help physicians resolve some of the tension between providing the best care to individual patients vs a group of patients, new ways to assess quality are required.

An article focusing on health system reform and quality of care may seem irrelevant in 1996, or at least too little, too late. Nevertheless, despite the failure to legislate health system reform at the federal level, the issues raised during the health care debate in 1993 and 1994 remain relevant and should continue to be addressed as the health system is "reformed" through market forces.

Even in the absence of national legislation, the health care delivery system in the United States is changing quickly and dramatically, dominated in particular by the shift from fee-for-service to managed care medicine and by the desire to contain the growth rate in medical expenditures. The emergence of managed care as the predominant force in the practice of medicine is virtually assured in the United States. Over 50 million people are currently enrolled in managed care organizations (approximately 20% of all Americans). Eleven managed care plans have more than 500 000 members, and one fourth of all managed care plans have at least 100 000 members. Predictions using reasonable rates of growth indicate that 40% to 65% of the US population will be enrolled in managed care plans in 5 years.[1]

The transition to managed care in the United States has been largely driven by a desire by employers, insurance companies, and the public to control soaring health care costs. Other countries have responded to similar economic pressure by cutting back on the supply of physicians or hospital beds. The curtailment of the growth of the health industry will continue to occur in the United States (and the rest of the world) even in the absence of national legislation.

Most of the literature related to health system reform has focused on macro-level issues such as the benefits of a single payer or whether a medical market can function efficiently. However, more fundamental issues occur at the micro level: As changes in health care payment and delivery systems occur, what are the clinical implications for the practice of medicine? More specifically, as the increase in health care resources is curtailed, how will the trade-off between cost and quality be affected?

Hopefully, this article provides new insights into the relationship between cost and quality, and the practice of medicine. We first present 8 critical questions that should be considered by everyone involved in the changing health care system. The questions are not meant to be exhaustive and critical questions are omitted. Our intent is not even to answer these questions. Rather, we use these questions to illustrate the importance of maintaining quality of care concerns on the policy agenda. The rest of this article provides information on what happens to quality when the system is changed, and how quality can be measured and maintained on the policy agenda. Finally, based on these questions and what we know about how quality can be measured, we suggest actions physicians as a group might pursue in order to ensure that quality remains a central value of the new American solution to the health care crisis of the 1990s.

❖ Eight Issues Related to the Cost Quality Trade-Off

(1) As the shift to managed care continues in response to cost pressures, will efforts focus solely on how to reduce expenditures, or will maintaining and even improving quality remain on the agenda? The principal concern at the employer and insurance company level has been the cost of health care. As health care delivery is transformed to a predominately managed care system, how can we ensure that quality of care remains part of the debate?

(2) How will the delivery of care change as a result of the shift from patient-based to population-based medicine? The emergence of managed care as the predominant health care delivery mode has resulted in a fun-

damental change in the paradigm of medical care. Previously, a physician's primary responsibility was to do everything possible for the patient who visited his or her office. Today, some physicians are responsible for a population of patients and for a budget that needs to be spent wisely. In other words, the physician in a managed care setting is responsible for the health of an entire enrolled population, not just those patients who actively use the health care system. This raises a number of questions: How do physicians made trade-offs between patients competing for limited resources? How much physician time should be invested in dealing with people who do not return to see a physician, or who never see a physician, as opposed to those who use the medical care system voluntarily? What strategies should be undertaken by the physician to track the patient population in terms of mental, physical, and social functioning? Should patients be required to be active participants in evaluating both their health care system and the effectiveness of the services that they receive (eg, provide written information on their physical functioning after receiving a new pair of knees, or provide information that will be used to determine if their physician provided an appropriate physical examination)?

(3) How will a potential reduction in contact time affect the quality of the physician-patient encounter? Since the amount of time afforded these contacts is being reduced, improving the productivity of such encounters becomes even more important. However, several questions surround this issue of productivity. For example, how can the information needed by the physician to make clinical decisions be transmitted quickly and inexpensively? How will we produce outcomes consistent with patient expectations if reduced time with the patient means we do not have an opportunity to assess patient values, or explain the implications of different treatment options? Exactly what level and mix of clinical training is needed to provide the most efficient and effective care to patients?

(4) Will cost containment be a clinically rational process? Will we, like the Dutch[2] and Swedes,[3] set clinically based priorities defining which services should be provided (eg, services for patients who cannot care for their basic needs due to physical or mental problems vs services to further life expectancy or control pain)? Or will care be cut without reference to its potential health benefits?

(5) Are we prepared as a society to take actions needed to improve the medical marketplace? Will we accept even minimal regulation of health plans? Will we require the public to provide or allow access to information necessary to assess both the quality and effectiveness of care?

(6) How much excess supply of health professionals is required to ensure that the level of quality of care is maintained? If we train only enough cardiac surgeons to meet specific demands, what happens if some fraction of them provide care below acceptable standards and the performance of these surgeons cannot be improved? Will the quest for efficiency eliminate a surplus of physicians, so that competition is reduced to a level that

sacrifices quality? If all hospital beds are full, and it takes years to build a new hospital, is there any external motive for a hospital to improve its quality?

(7) What role does public information have in helping ensure that medical care provides the best value to all patients? Until recently, patients have not had access to data about the quality or cost of a particular type of care prior to receiving that care. This has changed somewhat with the public release of 2 forms of information. First, data about provider outcomes and cost have been released by several state and private agencies.[4-6] Second, procedure-specific guidelines are beginning to be published by government and private organizations.[7,8] Both of these forms of information are meant to help patients with their medical care decisions. However, several questions still remain.[9,10] Are the publicly available data on quality of care valid enough to be used by consumers in making health care choices? Are case-mix adjusters adequate to protect against gaming and misuse of data in ways that might actually reduce quality? What method of presenting information is most likely to facilitate consumer use? Indeed, will patients use this information to help them achieve the best value for their medical care dollars?

(8) What will be the effect on society as the currently disadvantaged populations learn, through the public release of information, that they are receiving inferior care? Both access to care and technical quality of care is inferior for disadvantaged populations.[11-16] For example, socioeconomically disadvantaged persons have a higher chance of dying than nondisadvantaged patients when they are hospitalized with a condition that responds positively to medical care (eg, myocardial infarction).[16] In this time of cost containment, is society prepared to make high-quality resources available to all persons?

❖ Lessons From Research

Health services research over the past 25 years has resulted in a dramatic increase in our knowledge about how changes in the health care system affect quality of care and health status, and about how quality of care and health status can be measured. We summarize the findings of some of this research below.

Changes in the Health System and Quality

First, radical changes in health policy, whether produced by the marketplace or government, will profoundly affect the health of people. For example, access to care is dramatically increased if one has health insurance, and this increased access has in turn been shown to improve outcomes, such as whether one lives or dies.[17-20] The most significant action within the health system that we can take to preserve health and improve longevity is to provide health insurance to everyone.

Second, research has shown that changes in economic policy or the organizational structure of the delivery system, short of eliminating health insurance, result in relatively equal reductions in both care that is necessary and care that is less than necessary to maintain health.[21,22] If we want to ensure that such reallocation decisions result in eliminating only less than necessary care, then new, clinically based tools must be provided to physicians and patients.

Third, the current practice of medicine is far from perfect. One fourth of hospital deaths may be preventable,[23] and one third of some hospital procedures may expose patients to risk without improving their health. One third of drugs may not be indicated, and one third of laboratory tests showing abnormal results may not be followed up by physicians.[24]

Fourth, we know that efficacy (the outcome of a procedure performed under ideal circumstances) may not predict effectiveness (the outcome of a procedure performed under usual circumstances), so that results from controlled clinical trials may mislead clinicians weighting the health risks and benefits of an intervention. Two examples illustrate this problem.

The first example is that of carotid endarterectomy. Methodologically sound randomized trials have established the efficacy of carotid endarterectomy in a number of clinical circumstances, including for people who have had a transient ischemic attack and who also have a 70% to 99% obstruction of the carotid artery that is responsible for the attack.[25,26] However, work in community-based practices has shown that the effectiveness of this procedure is much lower than its efficacy, ie, that complication rates among community-based surgeons are not as low and outcomes are not as good as among those in sites participating in controlled clinical trials.[27] A primary care physician in a managed care organization, when faced with recommending either medical care or surgery to a patient for whom results from a controlled clinical trial would favor surgery, must have information about the complication rate and the experience of the surgeon to whom the patient is being referred. Without such information, making clinical decisions based solely on the results of the randomized controlled clinical trial may do more harm than good.

A second example concerns heart attack patients. Today it is believed that hospitalization in a modern coronary care unit results in better outcomes for patients with acute heart attacks than athome care. However, research has also demonstrated that, after controlling for patient severity at admission, hospital death rates for patients who suffer a myocardial infarction may vary by as much as 6 deaths per 100 patients admitted with this disease.[28] What are the implications for the physician who wants to optimize patient outcomes? First, the physician must have data about outcomes at hospitals to which the patient might be admitted. Second, he or she must know the risk of delay if the hospital with the best demonstrated outcomes is farther away than one with worse outcomes. Physicians must have a real-time system that enables them to assess the trade-off between better hospital care and the delay in obtaining it. Will such a system become available in the near future?

Measuring Quality of Care

Perhaps one of the greatest advances in health services research for facilitating the development of a clinically rational system for making resource allocation decisions has been what we have learned about measuring quality of care and health status.

First, we have learned that quality and health status can be measured.[29-34] Although instruments to measure quality of care and health status could, of course, be improved, they are as reliable and valid as the otoscope, the stethoscope, the x-ray, the medical history, and other tools currently used in medicine.[35,36]

Second, we know that the quality of both processes and outcomes of care can be evaluated. Process measures (what is done to a patient) are more sensitive measures of quality of care because poor outcomes (what happens to a patient) may not occur each time something is done incorrectly or something is omitted that should have been done. For example, a process criterion might state that all pregnant women should be screened for gonorrhea; however, omission of the test will result in a poor outcome only occasionally, because most pregnant women do not have the infection, and even if they do, it will not always result in harm. Similarly, failure to give appropriate myocardial infarction patients thrombolytic therapy will not result in the death of all of these patients.

Third, there are 5 different methods that can be used to evaluate quality.[37] The major differences between these methods are the aspect of care that is assessed (process, outcome, or overall) and whether criteria are established *a priori* to judge adherence to a standard (the explicit method) or if expert judgments are used (the implicit method). Although these 5 methods when applied will produce a different absolute value on a quality scale, the results from their application will correlate and an institution that is rated higher on one method will, in general, be rated higher on another.[38]

Fourth, we have determined that if one is to obtain a meaningful measure of quality of care, one usually cannot rely solely on administrative data. An exception to this general rule is the provision of many preventive services where administrative data are adequate to assess quality concerns. However, relevant clinical data to evaluate most aspects of acute and chronic care need to be collected, and this usually involves talking to the patient, observing the physician-patient encounter, or abstracting the medical record.[39-41]

Fifth, outcomes are multidimensional; a complete assessment of the out-

ᵈ ᵇ ꞊ ʰₐᵇⁱ ᵗ

come of care requires the measurement of general, physiologic, mental, physical, and social health and patient satisfaction. In addition, disease-specific outcome data must be collected to measure fully the outcome of care,[30,31] and patient preferences should be incorporated into these assessments. For example, in treating a patient for prostatic cancer one must ask questions about disease-specific outcomes, such as impotence or incontinence.[42]

Sixth, even though it is currently fashionable to measure outcomes other than mortality, such as functioning, we should not lose sight of the fact that mortality is a critical outcome when it comes to assessing quality of care. As stated above, perhaps one fourth of in-hospital deaths from some diseases could be prevented.

Seventh, data obtained by interviewing patients are not sufficient to assess technical quality. Treating a patient in a pleasant and respectful manner (ie, having a high "art" of care) can mask poor technical care. The result is that poor technical quality of care and patient satisfaction can occur simultaneously. For example, a patient undergoing an unnecessary operation (and not realizing the operation is unnecessary) might be satisfied if the art of the care were to his or her liking. It is much easier for the patient to judge if the phone is answered promptly and if he or she can talk with the physician than to judge the clinical appropriateness of a medical procedure.

Finally, procedure-specific or disease-specific guidelines are valuable tools available to physicians when deciding how to treat or refer patients. In addition, clinically based guidelines, which combine science and judgment, help the physician improve patient outcomes.[43-45] Because physicians who perform a procedure are likely to be more enthusiastic about its use than can be justified by the existing science, these guidelines should be developed by multispecialty physician groups that explicitly use the input from all the types of physicians who care for patients with the given disease.[46,47]

❖ Why Information On Quality Is Essential For An Effective System

Now that we have discussed some of the major issues facing the health system in a cost-containment era and some of the findings that can be reached from health services research, we turn to what physicians need to do, know, or lobby for to ensure that quality of care is kept on the agenda as the health care system changes.

First, physicians need to have access to information about the geographic distribution of health services. Where we reside determines to a large extent the procedures or services we receive, with use of many services varying more than 3-fold by geographic area.[48-51] There needs to be an interchange of information among physicians in different parts of the country and in different countries to address questions such as why a particular procedure is performed more in one place than in another. For example, the use of coronary artery bypass graft surgery in persons over 65 years of age is much lower in Canada than in the United States.[52] What is happening in Canada that enables this to occur? Based on clinical criteria and data, is there overuse of the procedure in the United States or underuse in Canada?[53] Is one's socioeconomic status a factor in the receipt of the procedure, regardless of where one lives? Practitioners need to know whether they practice in a low-use or high-use area, what policies or conditions motivate the level of use, and what the implications are for their patients.

Second, physicians (and their patients) need to know that where one receives care is the greatest determinant of the quality of care one receives. For example, quality of care for common medical conditions is worse in US rural hospitals than in urban hospitals.[38] Knowledge that quality varies as a function of hospitals and health systems needs to be disseminated among those who refer patients to hospitals as well as among the patients who receive that care.

Third, physicians need tools to coordinate their patients' care in a complex medical care system. As physicians increasingly practice in groups, the need to transfer information among providers will increase. Until electronic medical records become the standard, we must do better in making sure that patient information is transferred with the patient. For example, if a nursing home patient with a terminal illness arrives at the hospital emergency department, information should travel with that patient about his or her wishes for resuscitation. Similarly, hospital discharge summaries need to be available in the ambulatory setting in a timely fashion so that events and decisions made in the hospital can be incorporated into the patient's outpatient care.

Fourth, we need to recognize that practicing physicians need concise and immediate information about treating their patients. We need to recognize that although articles (such as this one) written for medical journals are useful to an interested audience, most physicians need real-time specific information in order to obtain the best value and quality of care for their patients. Guidelines, disease management strategies, and information on both the costs of different diagnostic strategies or different medications should all be accessible to physicians on a user-friendly computer. The development and implementation of this tool kit across the spectrum of medical care is certainly beyond the capability of individual physicians and most health care companies. It will require cooperation between the public and private sectors and between the producers and the users of clinical science. At a minimum, physicians should insist that the quality standards and criteria are in the public domain and the process by which the tools are produced uses a sufficient level of science to ensure the tools' validity. Evaluation of the adequacy of the science of the tool kit must include questions such as, "Was the scientific literature systematically collected and analyzed, and was expert judgment, when required, incorporated into the tool kit development process in a manner consistent with the best social science practices?"

Fifth, physicians must support the development of efficient, publicly accountable, quality-of-care reporting systems that incorporate the following:

❖ Results from quality-of-care systems should be consistent with economic incentives. Although physician or patient behavior can be changed by noneconomic means, this change is generally small and slow to occur.[54] Both physicians and patients respond strongly and quickly, however, to economic incentives. Patients assigned even a small coinsurance or deductible as part of the Health Insurance Experiment reduced their use of medical services to almost half that of patients with free care.[55] Changing the payment of hospitals from a cost-plus to a fixed-price system when prospective payment was introduced for Medicare resulted in lengths of stay being reduced by one fourth almost immediately.[56] Altering the amount of reimbursement to physicians in home care in Norway dramatically changed the number of home visits within a short period of time.[57] Providers (physicians and hospitals) need to be rewarded by an economic incentive, such as more money or higher market share, for producing better quality medical care.

❖ Quality-of-care reporting systems need to rely primarily on clinically valid process (vs outcome) measures. Outcomes often take too long to occur and can require very large samples to measure a statistically significant effect. For example, because the proportion of low-birth-weight babies delivered by women receiving poor prenatal care is very small, a large sample would be needed to observe differences in outcome (ie, low-birth-weight babies) in one plan or another.[58] One could use process measures that have been shown to improve this outcome in comparing the adequacy of the process of prenatal care among plans.[59]

❖ The reporting system should be based on a model of medically preventable morbidity or mortality, with emphasis on technical quality of care and on preventing underuse of necessary care.

❖ The measures of quality should focus on cost-effective interventions, so that very small improvements in health are not produced at a price that is exorbitantly high.

❖ The measures should cover the scope of outcomes we are prepared to manage and pay for. For example, process measures to deal with helping the elderly to be less lonely should not be included in such a system unless we are prepared to consider relieving loneliness as part of the medical mission of managed care organizations and to reflect that mission in premium prices.

❖ The application of quality-of-care measures should allow us to determine if a managed care organization provides good quality across all diseases and patient subgroups, or if a particular organization is best in handling a specific disease or procedure.

❖ Future Challenges

What does the future hold for managed care organizations? Unquestionably, their activities will be governed by a desire to be less expensive. But should they not also strive for high-quality care for their enrolled population?

One way that quality could be incorporated into the routine activities of a managed care organization would be to collect patient-level quality-of-care process data for use in a system designed to improve outcomes. For example, because managed care plans are responsible for enrolled populations, it would be possible for them to determine the proportion of patients who had died within the prior year. The organization could collect process data concerning each death from the plan's medical records and, by comparing those data to explicit models, or through the use of expert judgment, determine what fraction of deaths was preventable. Was a patient who died of lung cancer and who smoked given the opportunity to participate in a smoking cessation program? Was a heart attack patient who died and who was eligible for thrombolytic therapy given the drug in a timely manner in the emergency department? Disease-specific models could be developed and scores calculated that would indicate the proportion of deaths that could have been prevented by better primary, secondary, or tertiary care. A further analysis of what is needed to obtain better care could then be undertaken. Next, the cost of those actions could be calculated and the plan could decide whether or not to alter the care; and finally, the plan could evaluate its quality improvement strategies. A similar assessment of the potential for improving quality could be accomplished by having a sample of the enrolled population complete a functional status questionnaire. The plan could then determine, through record review or examination of the patient, which functional impairments might be preventable or correctable through the use of, for instance, hearing aids, treatment for depression, or walking aids. One could perform a cost-benefit analysis of proposed changes in process of care, implement changes, and then measure the extent to which those changes affected the population's functional status.

If quality stays on the agenda in a managed care environment, we will need to begin a dialogue about the reasonable limits of medicine. For example, how quickly must a nurse respond to the requests of a hospitalized patient? How often and how many at-home health services should be provided to discharged patients—many such services are labor-intensive, expensive, and may simply not be affordable. Is it the obligation of the physician to inform the patient of all potential options, or should the patient just be apprised of the options "most consistent" with available resources? If a physician does not offer a mammogram to a woman in her early 40s because the scientific evidence does not support the use of screening mammograms among her age group, must she be told of this deliberate decision? If a more expensive combination pill is available for the treatment of hypertension that allows the patient to take 1 pill a day instead of 3 at different times during the day, should that patient be offered the combination drug?

Finally, we need to address the tension between providing the best care to individual patients and providing the best care to a group of patients. How much in the way of resources should be invested in trying to provide quality care to patients who do not have regular recommended mammograms or flu shots, or who do not return to a physician for care for their chronic condition? Should we spend resources on assessing and improving the functional status of depressed patients who do not take their antidepressant medications? Or should resources be reserved for those who do participate in the medical system? As we move toward a combination of population- and patient-based medicine, we will need to address these issues.

These questions may provoke heated discussions between those who believe that quality should be optimized for the individual patient, and those who believe that resources should be allocated to maximize the health of a community. That is, in fact, our objective. No matter how one approaches the issues and no matter how (or if) the issues are resolved, it is very important that such discussions take place. If we do not experiment with new ways to address issues of quality, then it may be impossible to keep quality on the health system reform agenda and we will all be the worse off.

❖ About the Authors

Robert H. Brook, M.D., Sc.D., is Professor, Schools of Medicine and Public Health, University of California, Los Angeles, and is with the RAND Corporation, Santa Monica, California.

Caren J. Kamberg, M.S.P.H., is with the RAND Corporation, Washington, DC.

Elizabeth A. McGlynn, Ph.D., is with the RAND Corporation, Santa Monica California.

REFERENCES

1. *Managed Care Digest: HMO Edition.* Kansas City, Mo: Marion Merrell Dow; 1994.
2. Commission on Choices in Health Care. *Choices in Health Care.* Zoetermer, the Netherlands: Ministry of Welfare, Health, and Cultural Affairs; 1992.
3. Swedish Parliamentary Priorities Commission. *Priorities in Health*

Care: Ethics, Economy, Implementa-tion. Stockholm, Sweden: Swedish Parliamentary Priorities Commis-sion; 1995:5.

4. Pennsylvania Health Care Cost Containment Council. A Consumer Guide to Coronary Artery Bypass Graft Surgery: Pennsylvania's Dec-laration of Health Care Information. Harrisburg: Pennsylvania Health Care Cost Containment Council; 1991.

5. Colorado Health Data Commis-sion. Colorado Hospital Outcomes: Mortality, Length of Stay and Charges for Cardiovascular and Other Diseases. Denver: Colorado Health Data Commission; 1992. Clinical Data Project.

6. National Committee on Quality Assurance. Report Card Pilot Pro-ject. Washington, DC; National Committee on Quality Assurance; 1993. NCQA Technical Report.

7. Konstam M, Dracup K, Baker D, et al. Heart Failure: Evaluation and Care of Patients With Left-Ventricu-lar Systolic Dysfunction. Clinical Practice Guideline No. 11. Rock-ville, Md: Agency for Health Care Policy and Research, Public Health Service, US Dept of Health and Human Services; 1994: AHCPR publication 94-0612.

8. Department of Practice Parameters, American Medical Association. Di-rectory of Practice Parameters: Titles, Sources and Updates. Chicago, Ill: Department of Practice Parameters, American Medical Association; 1996.

9. US General Accounting Office. Re-port Cards Are Useful but Significant Issues Need to Be Addressed: Report to the Chairman, Committee on Labor and Human Resources, US Senate. Washington, DC: US General Ac-counting Office; 1994. Document GAO/HEHS-94-219.

10. US General Accounting Office. Employers Urge Hospital to Battle Costs Using Performance Data Sys-tems: Report to Congressional Re-questers. Washington, DC: US Gen-eral Accounting Office; 1994. Document GAO/HEHS-95-4.

11. Kasiske BL, Newlan JF, Riggio RR, et al. The effect of race on access and outcome in transplantation. N Engl J Med. 1991;324:302-307.

12. Yergan J, Flood AN, LoGerfo JP, Diehr P. Relationship between pa-tient race and the intensity of hos-pital services. Med Care. 1987;25: 592-603.

13. Burstin HR, Lipsitz SR, Brennan TA. Socioeconomic status and risk for substandard medical care. JAMA. 1992;268:2383-2387.

14. Wenneker MB, Epstein AM. Racial inequalities in the use of proce-dures for patients with ischemic heart disease in Massachusetts. JAMA. 1989;261:253-257.

15. Goldberg KC, Hartz AJ, Jacobsen SJ, et al. Racial and community factors influencing coronary artery bypass graft surgery rates for all 1986 Medicare patients. JAMA. 1992;267:1473-1477.

16. Kahn KL, Pearson ML, Harrison ER, et al. Health care for black and poor hospitalized Medicare patients. JAMA. 1994;271:1169-1174.

17. Lurie N, Ward NB, Shapiro MF, Brook RH. Termination from Medi-Cal: does it affect health? N Engl J Med. 1984;311:480–484.

18. Lurie N, Ward NB, Shapiro MF, Gallego C, Vaghaiwalla R, Brook RH. Termination of medical bene-fits: a follow-up study one year later. N Engl J Med. 1986;314:1266-1268.

19. Weissman JS, Epstein AM. Falling Through the Safety Net: The Impact of Insurance on Access to Care. Bal-timore, Md: Johns Hopkins Uni-versity Press; 1994.

20. Franks P, Clancy CM, Gold MR. Health insurance and mortality: evidence from a national cohort. JAMA. 1993;270:737-741.

21. Lohr K, Brook RH, Kamberg C. Use of medical care in the RAND Health Insurance Experiment: di-agnosis- and service-specific anal-

yses in a randomized controlled trial. *Med Care.* 1986;24:S1-S87.

22. Soumerai SB, McLaughlin TJ, Ross-Degnan D, et al. Effects of limiting Medicaid drug-reimbursement benefits on the use of psychotropic agents and acute mental health services by patients with schizophrenia. *N Engl J Med.* 1994;331:650-655.

23. Dubois RW, Brook RH. Preventable deaths: who, how often, and why? *Ann Intern Med.* 1988;109:582-589.

24. Brook RH, Kamberg CJ, Mayer-Oakes A, et al. Appropriateness of acute medical care for the elderly: an analysis of the literature. *Health Policy.* 1990;14:225-242.

25. North American Symptomatic Carotid Endarterectomy Trial Collaborators. Beneficial effect of carotid endarterectomy in symptomatic patients with high-grade carotid stenosis. *N Engl J Med.* 1991;325:445–453.

26. European Carotid Surgery Trialists Collaborative Group. MRC European Carotid Surgery Trial: interim results for symptomatic patients with severe (70-99) or with mild (0-29) carotid stenosis. *Lancet.* 1991;337:1235-1243.

27. Winslow CM, Solomon DH, Chassin MR, et al. The appropriateness of carotid endarterectomy. *N Engl J Med.* 1988;318:721-727.

28. Kahn KL, Rogers WH, Rubenstein LV, et al. Measuring quality of care with explicit process criteria before and after implementation of the DRG-based prospective payment system. *JAMA.* 1990;264:1969-1973.

29. Berzon RA, Simeon GP, Simpson RL, Jr, Donnelly MA, Tilson HH. Quality of life bibliography and indexes: 1993 update. *Qual Life Res.* 1995;4:53-74.

30. Meenan RF, Mason JH, Anderson JJ, Guccione AA, Kazis LE. AIMS2: the content and properties of a revised and expanded Arthritis Impact Measurement Scales health status questionnaire. *Arthritis Rheum.* 1992;35:1-10.

31. Guyatt G, Mitchell A, Irvine EJ, et al. A new measure of health status for clinical trials in inflammatory bowel disease. *Gastroenterology.* 1989;96:804-810.

32. Donabedian A. *Explorations in Quality Assessment and Monitoring, Volume 1: The Definition of Quality and Approaches to its Assessment.* Ann Arbor, Mich: Health Administration Press; 1980.

33. Donabedian A. *Explorations in Quality Assessment and Monitoring, Volume II: The Criteria and Standards of Quality.* Ann Arbor, Mich: Health Administration Press; 1982.

34. Donabedian A. *Explorations in Quality Assessment and Monitoring, Volume III: The Methods and Findings of Quality Assessment and Monitoring.* Ann Arbor, Mich: Health Administration Press; 1985.

35. Koran LM. The reliability of clinical methods, data and judgments, part 1. *N Engl J Med* 1975;293:642-646.

36. Koran LM. The reliability of clinical methods, data and judgments, part II. *N Engl J Med.* 1975;293:695-701.

37. Brook RH, Appel FA. Quality of care assessment: choosing a method for peer review. *N Engl J Med.* 1973;288:1323-1329.

38. Keeler EB, Rubenstein LV, Kahn KL, et al. Hospital characteristics and quality of care. *JAMA.* 1992;268:1709-1714.

39. Iezzoni LI. Monitoring quality of care: what do we need to know? *Inquiry.* 1993;30:112-114.

40. Iezzoni LI, Foley SM, Daley J, Hughes J, Fisher ES, Heeren T. Comorbidities, complications, and coding bias: does the number of diagnosis codes matter in predicting in-hospital mortality? *JAMA.* 1992;267:2197-2203.

41. Iezzoni LI, Restuccia JD, Shwartz M, et al. The utility of severity of illness information in assessing the quality of hospital care: the role of

the clinical trajectory. *Med Care.* 1992;30:428–444.

42. Litwin MS, Hays RD, Fink A, et al. Quality-of-life outcomes in men treated for localized prostate cancer. *JAMA.* 1995;273:129-135.

43. Feder G, Griffiths C, Highton C, Eldridge S, Spence M, Southgate L. Do clinical guidelines introduced with practice based education improve care of asthmatic and diabetic patients? a randomised controlled trial in general practices in east London. *BMJ.* 1995;311:1473-1478.

44. Kravitz RL, Laouri M, Kahan JP, et al. Validity of criteria used for detecting underuse of coronary revascularization. *JAMA.* 1995;274:632-638.

45. Lennox EL, Stiller CA, Morris Jones PH, Kinnier Wilson LM. Nephroblastoma: treatment during 1970-3 and the effect on survival of inclusion in the first MRC trial. *BMJ.* 1979;2:567-569.

46. Kahan JP, Park RE, Leape LL, et al. Variations by specialty in physician ratings of the appropriateness and necessity of indications for procedures. *Med Care.* 1996;34:512-523.

47. Scott EA, Black N. When does consensus exist in expert panels? *J Public Health Med.* 1991;13:35-39.

48. Chassin MR, Brook RH, Park RE, et al. Variations in the use of medical and surgical services by the Medicare population. *N Engl J Med.* 1986;314:285-290.

49. Wennberg J, Gittelsohn A. Variations in medical care among small areas. *Sci Am.* 1982;246:120-135.

50. McPherson K, Wennberg JE, Hovind OB, Clifford P. Small area variations in the use of common surgical procedures: an international comparison of New England, England, and Norway. *N Engl J Med.* 1982;307:1310-1314.

51. Bunker JP. Surgical manpower: a comparison of operations and surgeons in the United States and in England and Wales. *N Engl J Med.* 1970;282:135-144.

52. Anderson GM, Grumbach K, Luft HS, Roos LL, Mustard C, Brook RH. Use of coronary artery bypass surgery in the United States and Canada. *JAMA.* 1993;269:1661-1666.

53. McGlynn EA, Naylor CD, Anderson GM, et al. Comparison of the appropriateness of coronary angiography and coronary artery bypass graft surgery between Canada and New York State. *JAMA.* 1994;272:934-940.

54. Grimshaw JM, Russell IT. Effect of clinical guidelines on medical practice: a systematic review of rigorous evaluations. *Lancet.* 1993; 342:1317-1322.

55. Newhouse JP, Manning WG, Morris CN, et al. Some interim results from a controlled trial of cost sharing in health insurance. *N Engl J Med.* 1981;305:1501-1507.

56. Brook RH, Kosecoff JB. Competition and quality. *Health Aff (Millwood).* 1988;7:150-161.

57. Kristiansen IS, Holtedahl K. Effect of the remuneration system on the general practitioner's choice between surgery consultations and home visits. *J Epidemiol Common Health.* 1993;47:481-484.

58. Siu AL, McGlynn EA, Morgenstern H, Brook RH. A fair approach to comparing quality of care. *Health Aff (Millwood).* 1991;10: 63-75.

59. Chalmers I, Enkin M, Keirse MJN, eds. *Effective Care in Pregnancy and Childbirth.* Oxford, United Kingdom: Oxford University Press; 1989: vol I, *Pregnancy,* pt I-V and index; vol II, *Childbirth,* pt VI-X and index.

❖ Evidence Based Medicine: What It Is and What It Isn't

It's About Integrating Individual Clinical Expertise and the Best External Evidence

DAVID L. SACKETT, WILLIAM C. ROSENBERG,
J. A. MUIR GRANT, R. BRIAN HAYNES,
W. SCOTT RICHARDSON

Evidence based medicine, whose philosophical origins extend back to mid-19th century Paris and earlier, remains a hot topic for clinicians, public health practitioners, purchasers, planners, and the public. There are now frequent workshops in how to practice and teach it (one sponsored by the *BMJ* will be held in London on 24 April); undergraduate[1] and postgraduate[2] training programmes are incorporating it[3] (or pondering how to do so); British centres for evidence based practice have been established or planned in adult medicine, child health, surgery, pathology, pharmacotherapy, nursing, general practice, and dentistry; the Cochrane Collaboration and Britain's Centre for Review and Dissemination in York are providing systematic reviews of the effects of health care; new evidence based practice journals are being launched; and it has become a common topic in the lay media. But enthusiasm has been mixed with some negative reaction.[4-6] Criticism has ranged from evidence based medicine being old that to it being a dangerous innovation, perpetrated by the arrogant to serve cost cutters and suppress clinical freedom. As evidence based medicine continues to evolve and adapt now is a useful time to refine the discussion of what it is and what it is not.

Evidence based medicine is the conscientious, explicit, and judicious use of current best evidence in making decisions about the care of individual patients. The practice of evidence based medicine means integrating individual clinical expertise with the best available external clinical evidence from systematic research. By individual clinical expertise we mean the proficiency and judgment that individual clinicians acquire through clinical experience and clinical practice. Increased expertise is reflected in many ways, but especially in more effective and efficient diagnosis and in the more thoughtful identification and compassionate use of individual patients, predicaments, rights, and preferences in making clinical decisions about their care. By best available external clinical evidence we mean clinically relevant research, often from the basic sciences of medicine, but especially from patient centred clinical research into the accuracy and precision of diagnostic tests (including the clinical examination), the power of prognostic markers, and the efficacy and safety of therapeutic, rehabilitative, and preventive regimens. External clinical evidence both invalidates previously accepted diagnostic tests and treatments and replaces them with new ones that are more powerful, more accurate, more efficacious, and safer.

Good doctors use both individual clinical expertise and the best available external evidence, and neither alone is enough. Without clinical expertise, practice risks becoming tyrannised by evidence, for even excellent external evidence may be inapplicable to or inappropriate for an individual patient. Without current best evidence, practice risks becoming rapidly out of date, to the detriment of patients.

This description of what evidence based medicine is helps clarify what evidence based medicine is not. Evidence based medicine is neither old hat nor impossible to practice. The argument that "everyone already is doing it" falls before evidence of striking variations in both the integration of patient values into our clinical behaviour[7] and in the rates with which clinicians provide interventions to their patients.[8] The difficulties that clinicians face in keeping abreast of all the medical advances reported in primary journals are obvious from a comparison of the time required for reading (for general medicine, enough to examine 19 articles per day, 365 days per year[9]) with the time available (well under an hour a week by British medical consultants, even on self reports[10]).

The argument that evidence based medicine can be conducted only from ivory towers and armchairs is refuted by audits from the front lines of clinical care where at least some inpatient clinical teams in general medicine,[11] psychiatry (J R Geddes *et al*, Royal College of Psychiatrists winter meeting, January 1996), and surgery (P McCulloch, personal communication) have provided evidence based care to the vast majority of their patients. Such studies show that busy clinicians who devote their scarce reading time to selective, efficient, patient driven searching, appraisal, and incorporation of the best available evidence can practice evidence based medicine.

Evidence based medicine is not "cookbook" medicine. Because it requires a bottom up approach that integrates the best external evidence with individual clinical expertise and patients' choice, it cannot result in slavish, cookbook approaches to individual patient care. External clinical evidence can inform, but can never replace, individual clinical expertise, and it is this expertise that decides whether the external evidence applies to the individual patient at all and, if so, how it should be integrated into a clinical decision. Similarly, any external guideline must be integrated with individual clinical expertise in deciding whether and how it matches the patient's clinical state, predicament, and preferences, and thus whether it should be applied. Clinicians who fear top down cookbooks will find the advocates of evidence based medicine joining them at the barricades.

Some fear that evidence based medicine will be hijacked by purchasers and managers to cut the costs of health care. This would not only be a misuse of evidence based medicine but suggests a fundamental misunderstanding of its financial consequences. Doctors practicing evidence based medicine will identify and apply the most efficacious interventions to maximise the quality and quantity of life for individual patients; this may raise rather than lower the cost of their care.

Evidence based medicine is not restricted to randomised trials and meta-analyses. It involves tracking down the best external evidence with which to answer our clinical questions. To find out about the accuracy of a diagnostic test, we need to find proper cross sectional studies of patients clinically suspected of harbouring the relevant disorder, not a randomised trial. For a question about prognosis, we need proper follow up studies of patients assembled at a uniform, early point in the clinical course of their disease. And sometimes the evidence we need will come from the basic sciences such as genetics or immunology. It is when asking questions about therapy that we should try to avoid the non-experimental approaches, since these routinely lead to false positive conclusions about efficacy. Because the randomised trial, and especially the systematic review of several randomised trials, is so much more likely to inform us and so much less likely to mislead us, it has become the "gold standard" for judging whether a treatment does more good than harm. However, some questions about therapy do not require randomised trials (successful interventions for otherwise fatal conditions) or cannot wait for the trials to be conducted. And if no randomised trial has been carried out for our patient's predicament, we must follow the trail to the next best external evidence and work from there.

Despite its ancient origins, evidence based medicine remains a relatively young discipline whose positive impacts are just beginning to be validated,[12,13] and it will continue to evolve. This evolution will be enhanced as several undergraduate, postgraduate, and continuing medical education programmes adopt and adapt it to their learners' needs. These programmes, and their evaluation, will provide further information and understanding about what evidence based medicine is and is not.

❖ About the Authors

David L. Sackett, is Professor, National Health Service Research and Development Center for Evidence-Based Medicine, Oxford-Radcliffe NHS Trust, Oxford.

William C. Rosenberg, is Clinical Tutor in Medicine, Nuffield Department of Clinical Medicine, University of Oxford, Oxford.

J. A. Muir Grant is Director of Research and Development, Anglia and Oxford Regional Health Authority, Milton Keynes.

R. Brian Haynes is Professor of Medicine and Clinical Epidemiology, McMaster University, Hamilton, Ontario, Canada.

W. Scott Richardson is Clinical Associate Professor of Medicine, University of Rochester School of Medicine and Dentistry, Rochester, New York.

REFERENCES

1. British Medical Association, *Report of the working party on medical education.* London: BMA, 1995.
2. Standing Committee on Postgraduate Medical and Dental Education. *Creating a better learning environment in hospitals. 1. Teaching hospital doctors and dentists to teach.* London: SCOPME, 1994.
3. General Medical Council. *Education committee report.* London: GMC, 1994.
4. Grahame-Smith D. Evidence based medicine: Socratic dissent. *BMJ* 1995;310:1126-7.
5. Evidence based medicine; in its place [editorial]. *Lancet* 1995;346:785.
6. Correspondence. Evidence based medicine. *Lancet* 1995;346:1171-2.
7. Weatherall DJ: The inhumanity of medicine. *BMJ* 1994;309:1671-2.
8. House of Commons Health Committee. *Priority setting in the NHS: purchasing. First report 1994–95.* London: HMSO, 1995. (HC 134-1).
9. Davidoff F, Haynes B, Sackett D, Smith R. Evidence based medicine: a new journal to help doctors identify the information they need. *BMJ* 1995;310:1085-6.
10. Sackett DL. Surveys of self-reported reading times of consultants in Oxford, Birmingham, Mil Keynes, Bristol, Leicester, and Glasgow. In: Rosenberg WMC, Richardson WS, Haynes B, Sackett DL. *Evidence-based medicine.* London: Churchill Livingstone (in press).
11. Ellis J, Mulligan I, Rowe J, Sackett DL. Inpatient general medicine is evidence based. L. 1995;346:407-10.
12. Bennett RJ, Sackett DL, Haynes RB, Neufeld VR. A controlled trial of teaching critical approach of the clinical literature to medical students. *JAMA* 1987;257:2451-4.
13. Shin JH, Flaynes RB, Johnston ME. Effect of problem-based, self-directed undergraduate education on life-long learning. *Can. Med Assoc J* 1993;148:969-76.

❖ Future Directions for Small Area Variations

John E. Wennberg

Approximately 18 years ago, Alan Gittelsohn and I published an article in *Science* called "Small Area Variations in Health Care Delivery."[1] In that article, we set forth a strategy for measuring the health care experiences of populations and uncovered a number of issues that have driven my research ever since. Most remain relevant today. My plan is to (1) review briefly the strategies of small area analysis; (2) identify the major policy issues that emerged from approximately 20 years of variation research, and (3) suggest some priorities for the future. I will end by suggesting that small area analysis provides an important tool for the reform of health care markets because

- ❖ It poses and helps answer the "which rate is right?" question (this is helpful in the reform of the microeconomy).
- ❖ It provides information relevant to the control of capacity (this is helpful in the reform of the macroeconomy).

❖ Background

Small area analysis is distinguished by at least four important features. First, it provides population-based rates. Second, it focuses on local provider communities, usually hospital market areas, with the intent of measuring variability among providers. Third, it can provide a comprehensive description of the health care delivery system, i.e., the types and quantities of resources deployed, such as the numbers of hospital beds and physicians per capita; the per capita expenditures for care; the services produced, in the aggregate and specifically (such as the rates for specific procedures); and the health care outcomes that occur at the population level. Fourth, it seeks answers to policy-relevant questions. When variations occur, why do they occur? What is the role of consumers (patients)? What are the roles of suppliers and public policy? How does variability relate to productivity? When greater amounts of resources are deployed (such as hospital beds or neurosurgeons per capita), what additional services are provided? When more is provided, what are the consequences for health outcomes?

❖ The Current Status of Variations Research

A number of the articles presented at this conference are devoted to the first two features of small area analysis—the measurement of rates and the definition of geographic areas. I have little to add to this growing discussion. However, much less attention currently is being paid to the unfinished tasks of providing a comprehensive description of the health care delivery system. When Alan Gittelsohn and I first envisioned what a small area analysis would look like, we were guided by a practical concern. In the late 1960s, I went to Burlington, Vermont, as the director of Vermont's Regional Medical Program. The Regional Medical Program furnished the resources and the focus for developing the small area approach. The resources of this program made it possible for us to develop the strategy for the purpose of solving one of the major problems of regional planning, i.e., what is the distribution of resources? The solution we developed was the allocation strategy for assigning resources to the populations that used them. Our *Science* article described the inputs to populations of hospital and nursing home beds, home health agency resources, and most important, the numbers of full-time equivalent physicians and other health care providers that were allocated to specific populations. Using this approach, we learned that some regions had twice as many surgeons and three times as many family practitioners as did others.

Most of the subsequent work in small area methods has concentrated on the utilization of care, not the distribution of resources.[2] Perhaps, this is because, in the 1980s, the country abandoned the idea of planning and became enamored with the notion that market forces would somehow even out the distribution of resources, or, at least, make the distribution of resources sensitive to patient demand. This neglect is unfortunate. I think it is inevitable that there will be a return to the problems of how many resources there are and how much is enough.

I want to propose the development of descriptive statistics of resource allocation and capacity as a priority area for research in the 1990s. Progress in this area will be greatly facilitated by the Health Care Financing Administration's recent implementation of a single, uniform billing number for physicians. This makes it possible to develop indicators of physician labor inputs with much greater ease because, formerly, a physician could have multiple identification numbers and, conversely, could share a single identification number with other physicians.

Although additional methodologic work will be needed to determine the degree to which the utilization patterns of Medicare enrollees predict the pattern of geographic usage for all patients, previous work suggests that the method is useful.[3] A national data base describing hospital market area locations and physician labor inputs is a feasible goal.

Let me briefly summarize the progress that has been made in the descriptive epidemiology of the use of specific services. We know a good deal, particularly about the patterns of use of surgery and of hospitals. The variation phenomenon has been widely studied in many parts of the world.[2] Most operations and causes of admissions to the hospital exhibit highly variable patterns of use, demonstrating an intrinsic variability greater than that seen for our empiric standard for discretionary surgery, i.e., the hysterectomy. The patterns of variation tend to be consistent between geographic areas.[4] In the case of surgery, the variability represents different hypotheses for the management of specific conditions, in which one option is usually medical management. Thus, variation in bypass surgery rates reflects tradeoffs between drug management versus angioplasty versus surgery. In the case of admissions for medical conditions, the variability has its source in the tradeoff between inpatient and outpatient strategies for the handling of sick patients, usually those with chronic diseases. Descriptive statistics describing the variability for ambulatory services have been less well studied and deserve some attention in the years to come.

Let me next consider some of the policy uses of small area studies. When variations occur, why do they occur? A good deal of effort has been spent tracking this problem. Some may still hold to the neoclassic theory of economics that utilization is determined by medical progress and patient demand, mediated through the physician who serves as a rational agent for patients, but the tide seems to have turned. Policy makers, patients, and physicians increasingly recognize the importance of professional uncertainty about what works in medicine. They are also recognizing the flaws in the agency role, i.e., supplier-induced demand based on the entanglement of professional preferences with those of patients.

The evidence for the professional uncertainty hypothesis and supplier induced demand arises from many sources, not the least of which is the critical appraisal of the strength of the evidence that treatments work as postulated. The important studies to develop the knowledge base, more often than not, simply, have not been done.[5,6] Another line of evidence is the failure to find consistent correlations between illness rates or access rates and the use rates for care. Yet a third source is a seldom-studied and underrecognized factor as to why the distribution of resources does not relate to illness rates, i.e., resources such as hospital beds are built for all sorts of reasons, including religious and professional orthodoxies, educational needs, and competition. None has to do with the relative illness rates or hypotheses about the benefits of specific levels of supply. Moreover, given the lack of direct information on the size of a population served by a provider, decisions to add resources in the local economy are, even now, made without knowledge of how many resources there are already relative to the population being served. Thus, as we see from our studies in Maine, surgeons immigrating into the state are as likely to settle in an area already abundantly supplied with their specialty as one that is not. It seems to me that those who argue for neoclassic economics have an obligation at least to hypothesize mechanisms through which the deployment of resources is modulated by rational decisions made in the context of the doctor-patient relationship.

Among the more interesting questions which small area analysis can address are: (1) how resources are used and (2) with what effect on health.

As an example, take the market for surgery. In virtually every small area, the supply of surgeons seems to exceed the amount required to provide procedures to the local population for those conditions which most, if not all, physicians—surgeons and nonsurgeons—agree are needed. Principal among such conditions are hip fractures, colonic cancer, and inguinal hernia. It is no coincidence that, for these conditions, the rates of surgery vary little among most small areas, closely reflecting the incidence of disease. These conditions, however, are the exception. Most of the workload of surgeons in the United States is invested in treating conditions for which there is little consensus about the single correct method of treatment.[6,7] Most of the investment is in conditions for which there are valid nonsurgical alternatives. Again, it is no coincidence that the rate of surgery for these conditions tends to be higher in markets with more surgical specialists per capita.

The effect of the supply of surgeons on the rate for specific procedures is, however, somewhat idiosyncratic because the individual surgeon will tend to concentrate on one of several possible workloads. For example, although we cannot precisely predict which surgical rate will increase when a neurosurgeon moves into an area, the effect will most likely be an elevation in either the back surgery or the carotid endarterectomy rate, but not both. I believe this occurs because surgeons become comfortable with a small range of procedures and are able to find patients for whom these procedures are "appropriate," no matter what the supply.[8,9]

The relationship between the supply of beds and rate of admissions to the hospital is similar but not identical. Hospital use for medical admissions track the available bed supply, i.e., populations living in areas with higher per capita inputs of beds experience greater hospital use. However, the supply of beds exerts a ubiquitous effect on the rate of admission to a hospital for most acute and chronic conditions. The exceptions, again, are those few conditions that physicians seem to agree should almost always be treated in a hospital, such as heart attacks or hip fractures. However, such conditions account for less than 10% to 15% of medical patient days.[7]

The second question, the effect of variation in the resources and services used on the outcomes of care, has become a central priority of the Congress and Agency for Health Care Policy and Research. Most of the effort has concentrated on variations in treatment hypotheses for specific conditions, such as benign prostatic hyperplasia (surgery versus watchful waiting), back pain (surgery versus medical management), and angina (bypass surgery versus angioplasty versus medical management). Variations research has been instrumental in identifying the need for such assessments by raising the question, "which rate is right?" However, small area variation studies provide only an entry to the problem. The Patient Outcomes Research Team (PORT) approach is applying a variety of experimental and nonexperimental strategies to attack the outcome problem.

There is, however, an important and relatively neglected area at the juncture between variations and outcomes research that warrants considerable attention. This concerns the aggregate impact of health care services on health, i.e., whether it is safe and in the public interest to reallocate resources invested in high-cost high-use rate areas to more productive purposes. The uses made of hospitals when bed supply increases is a good example of a type of problem that may not yield to the PORT condition-specific approach. The reason is that hospital resources are allocated across broad and fuzzy sets of illnesses without clear hypotheses as to why more is better or even how resources might be used. It is not possible to open a textbook of medicine and find a debate about how many beds per capita are needed to treat sick people. Indeed, it is fair to say that the theoretic basis for deploying hospital resources against chronic and most acute medical conditions is implicit. Practice patterns emerge out of the matrix of supply. Physicians do not know the numbers of beds per capita that are used in their communities. Those practicing in high rate areas, like Boston, are not aware that they use more inpatient beds, nor are their theories of practice known to be different. Physicians practicing in low rate areas, such as New Haven, do not believe that they are rationing care, in the sense that they are withholding valuable services because they do not have enough beds. Medical reasoning and the supply of resources appear to be in equilibrium.

The contribution of variations research in such fuzzy zones seems most promising if the question of outcomes is kept global. Given the lack of an explicit hypothesis to test, is it possible to find any evidence that more is better? Correlations between age-adjusted utilization and mortality rates are a good place to start. Jean Freeman (personal communication) has been characterizing the propensity to admit terminally ill patients to the hospital, which varies substantially among market areas as a function of bed supply. Briefly, her results suggest that the greater the per capita bed supply, the greater the proportion of resident population who die in the hospital and the more days that are spent in the hospital during the last year of life. In this study, there is no suggestion that more is better in terms of greater life expectancy among area residents. Indeed, the correlation sometimes go vaguely in the opposite direction, raising the hypothesis that more invasive intensive hospital-based care of the elderly patient results in a decrease in the life expectancy.

We are also pursuing a cohort approach to studying the relationship between the propensity to intervene and the life expectancy. Elliott Fisher (unpublished data) has developed a strategy for identifying cohorts of patients according to the reason for their admission and place of residence. He found that patients living in areas with a greater availability of hospital resources experience greater probabilities for readmission to the hospital, no matter what their initial condition is. The relative risks of admission for these cohort members are exactly predicted by the relative risks for hospital use obtained in cross-sectional variations. Moreover, when the cohorts are further classified according to the hospital used during the initial admission it becomes clear that hospitals within an area differ in their propensity to treat intensively. We think this cohort strategy, which allows for life-table analysis, provides a good basis for examining the effects of variations in the intensity of care and life expectancy.

❖ Small Area Analysis and Health Care Reform

What about the role of small area variations in strategies to reform health care markets? I want to make explicit a distinction that I have already introduced between the microeconomy of the doctor—patient relationship (in which individual patient problems are evaluated and services produced) and the macroeconomy (i.e., the strategies and forces that determine the size of the national health care economy and the deployment of its resources among local markets).

The "which rate is right?" question, directed to the microeconomy asks the following. What is the rate of service that would occur if patients were fully and neutrally informed about the state of medical progress (what works and what are the uncertainties) and if they were free to choose the treatments they wanted, according to their own preferences? By raising the question of the insufficiency of the knowledge base in medicine and by pointing out that quality in medicine must include the principle that the choice of treatment should be free from supplier-induced demand, small area studies have helped set the agenda for reform of the doctor-patient relationship, for the replacement of delegated decisionmaking with shared decisionmaking, and a commitment by the profession to the ethic of evaluation. This is probably all it can do. Outcomes and preference research must do the rest.

At the level of the macroeconomy, however, I see an increasing role for small area studies as the nation struggles to learn how to redirect its health care priorities. The descriptive statistics of small area studies, particularly those concerned with resource allocation, stimulate policy makers to consider new options. The case of Oregon stands out. This state chose a strategy for containing capacity that required the explicit rationing of effective services, such as bone marrow transplantation. Small area studies challenge the necessity to ration services that are known to work and which patients want by pointing to the many examples of excess capacity in the supply of hospitals and physicians—a capacity above that required to produce services that work and patients want. It also offers an alternative. Oregon, like New England, has its Bostons and its New Havens, its examples of high and low rates of use of resource allocation. Their locations become known through small area studies. Elliott Fisher, Gil Welch, and I have shown where these areas are and estimated the resources that would be available if the resources allocated to hospitals were freed up.[10] The potential for reallocation is extraordinary. Three hundred million dollars would be available if the rates of use in New Haven were adopted in Boston. If the high rate areas in Oregon were reduced to the rate seen in Salem, the state capital, the resources needed to fund the entire Oregon Medicaid program would be realized.[10,11]

The research tradition of small area studies sets the stage for a public debate and, possibly, the emergence of a political consensus on the definition of excess capacity. It provides a technology that points to its location among the local hospital market areas of the nation. This may prove the most interesting and challenging use of this research.

❖ About the Author

John E. Wennberg, M.D., is Professor and Director of the Center for Evaluative Clinical Sciences, Dartmouth Medical School, Hanover, New Hampshire.

REFERENCES

1. Wennberg JE, Gittelsohn AM. Small area variations in health care delivery. Science 1973;183: 1102.

2. Paul Shaheen P, Clark JD, Williams D. Small area analysis, a review and analysis of the North American literature. J Health Polit Policy Law 1987;12:741.

3. Wennberg J, Jaffe R, Sola L. Some uses of claims data for the analysis of surgical practices. In: Proceedings of New Challenges for Vital and Health Records. Bethesda, MD: Public Health Service, publication no. (PHS) 81-1214, 1980.

4. Roos N, Wennberg J, McPherson K. Using diagnosis related groups for studying variations in hospital admissions. Health Care Financ Rev 1988;9:53.

5. Cochrane AL. Effectiveness and Efficiency: Random Reflections on Health Services. London: Nuffield Provincial Hospital Trust, 1972.

6. Wennberg JE, Bunker JP, Barnes B. The need for assessing the outcome of common medical practices. Annu Rev Public Health 1980;1:277.

7. Wennberg JE. Small area analysis and the medical care outcome problem. In: Agency for Health Care Policy and Research Conference Proceedings: Research Methodology: Strengthening Causal Interpretations of Nonexperimental Data. Bethesda, MD: Public Health Service, publication no. (PHS) 90-3454, 1990:177.

8. Chassin MR, Kosecoff J, Park RE, et al. Does inappropriate use explain geographic variations in the use of health care services? A study of three procedures. JAMA 1987;258:2533.

9. Wennberg JE. The paradox of appropriate care. JAMA 1987;258: 2568.

10. Fisher ES, Welch HG, Wennberg JE. Prioritizing Oregon's hospital resources: An example based on variations in discretionary medical utilization. JAMA 1992;267:1925.

11. Wennberg JE, Freeman JL, Culp WJ. Are hospital services rationed in New Haven or over-utilised in Boston? Lancet 1987;1:1185.

❖ Incremental Coverage of the Uninsured

KAREN DAVIS

Trends in today's health care marketplace are putting care for the uninsured at risk. The numbers of insured are growing,[1] and safety net providers such as public hospitals and community health centers are feeling the financial strain of the growth of Medicaid managed care. The uninsured have experienced difficulty obtaining needed care in the past,[2-7] and their ability to obtain such care in the future is in even greater jeopardy.

In the absence of attention to the aggregate problem of the uninsured, special focus on vulnerable subpopulations—children, low-income women, the unemployed, and older uninsured adults—should receive greatest priority. Incremental changes that would expand health insurance coverage to groups most likely to benefit from access to care would reduce the immediate burdens created by shrinking availability of free care.

❖ Incremental Options for Expanding Health Insurance Coverage

Building on existing programs and administrative structures offers a foundation for incremental expansions. Three strategies for expanding health insurance coverage for those most at risk deserve consideration: Medicaid expansions, permitting purchase of Medicare by older adults, and financing care for the unemployed.

Given the success of Medicaid in enrolling the most vulnerable populations in health insurance plans—including one third in managed care plans—expanding Medicaid to cover other low-income individuals is a relatively quick and administratively feasible strategy. Consider the following 3 options:

Accelerating Coverage of Children Aged 12 to 18 Years in Families With Incomes Up to the Federal Poverty Level

Currently, states are required to bring poor children into Medicaid 1 year at a time, so that all poor children will be eligible for Medicaid by the year 2002. Accelerating this timetable would bring 1 million poor, uninsured adolescents into coverage more quickly.

Coverage of Parents of Medicaid Children

Covering low-income women only during pregnancy makes little sense because it creates particular problems for managed care health plans and undermines continuity of care.[8] Giving states the option of covering poor parents of Medicaid children with federal matching funds or mandating coverage would reduce turnover in enrollment, promote continuity in relationships with primary care physicians, and permit greater emphasis on preventive care.

Subsidized Purchase of Medicaid for Near-Poor Families

For those low-income families with incomes above the poverty level who do not have access to health insurance coverage through their employment, permitting the purchase of Medicaid on a subsidized basis or sliding scale would encourage these families to move into jobs and take on increased hours by allowing them to keep Medicaid.

These options, while incremental and targeted on relatively healthy families, would require additional budgetary outlays at a time when budgetary pressures are particularly intense. There are approximately 9.4 million uninsured people with incomes below the poverty level in the United States, including approximately 3.3 million adult women, 4.0 million adult men, 1.1 million adolescents, and 1.0 million poor children younger than 13 years. The 1993 average Medicaid cost per child covered under Aid to Families With Dependent Children (AFDC) is $1057, while the average Medicaid cost per adult covered under AFDC is $1959.[9] At the outside, full coverage of all poor uninsured Americans under Medicaid might add $18 billion annually to the program (assuming that participation is 100% and health status is the same as and not better than currently covered Medicaid beneficiaries).

Options for financing expanded coverage include earmarking budget savings from changes in disproportionate share payments to hospitals under Medicare and Medicaid for this purpose (approximately $4.4 billion annually from Medicare[10(p.273)] and $16.9 billion annually from Medicaid[9]), increasing tobacco taxes ($10 billion annually[10(p.280)]), or assessing managed care plans, employer health insurance plans (including Employee Retirement Income Security Act plans), and Medicare 2% of revenues to contribute to a pool for expanding Medicaid coverage (over $10 billion annually).

❖ Financing Health Insurance for the Unemployed

Since most workers obtain health insurance through their place of employment, loss of a job also often triggers loss of health insurance coverage. While the Consolidated Omnibus Budget Reconciliation Act

(COBRA) provisions permit continuation of coverage, such an option is often not financially feasible at such an economically stressed time for families. Only an estimated 20% of eligible people participate.[11] Using unemployment compensation funds to pay COBRA premiums or partially subsidize premiums for unemployed workers would help many families maintain their financial equilibrium at times when money is scarce.

❖ Making Medicare Available to Older Adults

One approach to assuring the availability of health insurance to older adults (ie, those between the ages of 55 and 64 years) is to give them the option of purchasing Medicare. The policy option of permitting adults younger than 65 years to purchase Medicare could be extended on a subsidized basis.

Premiums for older adults could be based on expected average costs for older adults in "average" health. This would require additional federal revenues to subsidize the premium if, as would seem likely, the Medicare buy-in option attracts older adults in poorer health. Some higher costs of adverse risk selection may be offset by Medicare's lower administrative costs and provider payment rates. Coverage could be extended to the following: all adults 55 to 64 years of age not covered by an employer plan (8 million people); family members of Medicare beneficiaries not covered by an employer plan (0.6 million spouses and 0.3 million dependents); early retirees taking Social Security cash benefits at age 62 years not covered by employer plans (1 million people). All of these incremental policy options would reduce the numbers of older adults at risk—but at a cost. Coverage of older adults is expensive, since per capita costs are highest among this group. Moreover, the option of early buy-in to Medicare coverage might accelerate the trend for employers to drop retiree health coverage. Yet, employers are cutting back on such commitments in any event,[12] and only 31% of Medicare beneficiaries have employer-provided retiree benefits.[13] As the baby boom population hits the 55- to 64-year-old range at the turn of the century, the number of uninsured older adults will become an increasingly serious problem.

In the context of broader options to address the financial solvency of Medicare, including raising the age of eligibility, it makes some sense to consider permitting beneficiaries to buy in at an earlier age on a subsidized basis. Trading off higher premium contributions, for example, for those older than 65 years with coverage options for those younger than 65 would make it easier for people to pay for their out-of-pocket medical expenses over the course of their retirement. A portion of Medicare savings from reduction or elimination of Medicare disproportionate share payments and other budgetary proposals under consideration could be used to finance needed subsidies.

❖ Conclusion

Reengaging the issue of expanding health insurance coverage is a difficult task—both economically and politically. Yet seeing that expanded health insurance coverage gets back on the national agenda is especially urgent in the changing US health care system. With the ongoing erosion of employment-based coverage for workers and retirees and the fact that jobs are no longer as long-lasting or stable as they once were, linking health insurance to employment may work even less well in the future. Absent a new foundation on which to build toward universal coverage, more modest, pragmatic steps should be explored. Building on bases capable of insuring and, as necessary, subsidizing costs of coverage for the uninsured offers the opportunity to broaden access to care at a time when market forces threaten to close doors previously open to the uninsured.

❖ About the Author

Karen Davis, Ph.D., is Executive Vice President of the Commonwealth Foundation, New York City. She is former Professor and Chair, Department of Health Policy and Management, School of Hygiene and Public Health, The Johns Hopkins University, Baltimore.

REFERENCES

1. Fronstin P, Rheem E. *Source of Health Insurance and Characteristics of the Uninsured: Analysis of the March 1995 Current Population Survey.* Washington, DC: Employee Benefit Research Institute: February 1996. EBRI Issue Brief 170.

2. Berk ML, Schur C, Cantor JC. Ability to obtain health care. *Health Aff (Millwood).* 1995;14:139-146.

3. Bindman AB, Grumbach K, Osmond D, et al. Preventable hospitalizations and access to health care. *JAMA.* 1995;274:305-311.

4. Braveman P, Schaaf VM, Egerter S, Bennett T, Schecter W. Insurance-related differences in the risk of ruptured appendix. *N Engl J Med.* 1994;331:444-449.

5. Franks P, Clancy CM, Gold MR. Health insurance and mortality. *JAMA.* 1993;270:737-741.

6. Hafner-Eaton C. Physician utilization disparities between the uninsured and insured: comparisons of the chronically ill, acutely ill, and well nonelderly populations. *JAMA.* 1993;269:787-792

7. Weissman JS, Gatsonis C, Epstein AM. Rates of avoidable hospitalization by insurance status in Massachusetts and Maryland. *JAMA.* 1992;268:2388-2394.

8. Short PF. *Medicaid's Role in Insuring Low-Income Women.* New York, NY: The Commonwealth Fund; 1996:1-8.

9. Liska D, Obermaier K, Lyons B, Long P. *Medicaid Expenditures and Beneficiaries: National and State Profiles and Trends 1984-1993: A Report of the Kaiser Commission on the Future of Medicaid.* Washington, DC: The Kaiser Commission; July 1995: 1-140.

10. Congressional Budget Office. *Reducing the Deficit: Spending and Revenue Options.* Washington, DC:

US Government Printing Office; February 1995:273.

11. Claxton G. *Reform of the Individual Health Insurance Market: A Report for The Commonwealth Fund*. Washington, DC: The Lewin Group; 1996:1-44.

12. Pension and Welfare Benefits Administration, US Dept of Labor. *Retirement Benefits of American Workers: New Findings From the September 1994 Current Population Survey*. Washington, DC: US Dept of Labor, September 1995:1-119.

13. Health Care Financing Administration. *Profiles of Medicare—1996*. Washington, DC: Health Care Financing Administration; May 1996:chart H-11.

❖ Recommended Reading

Adler, N. E., Boyce, T., Chesney, M. A., Folkman, S., and Syme, L. (1993). Socioeconomic inequalities in health: No easy solution. *Journal of the American Medical Association, 269*(24): 3140–3145.

Abdelmonem, A. A., & Breslow, L. (1994). The maturing paradigm of public health. *Annual Review of Public Health, 15:* 223-35.

Aiken, L. H. (1995). The registered nurse workforce: Infrastructure for health care reform. *Statistical Bulletin, 76*(3):2-9.

Aguirre-Molina, M., & D. M. Gorman. (1996). Community-based approaches for the preventions of alcohol, tobacco, and other drug use. *Annual Review of Public Health 17:* 337-358.

Andrulis D.P., Acuff, K. L., Weiss. K. B., & Anderson, R. J. (1996). Public hospitals and health care reform: Choices and challenges. *American Journal of Public Health, 86*(2):162-165.

Berk, M. L., C. L. Schur, & J. C. Cantor. (1995). Ability to obtain health care: Recent estimates of the Robert Wood Johnson Foundation National Access to Care Survey. *Health Affairs, 14:* 138-146.

Bindman, A. B., K. Grumbach, D. Osmond, M. Komary, K. Vranizan, N. Lurie, J. Billings, and A. Stewart. 1995. Preventable hospitalizations and access to health care. *Journal of the American Medical Association, 274:* 305-311.

Blumenthal, D., (1991). The timing and course of health care reform. Abridged from *The New England Journal of Medicine, 325*(3):198-200, under "Sounding Board: The timing and course of health care reform." Copyright 1991 by the The New England Journal of Medicine. Reprinted by permission of the publisher in The Nation's Health (4th edition, pgs. 219-223).

Bodenheimer, T., & Estes, C. L. (1994). Long Term Care: Requiem for Commercial Private Insurance. (Published in the 4th edition of *The Nation's Health,* pgs. 350-358)

Bond, P., & Weissman, R. (1997, forthcoming). The costs of mergers and acquisitions.

Bortz IV, W. M., & Bortz II, W. M. (1996). How fast do we age? Exercise performance over time as a biomarker. *Journal of Gerontology: MEDICAL SCIENCES, 51A*(5):M223-M225.

Breslow, L. (1990). The future of public health: prospects in the United States for the 1990s. *Annual Review of Public Health, 11:* 1-28.

Brindis, C. (1995). Promising approaches for adolescent reproductive health service delivery: The role of school-based health centers in a managed care environment. *The Western Journal of Medicine, 163* (2)(suppl):50-56.

Brook, R. H., Kamberg, C. J., and McGlynn, E. A. (1996). Health system reform and quality. *Journal of the American Medical Association, 276*(6): 476-480.

Brown, J.R., Ye, H., Bronson, R.T., Dikkes, P., and Greenberg, M.E. (1996). A defect in nurturing in mice lacking the immediate earely gene fosB. *Cell, 86:*297-309.

Bunker, J.P. (1995). Medicine matters after all. *Journal of the Royal College of Physicians (London), 29:* 105-12.

Bunker, J.P., Frazier, H.S., and Mosteller, F. (1994). Improving health: measuring effects of medical care. *Milbank Quarterly, 2:*225-58.

Burke, T.A., Shalauta, N.M., Tran, N.L. (1994). The Environmental Web.

Identification of state environmental services. A profile of the state infrastructure for environmental health and protection. A report for the Health Resources and Services Administration. U.S. Public Health Service.

Clinton, W.J. (1992). "The Clinton Health Care Plan." *New England Journal of Medicine, 330*(1):75-79.

Collins, F.S. (1995). Positional cloning moves from perditional to traditional. *Nature Genetics* 9:347-50.

Collins, F.S. (1996). Advances in genetics research and technologies: challenges for public policy. Presented before the Senate Committee on Labor and Human Resources. Washington DC.

Commission on Risk Assessment and Risk Management. (1996). Risk assessment and risk management in regulatory decision-making. Draft report for public review and comment.

Culbertson, R. and Lee, P.R. (1997, forthcoming). Medicare and physician autonomy.

Davis, D.L., and Bradlow, H.L. (1995). Can environmental estrogens cause breast cancer? *Scientific American, 273*(4):166-172.

Davis, K. (1996). Incremental coverage of the uninsured. *Journal of the American medical Association, 276*(10:831-832.

Donelan, K., Blendon, R.J., Hill, C.A., Hoffman, C., Rowland, D., Frankel, M. and Altman, D. (1996). Whatever happened to the health insurance crisis in the United States? *Journal of the American Medical Association,* 276(16):1346-1350.

Donley, Sr. R. (1995). Advanced practice nursing after health care reform. *Nursing Economics,* 13(2):84-88, 98.

Duffy, J. (1990). *The sanitarians: a history of public health.* Unisersity of Illinois Press, Chicago, IL.

Dunlop. (1988). *Scientists, citizens, and public policy.* Princeton, NJ: Princeton University Press.

Enthoven, A.C. (1993). "The History and Principles of Managed Competition," *Health Affairs,* Supplement. 12: 24-48.

Enthoven, A.C. & Kronick, R. (1991). Universal health insurance through incentive reform. (Published in the 4th edition of *The Nation's Health,* pgs. 284-291).

Estes, C. L. (1992). Privatization, the Welfare State, and Aging: The Reagan-Bush Legacy. Abridged from a paper presented at the 21st Annual Conference of the British Society of Gerontology, University of Kent at Canterbury, September 19, 1992. Reprinted by permission of the author in *The Nation's Health* (4th edition, pgs. 138-148).

Estes, C. L., and Close, L. (1993). Public policy and long term care. In R.P. Abeles, H. C. Gift, & M. G. Ory (Eds.), *Aging and quality of life* (pp. 310-335). New York: Springer.

Evans, R.G., Barer, M.L., and Marmor, T.R. (eds). (1994). Why some people are healthy and others are not? The determinants of health of populations. New York: Aldine De Gruy.

Fagin, C.M. (1996). Improving nursing practice, education, and research. *Journal of Nursing Administration,* 26(3):30-37.

Fee, E. (1991). The origins and development of public health in the United States. In: *Oxford textbook of public health (2nd Edition).* W Holland, R Detels, G Knox 3:3-22. Oxford/New York/ Toronto: Oxford Medical Publications. 657 pp.

Friedman, E. (1991). The uninsured: From dilemma to crisis. Abridged from *Journal of the American Medical Association 265:* 2491-2495. Copyright 1991, American Medical Association.

Fuchs, V. R. (1996). Economics, values, and health care reform. *American Economic Review, 86:* 1-24.

Gershon, A. A. (1995). Present and future challenges of immunizations on the health of our patients. *Pediatric Infectious Diseases Journal 14:* 445-449.

Glantz, S.A. (1996). Preventing tobacco use—the youth access trap. *American Journal of Public Health, 86:* 156-158.

Guyer, M.S., and Collins, F.S. (1993). The Human Genome Project and the future of medicine. *American Journal of Diseases of Children, 147:* 1145-52.

Guyer, M.S., and Collins, F.S. (1995). How is the Human Genome Project doing, and what have we learned? *Oroceedings of the National Academy of Science. 92:*1841-8.

Halfon, N., Inkelas, M., and Wood, D. (1995). Nonfinancial barriers to care for children and youth. *Annual Review of Public Health 16:* 447-472.

Harrington, C. (1996). Nurse staffing: Developing a political action agenda for change. *Nursing Policy Forum,* 2(3):14-27.

Hubbard, R., and Lewontin, R. C. (1996). Sounding Board: Pitfalls of genetic testing. *The New England Journal of Medicine, 334*(18): 1192-1194.

Immershein, A. W., and Estes, C. L. (1996). From Health Services to Medical Markets: The Commodity Transformation of Medical Production and the Nonprofit Sector. *International Journal of Health Services, 26*(2): 221-238.

Institute of Medicine (IOM). (1988). The Future of Public Health: Summary and Recommendations. Washington DC: National Academy Press.

Jefferys, M. (1996). Social inequalities in health: Do they diminish with age? *American Journal of Public Health, 86:* 474-475.

The Kaiser Commission on the Future of Medicaid. (1996). Policy Brief: Medicaid and long-term care. Washington, DC: The Kaiser Commission on the Future of Medicaid.

Kassirer, J.P. (1994). Academic medical centers under siege. *New England Journal of Medicine, 331*(20):1370-1371.

Kaplan, G. A., Pamuk E. R., Lynch JW, Cohen RD, Balfour JL. (1996). Inequality in income and mortality in the United States: analysis of mortality and potential pathwyas. *British Medical Journal, 312:* 999-1003.

Kessler, D. A. (Jul 20, 1995). Nicotine addiction in young people. *The New England Journal of Medicine, 333:* 186-189.

Kessler, D. A., Witt, A. M., Barnett, Philip S., et al. (September 26, 1996). The Food and Drug Administration's regulation of tobacco products. *The New England Journal of Medicine, 335*(13):988-994.

McGinnis, J. M., and Lee, Philip R. (1995). Healthy People 2000 at mid decade. *Journal of the American Medical Association, 273:*(14)1123-1129.

Lee, Philip R. (1995). Keynote Address: State of the Nation's Health. *Bulletin of the New York Academy of Medicine,* 72(Winter Supplement 2):552-569.

Lee, Philip R., and Benjamin, A. E. (1993). Health policy and the politics of health care. Abridged from S. J. Williams & P. R. Torrens (Eds.) *Introduction to Health Services,* 4th edition. Copright 1993 by Delmar Publishers. Reprinted by permission of the Delmar Publishers in *The Nation's Health* (4th edition, pgs. 121-137).

Lee, P. R., and Estes, C. L. (1994). The nation's health(4th Edition). Boston: Jones and Bartlett.

Lee, P.R., Benjamin, A.E., and Weber, M.A. (1996). Policies and strategies for health in the United States. In Oxford Textbook of Public Health (3rd ed.). Oxford: Oxford University Press (in press)

Luft, H.S. (1996). Modifying managed competition to address cost and quality. *Health Affairs,* 15(1):23-48

M. G. Marmot, George Davey Smith, Stephen Stansfeld, Chandra Patel, Fiona North, Jenny Head, Ian White, Eric Brunner, and Amanda Feeney. (1991). Health inequalities and social class. Abridged from *The Lancet,* Vol.337:1387-1392, under the original title "Health inequalities among British civil servants: The Whitehall II Study." (Reprinted by permission of the publisher and authors in the 4th edition of *The Nation's Health,* pg. 34–40).

Max, W. and Rice, D.P. (1993). The cost of smoking in California, (1993.) *Tobacco Control 4(supplement 1):* s39-s46.

Mann, C. (1995). Women's health research blossoms. *Science, 269:* 766-770.

McGinnis, J.M., and Foege, W.H. (1993). Actual causes of death in the United States. *Journal of the American Medical Association, 270:*2207-12.

McGinnis, J.M., and Lee, P.R. (1995). Healthy People 2000 at mid decade. *Journal of the American Medical-Association, 273:*1123-9.

McKeown, T. 1978. Determinants of health. Abridged from Human Nature, April 1978. Copyright 1978 by Human Nature, Inc. (Reprinted by permission of the publisher in the 4th edition of The Nation's Health, pg. 6-13).

McKeown, T. (1979). The role of medicine: dream, mirage, or nemesis? Princeton, NJ: Princeton University Press.

Moon, M., and Davis, K. (1995). Preserving and strengthening Medicare. *Health Affairs, 14*(4):31-46.

Navarro, V. (1990). Race or class versus race and class: Mortality differentials in the United States. *The Lancet, 336:* 1238-1240.

Newacheck, P., Jameson, W.J., and Halfon, N. (1994). Health status and income: The impact of poverty on child health. *Journal of School Health 64:* 229-233.

Nestle, M. (1993). Food lobbies, the food pyramid, and U.S. nutrition policy. *International Journal of Health Services, 23*(3):483-496.

Nestle, M. (1995). Dietary guidance for the 21st century: New approaches. *Journal of Nutrition Education, 27*(5): 272-275.

Nestle, M. and Cowell, C. (1993). Health promotion for low-income minority groups: the challenge for nutrition education. *Health Education Research, 5:*527-33.

Paffenbarger, R. S., Hyde, R. T., Wing, A. L., et al. (1993). The association of changes in physical activity level and other lifestyle characteristics with mortality among men. *The New England Journal of Medicine 328:* 538-545.

Palley, H.A. (1995). The evolution of the FDA policy on silicone breast implants: A case study of politics, bureacracy, and business in the process of decision-making. *International Journal of Health Services, 25*(4):573-591.

Pate, R.R., Pratt, M. S., Blair, N. et al. (1995). Physical activity and public health: A recommendation from the Centers for Disease Control and Prevention and the American Colege of Sports Medicine. *Journal of the American Medical Association 273:* 402-407.

Phillips, K. A., and T. J. Coates. (1995). HIV counselling and testing: Research and policy issues. *AIDS CARE, 7:* 115-124.

Pappas, G. (1994). Elucidating the relationship between race, socioeconomic status, and health. *American Journal of Public Health, 84*(6):892-893.

Reinhardt, U. E. (1994). Providing access to health care and controlling costs: The universal dilemma. Reprinted by permission of the author in *The Nation's Health* (4th edition, pgs. 263-278).

Robinson, J.C. (1996). The dynamics and limits of corporate growth in health care. *Health Affairs, 15*(155-169).

Rother, J. (1996). Consumer protection in managed care: A third-generation approach. *Generations, 20*(2):42-46.

Sackett, D.L., Rosenberg, W. C., Muir Gray, J.A., Haynes, R.B., and Richardson, W.S. (1996). Evidence based medicine: What it is and what it isn't. *British Medical Journal, 312:* 71-72.

Task force on Genetic Testing. (1996). Interim Principles. Task force on genetic testing. NIH-DOE Working Group on Ethical, Legal, and Social Implications of Human Genome Research.

Thacker, S. B., Stroup, D. F., Parrish, R. G., and Anderson, H. A. (1996). Surveillance in environmental public health: Issues, systems, and sources. *American Journal of Public Health, 86*(5):633-637.

U.S. Department of Health and Human Service. (1977). Surgeon General's

Report on Health Promotion and Disease Prevention. Public Health Service, Washington DC.

U.S. Department of Health and Human Services. (1980). Surgeon General's Report on Promoting Health/Preventing Disease: Objectives for the Nation in the U.S. Public Health Service. Public Health Service, Washington DC.

U.S. Department of Health and Human Services. (1980). Ten Leading Causes of Death in the United States in 1977. Public Health Service, Centers for Disease Control and Prevention, Atlanta, GA.

U.S. Department of Health and Human Services. (1988). Surgeon General's Report on Nutrition and Health. Public Health Service. Public Health Service, Washington DC. 88-50210.

U.S. Department of Health and Human Services. (1988). The Health Consequences of smoking: Nicotine Addiction. A Report of the Surgeon General. Public Health Service, Washington DC. 88-8406.

U.S. Department of Health and Human Services. (1989). Reducing the Health Consequences of Smoking. A Report of the Surgeon General. Public Health Service, Washington DC. 89-8411.

U.S. Department of Health and Human Services. (1990). Healthy People 2000: National Health Promotion and Disease Prevention Objectives. Public Health Service, Washington DC.

U.S. Department of Health and Human Services. (1994). Preventing Tobacoo Use Among Young People: A Report of the Surgeon General. Atlanta, GA. Public Health Service. Centers for Disease and Prevention.

U.S. Department of Health and Human Services. (1994). Training and Education for Public Health: a Report to the Assistant Secretary for Health. U.S. Department of Health and Human Services, Washington DC.

U.S. Department of Health and Human Services. (1995). For a Healthy Nation: Returns on Investment in Public Health. Public Health Service, Washington DC.

U.S. Department of Health and Human Services. (1995). Integrating Public Health and Surveillance Systems. A report and recommendations from the CDC/ATSDR Steering Committee on Public Health Information and Surveillance System Development.

U.S. Department of Health and Human Services. (1995). 1992-1993 National Profile of Local Health Departments. National Association of City and County Health Officials. Centers for Disease Control and Prevention, Atlanta, GA.

U.S. Department of Health and Human Services. (1996). Health Care Financing Administration.

U.S. Department of Health and Human Services. (1996). Surgeon General's Report on Physical Activity and Health. Public Health Service.

U.S. Congress, Office of Technology Assessment. (1994). Researching Health Risks. OTA-BBS-570. Washington DC: U.S. Government Printing Office.

U.S. Environmental Protection Agency. (1986). Guidelines for carcinogen risk assessment. *Federal Register, 51:* 34028-40.

Varmus, H. (1995). Shattuck Lecture— Biomedical Research Enters the Steady State. *New England Journal of Medicine, 333:* 811-5.

Vladeck, B. C. (1995). Medicaid 1115 demonstrations: Progress through partnership. *Health Affairs, 14:* 217-220.

Waitzman, N.J., and Smith, K.R. (1996). Phantom of the area: poverty, residence and mortality in the U.S. Presented at the Forum on Social and Economic Disparities in Health and Health Care, Salt Lake Cit, UT.

Wennberg, J.E. (1993) Future directions for small area variations. *Medical Care, 31*(5):YS75-80, Supplement.

Wilkinson, R. G. (1992). Income distribution and life expectancy. *British Medical Journal, 304:*165-8.

❖ Index